Immunology of the Male Reproductive System

IMMUNOLOGY SERIES

1. Mechanisms in Allergy: Reagin-Mediated Hypersensitivity
   Edited by Lawrence Goodfriend, Alec Sehon and Robert P. Orange
2. Immunopathology: Methods and Techniques
   Edited by Theodore P. Zacharia and Sidney S. Breese, Jr.
3. Immunity and Cancer in Man: An Introduction
   Edited by Arnold E. Reif
4. *Bordetella pertussis:* Immunological and Other Biological Activities
   J.J. Munoz and R.K. Bergman
5. The Lymphocyte: Structure and Function (in two parts)
   Edited by John J. Marchalonis
6. Immunology of Receptors
   Edited by B. Cinader
7. Immediate Hypersensitivity: Modern Concepts and Development
   Edited by Michael K. Bach
8. Theoretical Immunology
   Edited by George I. Bell, Alan S. Perelson, and George H. Pimbley, Jr.
9. Immunodiagnosis of Cancer (in two parts)
   Edited by Ronald B. Herberman and K. Robert McIntire
10. Immunologically Mediated Renal Diseases: Criteria for Diagnosis and Treatment
    Edited by Robert T. McCluskey and Giuseppe A. Andres
11. Clinical Immunotherapy
    Edited by Albert F. LoBuglio
12. Mechanisms of Immunity to Virus-Induced Tumors
    Edited by John W. Blasecki
13. Manual of Macrophage Methodology: Collection, Characterization, and Function
    Edited by Herbert B. Herscowitz, Howard T. Holden, Joseph A. Bellanti, and Abdul Ghaffar
14. Suppressor Cells in Human Disease
    Edited by James S. Goodwin
15. Immunological Aspects of Aging
    Edited by Diego Segre and Lester Smith

16. Cellular and Molecular Mechanisms of Immunologic Tolerance
Edited by Tomáš Hraba and Milan Hašek

17. Immune Regulation: Evolution and Biological Significance
Edited by Laurens N. Ruben and M. Eric Gershwin

18. Tumor Immunity in Prognosis: The Role of Mononuclear Cell Infiltration
Edited by Stephen Haskill

19. Immunopharmacology and the Regulation of Leukocyte Function
Edited by David R. Webb

20. Pathogenesis and Immunology of Treponemal Infection
Edited by Ronald F. Schell and Daniel M. Musher

21. Macrophage-Mediated Antibody-Dependent Cellular Cytotoxicity
Edited by Hillel S. Koren

22. Molecular Immunology: A Textbook
Edited by M. Zouhair Atassi, Carel J. van Oss, and Darryl R. Absolom

23. Monoclonal Antibodies and Cancer
Edited by George L. Wright, Jr.

24. Stress, Immunity, and Aging
Edited by Edwin L. Cooper

25. Immune Modulation Agents and Their Mechanisms
Edited by Richard L. Fenichel and Michael A. Chirigos

26. Mononuclear Phagocyte Biology
Edited by Alvin Volkman

27. The Lactoperoxidase System: Chemistry and Biological Significance
Edited by Kenneth M. Pruitt and Jorma O. Tenovuo

28. Introduction to Medical Immunology
Edited by Gabriel Virella, Jean-Michel Goust, H. Hugh Fudenberg, and Christian C. Patrick

29. Handbook of Food Allergies
Edited by James C. Breneman

30. Human Hybridomas: Diagnostic and Therapeutic Applications
Edited by Anthony J. Strelkauskas

31. Aging and the Immune Response: Cellular and Humoral Aspects
Edited by Edmond A. Goidl

32. Complications of Organ Transplantation
Edited by Luis H. Toledo-Pereyra

33. Monoclonal Antibody Production Techniques and Applications
Edited by Lawrence B. Schook

34. Fundamentals of Receptor Molecular Biology
Donald F. H. Wallach

35. Recombinant Lymphokines and Their Receptors
Edited by Steven Gillis

36. Immunology of the Male Reproductive System
Edited by Pierluigi E. Bigazzi

Additional Volumes in Preparation

Immunology of the Male Reproductive System

edited by
PIERLUIGI E. BIGAZZI
The University of Connecticut Health Center
Farmington, Connecticut

MARCEL DEKKER, INC. New York and Basel

Library of Congress Cataloging-in-Publication Data

Immunology of the male reproductive system.

(Immunology series ; 36)
Includes index.
1. Testis--Diseases--Immunological aspects.
2. Antoimmune diseases. 3. Human reproduction--
Immunological aspects. 4. Generative organs, Male--
Diseases--Immunological aspects. 5. Vasectomy--
Immunological aspects. I. Bigazzi, Pierluigi E.
II. Series. III. Series: Immunology series ; v. 36.
[DNLM: 1. Genitalia, Male--immunology. W1 IM53K v.36 /
WJ 700 I33]
RC898.I46 1987 616.6'5079 87-9269
ISBN 0-8247-7648-8

MARCEL DEKKER, INC.
270 Madison Avenue, New York, 10016

Current printing (last digit):
10 9 8 7 6 5 4 3 2 1

PRINTED IN THE UNITED STATES OF AMERICA

Series Introduction

One of the most intriguing areas of modern medical research is the interdigitation of the immunological and reproductive systems. We see two-way interactions at many levels: Peptide hormones of the pituitary act upon the thymus, which regulates the immune response; similarly, the immune response can alter the function of the testes and ovary, while steroid hormones affect lymphocyte levels. Pregnancy requires suspension of the usual laws of allo-rejection and, in turn, significantly alters the course of immunological diseases.

These interactions between the reproductive and immunological systems have attracted the interest of many investigators. A number of books have appeared recently to deal with the effects of pregnancy on the immune response and the immunology of the female reproductive system. It is ironic, therefore, that there has not been sufficient attention to the male reproductive system from an immunological viewpoint. The deficiency is particularly striking because of the historical connection between studies of the testes and the immune response, as described by Professor

Voisin in the foreword. It is, therefore, especially appropriate that Dr. Bigazzi and his colleagues have assembled an up-to-date and comprehensive review of this important field. A review of the table of contents emphasizes the broad spectrum of topics encompassed, ranging from the unique antigenic structures of the testes and genital tract, to the role of antibodies in regulating fertility, and the immunology of testicular and prostatic tumors. This book will fill a serious void in the immunological library and will attract many new investigators to this challenging field.

Noel R. Rose
Professor and Chairman
Department of Immunology and
Infectious Diseases
The Johns Hopkins University
School of Hygiene and Public Health
Baltimore, Maryland

Foreword

The immunology of the male reproductive tract was, by more than 50 years, the first of several fields presently embraced by the growing domain of the immunology of reproduction. Actually, investigations were begun by Metchnikoff in 1899 (spermatoxins = spermotoxic antibodies) and Metalnikoff in 1900 (autosperma-toxins = spermotoxic autoantibodies). Then, several experimenters and clinicians injected females with sperm in order to control fertility by this type of antibodies, but it was not before half a century had passed that immunopathology—a word we coined first in 1952 to name our laboratory, one year after having described guinea pig autoimmune aspermatogenic orchitis—of the male system was first investigated. Since then there has been growing interest regarding autoimmune reactions to spermatozoa and various antigens of the reproductive tract and, for females, isoimmune reactions to spermatozoa and seminal plasma antigens.

Other aspects of the immunology of reproduction (materno-fetal immune relationship, fertility-related hormone immunology, and breast-feeding-related immunologic events) have been, for the most part, covered during recent meetings and in several books.

Gamete immunology—more particularly male antigens and the immune reactions built up against them by males and females—seems to have been relatively neglected these past few years; however, it is a major field of reproduction immunology and bears on several important consequences, both practical and theoretical.

From a practical point of view, we are concerned with the diagnosis and treatment of immunologic forms of infertility in males and females, as well as with aspects of immunologic control of fertility in human beings. (The sharply rising population of the world is expected to reach 10 billion by the year 2100.) A related aspect of great interest is the necessity to increase cattle production and to detect infertile animals, as stressed by the late Kyril Bratanov. The techniques and problems encountered with farm animals are closely related to those described for humans. Fertilization in vitro and embryo transplantation have immunologic aspects in that they may evoke immune responses or be used to bypass a fertility problem.

From a theoretical point of view, male tract immunology, especially of spermatozoa and testis, has far-reaching implications, touching on several domains: autoantigens and autoimmune diseases due to the induction of the autoimmune reaction (induced experimentally or by vasectomy); the effector pathways of organ-specific autoimmune damage; and the reasons autoimmune reactions, which are among the most physiological of phenomena (simply consider the idiotype/anti-idiotype network), sometimes become highly pathologic. Male tract immunology also involves problems in self-recognition and self-tolerance: These are far from having been solved for autologous substances. Clonal elimination for antiself-reactive clones certainly does not apply to spermatozoal autoantigens in spite of the high probability that—like thyroglobulin—highly soluble and diffusible acrosomal autoantigens diffuse systemically. The local immune response in the genital tract demonstrates an aspect of the relative compartmentalization of the immune reaction, at variance with homogeneous test tube mixtures. The fields of tumor immunology and differentiation themselves will benefit from studies of testicular tumors with their embryonal antigens and the still mysterious F9 shared by spermatozoa and early embryo. This book therefore comes in time to respond to a need.

Guy André Voisin, M.D. Sci.D.
President
The International Society for the
Immunology of Reproduction

Preface

Investigation of spermatozoal antigens was initiated at the end of the last century by Landsteiner and Metchnikoff. In the years following those landmark studies, the literature on reproductive immunology grew at such a rapid pace that it is now difficult to present in a single book an in-depth review of the immunology of the male reproductive system together with that of pregnancy and the female reproductive tract. These considerations led to the preparation of the present book, aiming at comprehensive coverage of the immunology and immunopathology of the male reproductive system, in order to provide a more extensive analysis than is currently available in other publications on reproductive immunology.

The opening chapter is focused on the numerous antigens of the testis and the excurrent tract, an area that is also addressed in many of the following chapters because of its importance and the rapid expansion of data through the use of monoclonal antibodies, SDS-PAGE, Western blotting, and other technologic advances. The various methods to detect antisperm antibodies are explained at length in the second chapter, also covering the choices among the techniques currently available, as well as the problems still unsolved. This is followed by a review of the immunologic regulation of fertility with spermatozoal antigens, stressing the development of synthetic peptides that may eventually be used as vaccines for birth control. The role of autoimmune responses to testicular antigens in male infertility is discussed in the next chapter, on the basis of experimental data and clinical observations. A review of the immunologic effects of vasectomy in men, including the useful lessons derived from the study of the autoimmune consequences of this sterilization procedure, is presented in the following chapter. The histopathology of immunologic lesions observed in testicular biopsies from infertile men is illustrated in the next section, together with an outline of the staging of human immune-complex orchitis. In logical sequence this is followed by a summary of the various treatments of immunologic infertility in men, a topic of obvious practical importance. The numerous animal models of testis autoimmunity, experimentally induced or naturally occurring, are then examined in detail, in an attempt to elucidate both the pathogenesis and etiology of autoimmune disorders of the male reproductive system. A subject not often covered in books on reproductive immunology, i.e., the immunobiology of testicular tumors as it relates to host-tumor interactions, is dealt with in the next chapter. Finally, two separate reviews elucidate the antigens of the normal prostatic gland as well as the immunology of prostatic tumors.

In all these chapters, a certain degree of overlap was unavoidable and perhaps to be encouraged, since it helps provide different perspectives on some issues, primarily the purification of antigens of spermatozoa and other constituents of the male reproductive tract, a field where we are anticipating rapid progress. Overall, the present book provides extensive coverage of male reproductive immunology and will stimulate interest and additional investigations in this field.

I thank all the contributing authors for their excellent collaboration and great patience during the long gestation of this book.

In addition, I wish to thank Dr. Noel R. Rose and Dr. Giuseppe A. Andres for their generous help and advice during my studies on autoimmunity of the testis.

Pierluigi E. Bigazzi

Contents

Contributors

Pierluigi E. Bigazzi, M.D.
Department of Pathology, University of Connecticut Health Center, Farmington, Connecticut

*B. K. Choe**
University of Toronto and Toronto General Hospital, Toronto, Ontario, Canada

A. B. Czuppon
Department of Obstetrics and Gynecology, Christian Albrecht's University, Kiel, Federal Republic of Germany

Franco Dondero, M.D.
University of Rome, Rome, Italy

Jan Friberg, M.D., Ph.D.
Department of Obstetrics and Gynecology, Mount Sinai Hospital Medical Center and Rush Medical College, Chicago, Illinois

---

**Present affiliation*: The University of Illinois College of Medicine, Chicago, Illinois

Christoph E. Hedinger, M.D.
Institute of Pathology, University of Zurich, Zurich, Switzerland

Tage Hjort, M.D.
Institute of Medical Microbiology, University of Aarhus, Aarhus, Denmark

Linda L. Kosuda, Ph. D.
Department of Pathology, University of Connecticut Health Center, Farmington, Connecticut

Professor Doctor L. Mettler
Department of Obstetrics and Gynecology, Christian Albrecht's University, Kiel, Federal Republic of Germany

Bijay Mukherji, M.D.
Department of Medicine (Oncology), University of Connecticut School of Medicine, Farmington, Connecticut

Noel R. Rose, M.D., Ph.D.
Department of Immunology and Infectious Diseases, School of Hygiene and Public Health, The Johns Hopkins University, Baltimore, Maryland

*Franco Salomon, M.D.**
Institute of Pathology, University of Zurich, Zurich, Switzerland

Sidney Shulman, Ph.D.†
Departments of Microbiology, Virology, and Obstetrics and Gynecology, New York Medical College and Metropolitan Hospital, New York, New York

---

**Present affiliation*: St. Thomas's Hospital Medical School, London, England
†Present affiliation: Fertility Antibody Diagnostics, Inc., New York, New York

Immunology of the Male Reproductive System

1
Antigens of the Testis and the Excurrent Duct

SYDNEY SHULMAN*

New York Medical College and Metropolitan Hospital, New York, New York

**Present affiliation*: Fertility Antibody Diagnostics, Inc., New York, New York

The testis contain antigens related to spermatozoa and to the germinal cells that develop into the spermatozoa. There have been many investigations of these systems. The testis must also contain antigens related to other structures, such as Sertoli cells and Leydig cells, but these have not been much studied. We shall concentrate on sperm cells and their progenitors in this discussion. There have been two major approaches to these antigens, namely, the reactions of autoimmune aspermatogenesis or orchitis, mostly in guinea pigs but also in other species, and the reactions of human autoantibodies to spermatozoa in certain cases of spontaneous infertility and vasectomy. In both areas of study, efforts have been made to characterize and to isolate the responsible antigens.

The excurrent duct consists of the epididymis, vas deferens, and urethra, along with the attached major glands, the prostate and seminal vesicle. All these structures have been given antigenic analysis; also, the prostatic fluid and the seminal plasma have been studied, being major secretions of these glands.

I. AUTOIMMUNE ORCHITIS

The destruction of testicular function by means of immune mechanisms has been investigated in experimental animals over the past 25 years. These observations may be of interest for several reasons. First, there may be human disorders that resemble this type of gonadal malfunction; in such cases, similar mechanisms may be involved. Second, new information on the various antigens of sperm cells has been obtained from studies of this phenomenon in experimental animals. Third, this kind of study has served to illustrate many of the features of autoimmunity. Fourth, a possible method for male contraception may be derived from such procedures.

A. Status in the Experimental Animal

The first significant steps in the study of antoantibodies and autoimmunity to sperm and testis were taken in the work of Voisin et al. (1951) and of Freund et al. (1963). Voisin et al. (1951) showed that guinea pigs that were injected with testicular tissue derived from guinea pigs, along with certain adjuvants, developed tissue damage in the testis, which was described as orchitis and epididymitis. Freund et al. (1963) independently made studies of the results of immunization with suspensions of guinea pig testicular tissue, obtaining them either from the same animal or from other members of the species. They showed that when these were injected in combination with a paraffin oil and heat-killed tubercle bacilli into guinea pigs—the subsequently named Freund's complete adjuvant—two kinds of immunologic consequences were produced: (1) the development of aspermatogenesis and (2) the formation of specific antibodies against testicular tissue and against spermatozoa, as demonstrated by complement fixation tests. These investigators provided convincing evidence that the response was a specific immune response. It may well be that these same antigens may manifest themselves in some of the other immunologic phenomena related to the spermatozoa.

This phenomenon of experimental aspermatogenesis has served as a model system for autoimmune responses and experimental autoimmune diseases in general. The use of incomplete Freund's adjuvant (omitting the bacilli) leads to the production of specific antibodies only, but the use of complete Freund's adjuvant leads to the additional production of atrophic tissue damage. These responses may also follow the injection of sperm suspensions in place of testicular homogenate; the spermatozoa that have been used have invariably been epididymal spermatozoa, a point that may have some significance in light of the antigenic distinctions between epididymal and ejaculated spermatozoa, at least in some animal species. Purified or modified preparations from testicular tissue are also effective, as shown in the work of Katsh, Bishop, Mancini, and their colleagues (Bishop et al., 1961; Katsh and Aguirre, 1968; Katsh and Bishop, 1958; Mancini et al., 1966). Immunization with seminal plasma in rabbits has also been utilized (Wentworth and Mellan, 1964; Yantorno et al., 1971).

It has also proven possible to induce this effect by freezing the tissue, and such studies have been reviewed elsewhere (Shulman and Zappi, 1972). This procedure of cryosurgical induction, omitting all use of adjuvant, was first described by Zappi and Shulman (1971,1972) and Ablin and Soanes (1972). As another alternative, the possibility of autoimmune injury following trauma to the testis has been discussed by Raitsina and Nilovsky (1967).

The majority of these various studies have been made on the guinea pig, However, similar studies have been made on several other species of animal. Freund et al. (1954) showed in their early work that rats were readily susceptible to this type of autoimmunogenic stimulation. Early findings that the disease could be transferred between strains of rats by the transfer of leukocytes (Laurence and Perlbachs, 1962; Laurence et al., 1965) were followed by the work of Kantor and Dixon (1972) and Tung et al. (1971). These later studies utilized a syngeneic strain of guinea pig. The disease was successfully transferred to healthy recipients by transfer of either lymph node cells (Tung et al., 1971) or peritoneal exudate cells (Katsh, 1964). The former were mostly lymphocytes, whereas the latter were primarily macrophages with relatively few lymphocytes. These investigators found that many fewer lymphocytes were needed when a large number of macrophages were present.

A useful system was later developed in the mouse. This finding opened many interesting possibilities for the distinctions that might exist among inbred strains. Pokorná et al. (1963) found that aspermatogenesis could be induced in mice by immunization with testicular homogenate and complete Freund's adjuvant from the same strain. In addition to the finding of histological damage, circulating antibodies were detected. Later work with mice introduced the use of pertussis vaccine as an adjuvant (Hargis et al., 1968). Genetic factors of susceptibility and resistance have been studied in mice (Boehme, 1965). A similar autoimmune system was reported in bulls (Losos et al., 1968; Menge and Christian, 1971) and also in the Japanese quail (Wentworth and Mellen, 1964). Eyquem and Krieg (1965) even produced testicular lesions in rabbits and monkeys, but only by means of direct injections of Freund's adjuvant into a testis. The difficulty of showing that rabbit spermatozoa can be antigenic within the same species has generally been a disturbing problem (Yantorno et al., 1971; Zappi and Shulman, 1974).

B. Status in the Human

A report dealing with the induction of aspermatogenesis in the human species was published by Mancini et al. (1965). They studied patients who had carcinoma of the prostate and who were injected with testicular homogenate plus Freund's adjuvant. The usual antigen was a preparation of washed and sonicated homologous spermatozoa or testicular homogenate. Immune responses were seen at 2–8 weeks after injection, consisting of circulating antibodies, although of low titer, as detected by complement fixation tests, as well as by precipitation, antiglobulin consumption, and passive cutaneous anaphylaxis. A positive skin test, indicating delayed hypersensitivity, was seen at the same time. In the testes of the men, patchy lesions developed, consisting of congestion, serous edema, and the sloughing of germinal cells; this tissue damage occurred in two of four men. Hence, lesions and circulating antibodies were produced that were very similar to the well-established phenomena in the guinea pig species.

Even without any immunization procedure, some kinds of antitesticular immunity with some damage in the human have been found (Dondero and Isidori, 1972; Isidori et al., 1970). Hendry et al. (1983) studied a large group of azoospermic men who had an obstruction in the sperm passage. After surgical reconstruction, a number of them had spermatozoa in the ejaculate but many also had sperm antibody. The antibody activity was found less often in the group of males whose female partners become pregnant than in those who did not produce pregnancies.

C. Purification of the Aspermatogenic Antigens

Many efforts have been made to purify the aspermatogenic substance(s). The earliest important work was done by Voisin and his group, as described in detail elsewhere (Shulman, 1974) and summarized briefly below. They claimed that there were four aspermatogenic factors, rather than just one; they were termed S, P, Z, and T. These components were isolated from guinea pig sperm (Voisin and Toullet, 1968, 1969).

All but compound Z have been obtained in moderately well purified condition; each has different antigenic and biochemical properties. They show different degrees of pathogenicity in the ease of inducing experimental aspermatogenesis or, as Voisin has termed it, autoimmune aspermatogenic orchitis (AIAO). The fractionation procedure started with the treatment of an extract of guinea pig spermatozoa with 5% trichloroacetic acid. The supernatant contained mostly antigen S, with some antigen P. The sediment contained mostly P, and it was agitated with chloroform to give a better preparation of P in the aqueous phase. Each of the preparations was filtered on a column of Sephadex G-100, giving S and P preparations free of each other. The major properties of these and the other two antigens can be summarized as follows (Voisin and Toullet, 1968, 1969).

1. Antigen S is a glycoprotein that is very rich in sugar. It is thermostable, water soluble, and soluble in trichloroacetic acid, and it is sensitive to proteolytic enzymes and to periodic acid. This component is highly autoantigenic, It elicits hypersensitivity of the delayed, anaphylactic, and Arthus types and also antibodies giving anaphylaxis and passive hemagglutination, but not precipitation or sperm immobilization. It is potently orchitogenic and aspermatogenic.
2. Antigen P is a protein that is poor in sugar. It is thermostable and water soluble but it is precipitated by trichloroacetic acid. It is less sensitive than S to the action of periodic acid and proteases. It also elicits hypersensitivity of the three types. It provokes the formation of antibodies that are able to precipitate and to give anaphylaxis, but not to be immobilizing. It can also induce lesions of AIAO.
3. Antigen T may be a proteolipid. It is thermolabile and water insoluble, and it is destroyed by trichloroacetic acid. It elicits the formation of immobilizing antibodies and can bring about testicular lesions of the AIAO type.
4. Antigen Z is a labile and nonabundant component. It is thermolabile, water soluble, and soluble in trichloroacetic acid. It has not been much studied.

More recent studies on purification have been published by Eylar and his colleagues (Hagopian et al., 1975, 1976; Jackson et al., 1975, 1976) and by Teuscher et al. (1983). In the first report from Eylar's group (Jackson et al., 1975), a purified aspermatogenic protein was isolated and termed AP1. For this very important achievement, they used the following series of steps; starting with homogenized guinea pig testes: delipidation with chloroform-methanol, acid extraction, precipitation with 85% saturated ammonium sulfate, extraction with trichloroacetic acid, gel filtration, column chromatography, and, finally, preparative gel electrophoresis at low pH. They obtained a yield of only 20 mg of this AP1 from 5000 g wet guinea pig testes. This final product was shown to be homogeneous by several analytic procedures, and it was also very potent in orchitogenic and aspermatogenic effects. In fact, Jackson et al. (1975), using as little as 0.2 μg for the injection (with complete Freund's adjuvant), showed that mild lesions were observed, and that with 0.5 μg or more, severe lesions occurred; these lesions consisted of intertubular and intratubular infiltration of mononuclear cells (orchitis) and damage and desquamation of the germinal cells (aspermatogenesis). Hence, the AP1 was much more active than any previously reported material. These workers also localized the site of this component, finding it to be in the spermatozoal acrosome.

For comparison with the work of Voisin and his colleagues, we can note that AP1 contains no carbohydrate and is thus quite different from antigen S. Further, it is soluble in trichloroacetic acid and is thus different from antigens T and P. These comparisons and others are the basis for claiming that this is an aspermatogenic substance that is distinct from these in the reports of earlier workers. It may be of considerable interest to note that the injected animals did not show any lesions in the liver, kidney, brain, spleen, or lung, showing, as with crude testicular extracts, that there is specificity for testicular damage.

In their chemical analyses, Jackson et al. (1976) then showed that the AP1 protein is a single polypeptide chain of 136 amino acids. It has a molecular weight of 15,000, with no sugar residues; in fact, their tests specifically excluded galactose, mannose, fucose, glucose, and hexosamine. The molecule seems to be very compact and stable, its activity being resistant to trypsin, to high temperature, to low pH, and to 8 M urea. This high resistance to denaturation may well be the result of its half-cystine content, thus allowing the occurrence of many disulfide linkages in the tertiary structure.

In their related work, Hagopian et al. (1975) isolated and purified four more components from guinea pig testes; these components, in contrast to AP1, were indeed glycoproteins, and they were termed GP1, 2, 3, and 4. It was found that GP1 and GP4 could induce aspermatogenic orchitis, whereas the other two glycoproteins could not. The potency of GP1 and of GP4 was somewhat less than that of AP1. In further studies, Hagopian et al. (1976) provided detailed analyses of amino acid and carbohydrate contents for these four glycoproteins. All of them had a carbohydrate content over 40%. The monosaccharide compositions of GP1 and GP4 are very similar, except that GP1 contains some sialic acid, whereas GP4 does not. Hence, it was speculated that GP4 is a subunit or a fragment of GP1; the estimated molecular weights are 28,000 for GP1 and 13,000 for GP4. The amino acid contents, although different, were considered to be unremarkable. Nonetheless, one can note very low contents of half-cystine, in contrast to that in AP1 protein. All four glycoproteins had different patterns of amino acid composition. GP1 and GP4, like AP1, were found in the sperm cell acrosome.

In more recent work from another group, Teuscher et al. (1983) have claimed to isolate another aspermatogenic substance from the guinea pig; they emphasized its preparation from spermatozoa instead of from testis, but the meaning of this distinction is not clear. Their starting material was the soluble acrosomal contents of cauda epididymal sperm. This was treated with trichloroacetate, frozen and thawed several times, and then subjected to gel filtration, to isoelectric focusing, and finally to SDS-PAGE (sodium dodecyl sulfate–polyacrylamide gel electrophoresis). The product seemed homogeneous, and it was named AP2. The product was very potent, with as little as 0.5 μg causing mild lesions and 5 μg causing severe damage. The molecular weight was estimated to be 9500. Amino acid analysis revealed that it is a polypeptide with no unusual features; it showed no carbohydrate. The authors pointed out that the composition was thus different from that of AP1, GP1, and GP4, the other aspermatogenic antigens.

D. Surface Sperm Antigens

Among the studies that have been made concerning human antigens of human sperm, not related to aspermatogenesis, efforts were made earliest by Kolk et al. (1974), Mettler and Gradl (1975), and Mettler and Skrabei (1979) and somewhat later by Poulsen and Hjort (1981) as well as by Shulman and Keane (1981).

The following study be De Almeida and her colleagues (1981) is of interest to consider in some detail. To identify human spermatozoal surface autoantigens, suspensions of previously frozen washed sperm were ground in a homogenizer and ultracentrifuged (170,000 × *g* for 60 min). The antigenicity of the fast supernatant (FS) and the fast pellet (FP), as produced by this fast centrifuging, were defined by specific inhibition of sperm-immobilizing and various sperm-agglutinating activities of autoimmune human sera. The FS and the urea-soluble extract of FP were fractionated on Sephadex G-200 columns, and the antigenicity of these fractions was similarly defined. Both FS and FP inhibited antispermatozoal activities, but to no variable extents. Inhibition of head-to-head (H-H) agglutination by FS was twice as strong as by FP. The reverse was observed with tail-to-tail (T-T) agglutination. To inhibit immobilization by all tested sera, 10 times more FS and FP was necessary. After FS filtration on Sephadex G-200, four fractions were collected. F_1 was a homogeneous protein, and it inhibited immobilization and H-H agglutination. F_2 inhibited all activities (including T-T agglutination). F_3 was a low-molecular-weight fraction, and it selectively inhibited H-H agglutination. F_4 was inactive. Treatment by 8 M urea allowed partial solubilization of FP antigenicity. Urea-soluble fractions inhibited immobilization and H-H, but not T-T, agglutination. The antigen(s) involved in T-T agglutination is (are) destroyed by urea, since the urea-treated FP was no longer able to significantly decrease T-T agglutination. These results suggested that at least three different autoantigens are responsible for the three activities of H-H sperm agglutination, T-T sperm agglutination, and immobilization.

In more recent studies, Lee et al. (1982) have prepared and used monoclonal antibodies to human spermatozoa. After successive immunizations with the particulate fractions of human sperm extract into BALB/c mice, the spleen cells were fused with appropriate myeloma cells. Several clones and their subclones were obtained and shown to produce antibodies against human sperm antigens. All three independently derived clones were shown to produce antibodies that cross-reacted with the same two human sperm antigens with a molecular weight of about 10,000. Using an indirect immunofluorescence assay, antibodies produced by these clones were shown to react with antigens localized on the acrosomal regions of human spermatozoa. Monoclonal antibodies produced by other clones, however, showed no cross-reactivity with any of the blotted proteins from SDS gels of human spermatozoa. This work is valuable, but it has yet to be shown that the *same* antigens are involved with these monoclonal antibodies and with the humn polyclonal antibodies found in certain sera from infertile people.

Poulsen (1983) has gone further with his early work and has isolated an isoantigen from human spermatozoa by detergent solubilization, lectin affinity chromatography, and indirect immunoprecipitation using human antisera for the testing. The isolated material was characterized by SDS–polyacrylamide gel electrophoresis. With these antisera it was possible to isolate four different polypeptide chains: one of molecular weight 41,000, two around 77,000, and one about 120,000. Young and Goodman (1980) have also studied the surface of human spermatozoa. They characterized four major components.

Recent studies on nonhuman spermatozoal antigens have repeatedly featured the use of monoclonal antibodies. For example, four surface regions were labeled on the surface of guinea pig spermatozoa (Myles et al., 1981). Similarly, four antigenically distinct antigenic regions were mapped on the surface of mouse spermatozoa (Feuchter et al., 1981). Another mouse study revealed a particular sperm antigen that was also associated with a polypeptide of molecular weight 28,000 (Gaunt, 1982). In this work, differentiation and specificity studies were also made. This antigen was detected only on testicular cells and spermatozoa. The antigen appeared on the cell surface at a specific state in spermatogenesis; it was not found on cells of the prepubertal, 8-day mouse testis but was first seen on pachytene primary spermatocytes arising at 14 days. The antigen was then retained on all postpachytene cells within the tests. By immunofluorescence, it was seen to be present over the entire cell surface of spermatozoa within the testis and caput epididymis, but cauda epididymal and vas deferens spermatozoa showed fluorescent labeling only upon the anterior tip of the head. Although it is tissue specific, the antigen is not species specific, for it was found on testicular cells of rat, rabbit, vole, and guinea pig, but not of the rhesus monkey. Subsequently, the same investigative group used monoclonal antibodies to study the mobility and distribution of three different antigens on the cell surface of rat spermatozoa (Gaunt et al., 1983). Of the antigens, two (designated 2B1 and 2D6) were classified as "mobile," since when detected by indirect immunofluorescence they were situated over the entire sperm flagellum and they were susceptible to antibody-induced patching. Patching was critically dependent upon antibody concentrations and was much reduced at 4°C. Patching of the 2B1 antigen was not induced by the 2B1 monoclonal antibody alone. Thus, 2B1 antibody labeled directly with fluorescein bound with a uniform distribution over the sperm flagellum, but this uniform fluorescence was made patchy on subsequent incubation in an unlabeled second antibody layer of anti-mouse IgG antiserum. The 2B1 antigen was found to be located on a 40,000 molecular weight polypeptide. The remaining "fixed" antigen (designated 1B6) was not susceptible to antibody-induced patching; it was restricted to a discrete domain on the postacrosomal region of the sperm surface.

Surface antigens of mouse sperm cells have also been studied by the use of a group of six monoclonal antibodies (Schmell et al., 1982). Quantitative assessment of antibody binding, using a solid-phase antibody-protein A assay, indicated that four antibody specificities bound to integral, sperm surface antigens; two others bound to nonintegral sperm antigens or epididymal fluid components. Immunofluorescence studies showed specific binding of individual antibodies to localized regions: acrosome, midpiece, and tail. All these antibodies inhibited sperm-egg binding, and those to the midpiece and/or tail immobilized sperm cells.

Even a nonmonoclonal approach has been used with mouse sperm, identifying seven surface antigens (Herr and Eddy, 1980). Again with polyclonal antibody, with rabbit sperm in this instance, O'Rand and Porter (1982) described a relatively simple preparative procedure for isolating sperm autoantigens using an SDS-polyacrylamide gel gradient column. The rabbit sperm membrane autoantigen, RSA-1, has been isolated without the use of an immunoadsorbent column, giving an almost 10-fold greater yield than with the previous immunoadsorbent column method. A second autoantigen (RSA-2) has been isolated. Both RSA-1 and RSA-2 retain their antigenic activity after isolation from the gel. The carbohydrate and amino acid content of RSA-1 was determined; RSA-1 is 9.1% carbohydrate and contains xylose, galactose, mannose, glucose, and glucosamine. The average hydrophobicity of RSA-1 indicates that it is a relatively nonpolar, asymmetric protein in the general category of fibrous or tropomyosinlike proteins. Oliphant and Singhas (1979) have also studied rabbit spermatozoa. They related the surface components to the capacitation process.

II. PROSTATE GLAND AND PROSTATIC FLUID

A. Rabbit Prostate

The prostate-related antigens have been explored in the rabbit; most of these studies have been performed on tissue extracts, and some were made on prostatic fluid. Many studies have been related to the formation of autoantibodies; there has also been an effort to demonstrate the existence of tissue-specific antigens. Figure 1 shows the anatomy of the urogenital system of the rabbit. In an early investigation, extracts were prepared from the prostate gland itself or from the total cluster of the accessory glands of reproduction, and rabbits were then immunized with these extracts of tissue incorporated into complete Freund's adjuvant plus additional killed tubercle bacilli, a preparation that was called fortified adjuvant. The series of bleedings was then examined by means of passive hemagglutination tests and gel diffusion plates. It was then established that antibody responses are obtained after several weeks of repeated injections and that these antibodies are actually autoantibodies. These antisera could then be used for tissue and species comparisons. Strong reactions were given by each of the accessory tissues, even with the use of an antiserum that was ob-

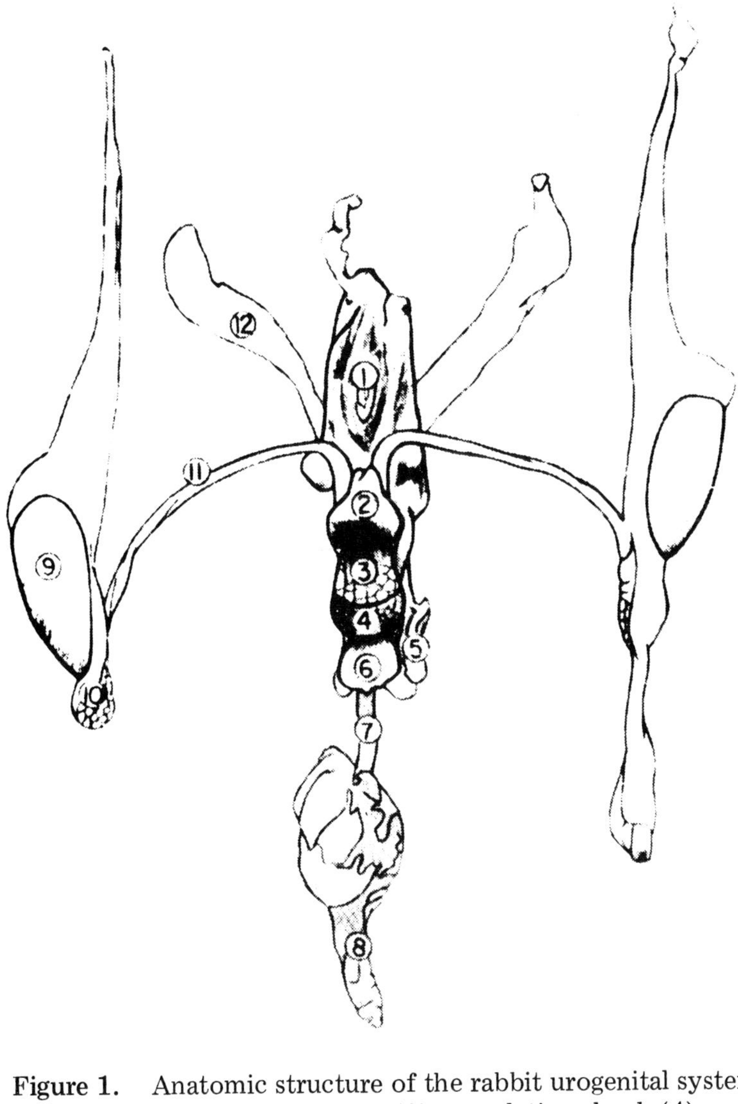

Figure 1. Anatomic structure of the rabbit urogenital system: (1) bladder, (2) seminal vesicle, (3) coagulating gland, (4) prostate gland, (5) paraprostate gland, (6) bulbourethral gland, (7) urethra, (8) penis, (9) testis, (10) epididymis, (11) vas deferens, (12) fat. (From Shulman et al., 1965b).

tained from a rabbit that was immunized with an extract of the prostate gland itself, carefully separated from the other tissues. This showed that there is a common antigen in all these related tissues. Reaction was also obtained with this rabbit's own autologous prostate. Inhibition was *not* produced, however, by bladder, liver, serum, or testis of rabbit. Other experiments showed that prostatic fluid from human or dog origin did not react, indicating the species specificity of the antigen. Gel diffusion experiments gave results in complete concurrence with these observations. Negative results were obtained with rabbit liver, kidney, adrenal, heart, thyroid, testis, bladder, uterus, and vagina. The gel diffusion experiments indicated that this reaction may involve two antigens. Many results were published in detail (Shulman and Yantorno, 1971; Shulamn et al., 1965b, 1966).

Other studies of autoimmune damage to rabbit male accessory glands have been reported by Yantorno and his colleagues (Vottero-Cima et al., 1973; Yantorno et al., 1973).

A quite different approach was also developed to the experimental production of autoantibodies to the accessory glands. This method replaces the customary adjuvant by an intensive freezing treatment of the tissue in situ. This cryosurgical procedure has led to a group of studies that were called cryoimmunology (Jagodzinski et al., 1967; Shulman, 1968, 1969; Shulman et al., 1968c; Shulman and Zappi, 1973; Yantorno et al., 1967; Zappi and Shulman, 1971, 1972; Zappi et al., 1972a). The fundamental procedures in regard to the accessory glands were first outlined in some detail by Yantorno et al. (1967). A large number of rabbits were subjected to tissue freezing, and they exhibited a rapid antibody response, achieving a maximum titer in 7–10 days, followed by a decline. The autoantibody response was tissue specific, and it showed many points of similarity to the autoantibody formation that followed isoimmunization by means of injection of tissue homogenate combined with complete Freund's adjuvant (Shulman et al., 1968a). It was also highly species specific. Although the same autoantigen seemed to be involved, the autoantibody response to the freezing of tissue was initiated much more quickly, and it rose to a maximum in a much shorter period than did the analogous autoantibody response that followed repeated intradermal injections.

In another study (Shulman et al., 1968c) antisera were fractionated. There was a predominant 19S (IgM) activity in the early bleedings. The presence of 7S (IgG activity) could be observed in the later bleedings, and this was found to be the major form at these later stages in the immune response.

It was also learned (Riera et al., 1968) that freezing stimulation could be applied at some time after sensitization by injection of extract and adjuvant and that this two-stage process elicited the formation of IgG antibody; this therefore constituted a booster type of antigenic stimulation in these animals. These studies provided additional evidence that the same autoantigen was involved in the freezing process and in the injection process. Booster responses could also be demonstrated by the other two-stage processes, that is, procedures in which there is cryoimmunization followed by isoimmunization or those in which there is freezing followed by a second episode of freezing (Shulman, 1969).

B. Canine Prostate

Canine prostatic fluid (CPF) can be obtained by means of pilocarpine stimulation, using prepared animals in which the prostate and urethra are isolated from the rest of the urologic system (Huggins and Sommer, 1963; Mason et al., 1961). These dogs can be stimulated to elaborate a product that is essentically pure prostatic fluid, and they can yield about 40–60 ml during an hour.

Antigenic analyses have also been made, revealing that canine prostatic fluid contains strong antigenic activity as judged from the antibody responses in rabbits (Yantorno et al., 1966). A significant part of this antigenic mixture represented prostate-specific antigens. Hence, there was no cross-reaction with other canine tissues, such as bladder, testis, kidney, liver, spleen, heart, muscle, and brain. Reactions occurred with prostate extract or seminal plasma, but this would be expected from the prostatic fluid component in these tissues, The lack of reaction of other tissues could not be ascribed to any failure in coating the cells, because there was identical information provided by the method of inhibition of hemagglutination. A tissue-specific antigen is thus present, and this is a major component in the mixture.

We have described the purification and study of this major antigen and of a minor antigen (Ahmed and Shulman, 1972, 1974; Shulman and Ahmed, 1971). Canine prostatic fluid was fractionated into three components, referred to as fraction A, S, and F, in order of elution; their relative proportions were 1, 9, and 90%, respectively, of the total recovered protein. Antigenic analysis was conducted with the use of rabbit antisera prepared against CPF. Gel diffusion studies showed three lines of precipitation. The antigenic analysis revealed a reaction of identity between the major components of fraction S and F, and these components were shown to be prostatic fluid specific (Ahmed and Shulman, 1972). Fractions S and F were further purified by recycling them through Sephadex G-100. These purified subfractions, S_1 and F_2, again showed a reaction of identity in gel diffusion precipitation, suggesting an antigenic similarity between the tissue-specific components of these fractions. However, the components are not really identical, as was shown by their having different points of elution from the column and by immunoelectrophoretic analyses. The interaction could also be shown by the inhibition of the line of precipitation of fraction S_1 by the adjacent fraction F_2. Apparently, there is an antigenic similarity between the components of fractions S and F. It is therefore possible that inhibition results from a zone of antigen excess provided by a high concentration of fraction F. Quantitative precipitation studies were made on each of these major fractions (Ahmed and Shulman, 1974). Caseinolytic activity was also measured in these fractions. The precipitation curves were quite different, whereas the proteolytic activities were essentially the same. It was concluded that CPF contains a single major antigen that exists in both the polymeric form (fraction S_1) and the monomeric form (fraction F_2), perhaps as a result of proteolysis of the original antigen molecule. The smaller molecules that were present in fraction F_2 could cause the inhibition of the precipitin line that was formed by their polymeric counterparts. Our terminology reflected the concept of a substrate (S) and a fragment (F) derived from it.

In a different approach, the influence of antiprostatic antibodies, as introduced by passive transfer, was explored in other studies, using rabbit anticanine prostatic fluid and injecting it into normal dogs. Degenerative changes in the recipient's prostate gland were described, and a number of immunologic interactions were studied (Macalalag and Prout, 1967; Peel, 1968), but the reactions were very complex and far from fully clarified.

C. Human Prostate

The immunologic properties of human prostatic fluid have been described in some considerable detail in an early study using antisera from intensively immunized rabbits (Barnes et al., 1963, 1965). It was shown that at least four or five antigens were distinctive for this fluid itself, in addition to another three or four antigens that were shared with the blood serum. Immunoelectrophoresis and immunofluorescence were used to characterize the specific antigens and to distinguish them from serum antigens. These antigens were also found in male urine, but not in female urine; the proteins in male urine may well represent prostatic secretion, and their presence may vary from time to time.

The biochemical nature of the substances responsible for this tissue specificity has also been studied. Human prostatic fluid has thus been analyzed and found to be a complex mixture when examined electrophoretically (Soanes et al., 1963), ultracentrifugally (Shulman et al., 1968b), and enzymatically (Shulman and Ferber, 1966; Shulman et al., 1964, 1965a). There have been many studies on the phosphatases and other enzymes, but the more recent approach has been to measure and characterize enzymes by means of a combination of enzymatic and antigenic properties (Dufour et al., 1965a, b, 1966; Moncure and Prout, 1970; Pfeiffer et al., 1970; Shulman et al., 1964, 1965a).

One particular method was based on a procedure of special staining of a gel diffusion reaction pattern (Shulman et al., 1964), and it is presented here as an example, in some detail. Gel diffusion and immunoelectrophoretic plates, containing reaction wells between samples of human prostatic fluid and rabbit antiserum to human prostatic fluid, were allowed to develop their precipitation reactions and then were stained by either the routine procedure for protein or a special staining procedure. The staining of total protein was done by amido Schwartz, followed by washing in the solvent mixture until the background was clear. Those slides that were to be stained for the acid phosphatase activity were treated with the buffer substrate, containing lead nitrate and sodium glycerophosphate. They were then rinsed in distilled water and then acetic acid and water and then briefly immersed in 2% ammonium sulfide. If the slides were to be counterstained after the phosphatase staining, to emphasize the other proteins, then light green SF stain was used. It was thus possible to see one major and one minor line of phosphatase-stained antigen-antibody precipitate in the reactions for human prostatic fluid. It was also found that the reaction of specific staining was inhibited by tartaric acid; this was additional evidence that this was really a staining of the phosphatase activity, since tartaric acid is known to inhibit the activity of prostatic acid phosphatase, although not of the plasma or erythrocyte phosphatases. A typical picture, including the results of making some dilutions of the prostatic fluid, is shown in Figure 2.

Figure 2 Part 1. Gel diffusion precipitation patterns of human prostatic fluid (PF) tested against rabbit antiserum to human prostatic fluid (aPF) and normal rabbit serum (NRS). The wells were filled as follows: (1) PF 1, (2) PF 2, (3), NRS, (4) aPF. Part 2. Gel diffusion precipitation patterns of human prostatic fluid tested against rabbit antiserum to human prostatic fluid. Staining has been done first for acid phosphatase and then for other proteins (using light green SF). The prostatic fluid had a protein concentration of 2.5%. The wells were filled as follows: 1-6, PF at the following dilutions, respectively: 1:1, 1:4, 1:8, 1:16, 1:32, and 1:64; 7-9, rabbit antiserum; 10, normal human serum. (From Shulman et al., 1965a).

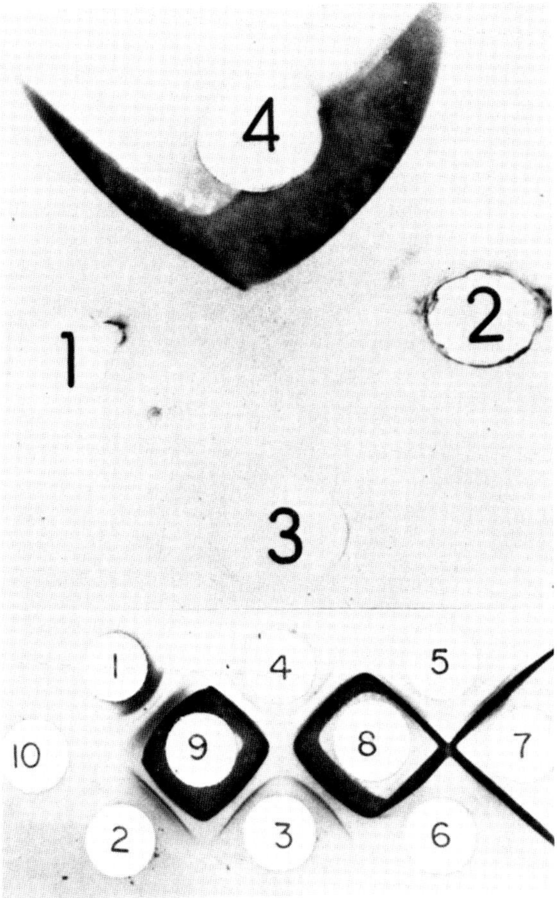

Figure 2

The sensitivity of the method of staining described above was evaluated by dilution studies. The limiting value that was attainable for the more prominent band varied with the individual sample. The presence of two stainable bands, especially since they had different mobilities in immunoelectrophoresis, indicated that there were two different molecular forms of prostatic acid phosphatase. Different samples of prostatic fluid, coming from different men, could be titrated in this gel diffusion procedure to various degrees (Shulman et al., 1965a). These titers ranged from 64 to 16,000. A set of such comparisons is shown in Figure 3. Furthermore, there was a good parallel between these titer values and the traditional King-Armstrong assay results for the phosphatase enzyme activity. In a third study, extracts of human prostate gland were also studied along with prostatic fluid. Several additional bands of precipitation were stained for phosphatase activity (Shulman and Ferber, 1966). The increased number of detected components in this study was the successful result of testing a number of different bleedings from each of several rabbits under long-term immunization. There were three major bands and two minor bands of this sort. The important conclusion of the whole study was that four or five different forms of acid phosphatase exist in prostatic tissue and secretion. An alternative enzymatic staining method was subsequently used by Pontes and colleagues (Choe et al., 1978; Pontes et al., 1977, 1981). They made use of the method for staining prostatic acid phosphatase as a method for identifying prostatic cells. Another specific antigen of prostate was identified and studied by Murphy and colleagues (Nadji et al., 1981; Papisero et al., 1981;

Figure 3. Gel diffusion precipitation patterns of human prostatic fluid tested against rabbit antiserum to human prostatic fluid. Each numbered row contains a dilution series from a different individual; the dilutions are 1:1, 1:4, 1:8, 1:16, 1:32, 1:64, 1:128, 1:256, 1:512, 1:1024, 1:2048, and 1:4096. Each row labeled a contains portions of the undiluted antiserum. (From Shulman et al., 1965a.)

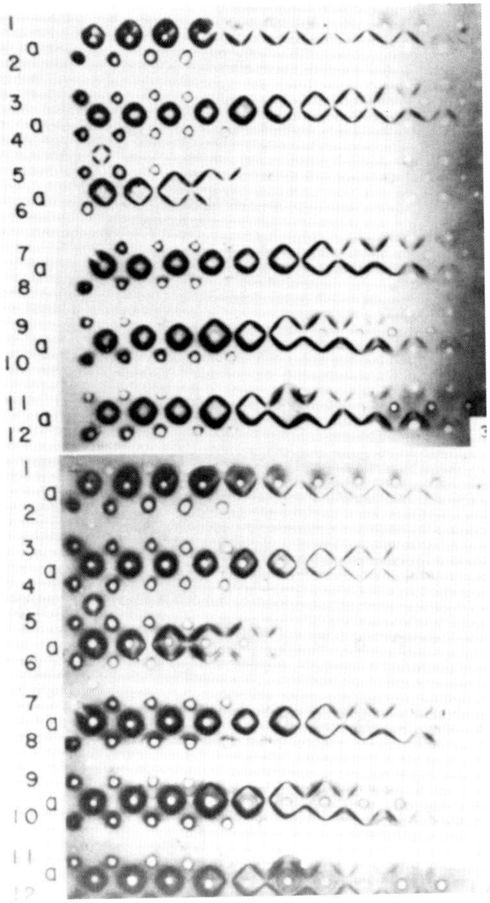

Figure 3.

Wang et al., 1979, 1981). More recently, Prout and colleagues made use of both these antigen-antibody systems to identify prostatic cells in cancer tissues, both primary and metastatic (Allhof et al., 1983). They found it very useful to stain the suspect sections from patients, to locate, if present, both the prostate-specific acid phosphatase (PSAP) and the prostate-specific antigen (PSA).

Another antigen—a carcinoembryonic antigen—like substance—has also been found to be associated with prostatic secretion (Aumüller et al., 1983). This component may become another useful marker of prostatic cells.

III. SEMINAL VESICLE

Studies have been made on the guinea pig in which the components of the seminal vesicle have been analyzed (Shulman, 1970; Shulman and Orsini, 1970). Figure 4 shows the anatomy of this gland, a remarkably large structure in this species of animal. A number of studies have been made on the vesicular fluid. If the fluid of the guinea pig seminal vesicle is used in isoimmunization, antibodies are produced. The major components have been termed I, II, and III, and minor components were additionally seen when large sample sizes were applied. By ultracentrifugal examination, this material looked quite homogeneous, with only a single symmetrical peak seen, with a sedimentation coefficient of about 1.5S. Starch block electrophoresis at pH 8.6 was used to separate the three major components, which were then studied by gel diffusion analysis (Orsini and Shulman, 1971). The isolated fractions were reasonably pure, judging from the patterns in cellulose acetate electrophoresis performed on each isolated sample and compared with the pattern for the whole material. Immunochemical studies were carried out by injecting rabbits with the whole guinea pig vesicular fluid; each rabbit antiserum showed a strong precipitation line in gel diffusion when tested with the vesicular fluid. These results are illustrated in Figure 5, which also shows additional comparisons, namely, the reactions of this antiserum with vesicular fluid, seminal plasma, prostate-coagulating gland extract,

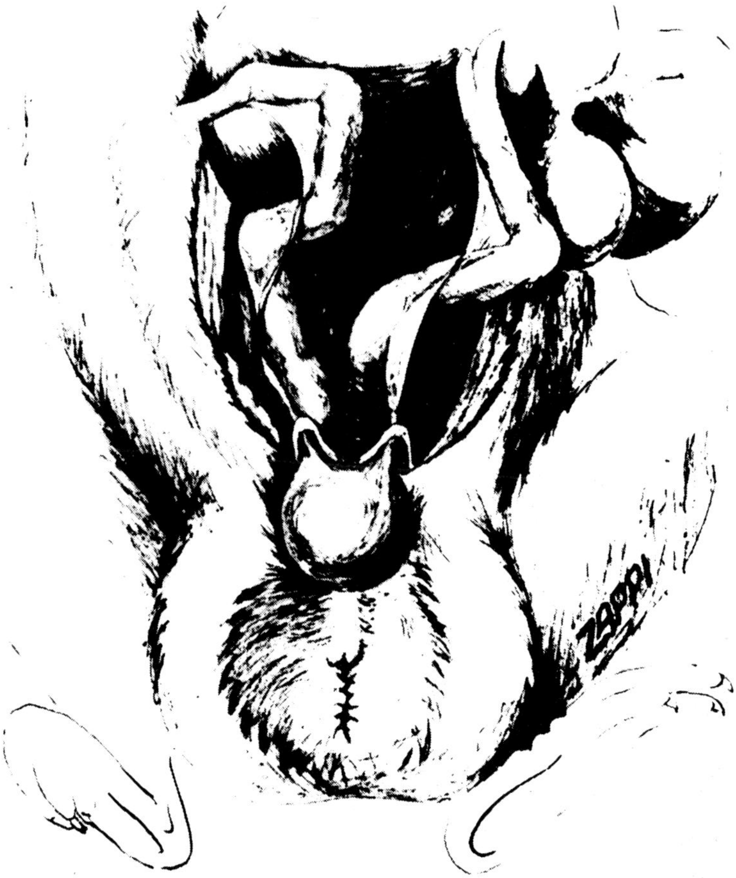

Figure 4. Anatomic structure of the seminal vesicles of the guinea pig showing their abdominal setting. (From Shulman, 1974.)

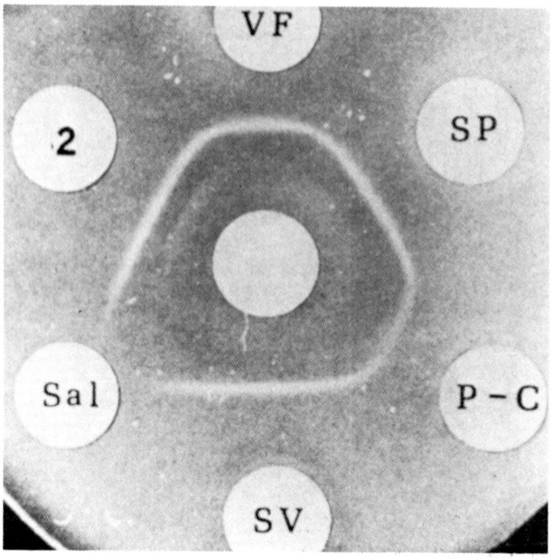

Figure 5. Gel diffusion precipitation pattern of guinea pig seminal vesicle and other preparations tested against a rabbit antiserum. Central well: rabbit anti-guinea pig vesicular fluid. Peripheral wells: VF, vesicular fluid; SP, seminal plasma; P-C, prostate-coagulating gland extract; SV, seminal vesicle extract; Sal, saline; 2, component II. (From Orsini and Shulman, 1971.)

and seminal vesicle extract. Each of these tissue preparations showed a strong precipitation line, and they all merged to indicate a common antigen. Well 6 contained a preparation of component II, isolated from the starch block. It clearly showed a positive reaction. When components I and III were tested, however, they completely failed to precipitate (Orsini and Shulman, 1971). Hence, there are interesting differences in properties among the components.

These antisera failed to give any precipitation with guinea pig serum or with other guinea pig organ extracts tested at various dilutions. These included testis, epididymis, and kidney; all of these were completely negative. The only organ extracts that contained antigenic material in common with the vesicular fluid were seminal plasma, prostate-coagulating gland, and seminal vesicle extract, as already mentioned.

Similar studies have been reported on the vesicular fluid of the rabbit (Shulman and Orsini, 1975). In contrast to the guinea pig, the rabbit has a vesicular fluid that contains only one major electrophoretic component. This component was isolated by starch block electrophoresis, and it was found to have a molecular weight of approximately 17,300, as determined by sedimentation and diffusion in the ultracentrifuge. It was highly tissue specific, that is, accessory gland specific, and it was also species specific. This fraction was also an effective antigen in procedures of iso-immunization, for these procedures led to the production of auto-antibodies. When rabbit vesicular fluid was ejaculated as part of the seminal plasma, its molecules were still able, in the subsequent mixture, to induce an autoantibody response by means of iso-immunization, and the response was the same as that induced by used of the vesicular fluid itself.

A different area of investigation of vesicular fluid has been developed by Matoušek and his colleagues (Dostal and Matoušek, 1973; Matoušek, 1973; Matoušek et al., 1973). They have studied a different species of animal and a variation of the aspermatogenesis phenomenon. They found that seminal vesicle fluid from the bull contained an aspermatogenic substance (AS), as tested by injection into mouse testes. This bovine vesicular component has been purified by several steps of gel filtration. It has a molecular weight of 22,000, and it also occurs as a dimer (of 44,000 molecular weight). Amino acid analyses were done, and the N-terminal amino acid was found to be lysine. No enzymatic activities (other than ribonuclease) could be found associated with the AS; however, it did exhibit high RNase activity. The AS was therefore renamed AS RNase.

IV. SEMINAL PLASMA

Although related to some of the other studies already discussed, the exploration of the components, especially the antigens, of seminal plasma has been a large area of study in its own right.

A. The Sperm-Coating Antigen

The antigenic properties of seminal plasma were first studied by Weil and his associates in pioneering investigations. They demonstrated a number of strong antigens in rabbit seminal plasma (Weil and Finkler, 1958) and three antigens (or groups of antigens) in human seminal plasma (Weil et al., 1956).

The antisera that had been prepared against human seminal plasma or against whole semen or washed spermatozoa reacted in complement fixation or in precipitation with seminal plasma in quite high titer and also reacted with well-washed spermatozoa (Weil et al., 1956). This cross-reaction with ejaculated spermatozoa was the first hint that at least one of the dominant antigenic components of the spermatozoa might derive from the fluid constituents of the semen rather than from the spermatozoa themselves. Later work showed the existence of an antigen of seminal plasma, which was called the spermatozoa-coating antigen (SCA). This was found in both rabbit (Weil, 1960) and human (Weil and Rodenburg, 1960). They showed, for example, that antisera against ejaculated spermatozoa, although showing strong positive reactions with ejaculated spermatozoa, did not react at all when tested with epididymal spermatozoa. Second, antisera against seminal plasma also gave strong positive reactions with ejaculated spermatozoa and were negative with epididymal spermatozoa. These studies indicated quite strongly that (1) the antigenic natures of epididymal spermatozoa and ejaculated spermatozoa are significantly different, (2) the epididymal spermatozoa acquire an additional antigenic property while they pass through the urethra, and (3) there is a component of the seminal plasma that interacts with and coats these spermatozoa. Weil and his co-workers gave good evidence that this spermatozoa-coating antigen originated in the seminal vesicle (Weil and Rodenburg, 1962). This was a portion of their study of seminal plasma antigenicity (Weil, 1961; Weil and Finkler, 1959; Weil et al., 1961).

B. Seminal Plasma Autoimmunity

In a later study (Riera et al., 1967; Shulman et al., 1968d), in which the approach to isoimmunization was again undertaken but from a different point of view, rabbits were injected with three different types of preparation for comparison—whole semen, seminal plasma, and extract of epididymis. The epididymal material did not elicit autoantibody, but the seminal plasma and semen injections did. This provided autoantibodies as reagents for the evaluation of tissue specificity. In hemagglutination tests, some tissues gave negative results when tested with this autoantibody. including testis, epididymis, kidney, and serum, but the results with extracts of the accessory glands and the seminal plasma were positive. This strong degree of cross-reaction between the seminal plasma and the accessory glands of reproduction was not surprising, since it had already been shown that at least some antigens are common to semen and accessory reproductive tissue, although they are absent from blood and from other tissues of the body.

Gel diffusion studies were of interest. When the antiseminal plasma was tested in gel diffusion against rabbit seminal plasma, one band of precipitation was seen for each early bleeding, but after several injections an additional line appeared. The first line, or main line, was shown to merge in a reaction of identity with the line that was characteristic of the organs in the accessory gland complex, so this must represent the characteristic antigen of the accessory glands discussed above and studied in the semen. The other, fainter line was found to be associated with an antigen of seminal plasma that was not connected with the accessory glands and was apparently characteristic of seminal plasma itself. It was shown in other experiments to be present in extracts of epididymis. As mentioned earlier, epididymal constituents did not cross-react with accessory gland constitutents. Seminal plasma was also seen to contain two distinctive antigens in this type of immunization, one of which is shared by the accessory glands but not the epididymis, and the other is shared by the epididymis but not the accessory glands (Shulman et al., 1968d).

These studies in the rabbit suggest that human seminal plasma constituents might also have the propensity for stimulating autoantibody formation and thus lead to pathologic conditions.

C. Composition of Human Seminal Plasma: Physicochemical Properties

The physicochemical analysis of the protein components of seminal plasma from various species has been widely described in the literature. Some techniques have utilized the ultracentrifuge (Boursnell et al., 1962; Larson et al., 1954), and others have been based on electrophoresis (Gray and Huggins, 1942; Larson and Salisbury, 1954; Ross et al., 1942, 1943; Rozin et al., 1963), including zone electrophoresis (Camba, 1957; Ekbom and Wetterdal, 1961; Mischler and Reineke, 1966; Paolella, 1957; Raboch, 1961), and more recently immunoelectrophoresis has been used with increasing frequency (Hermann, 1960; Herrmann and Schirren, 1961; Klopstock et al., 1963; Searcy et al., 1964).

A problem with many of these reports is that the condition of the semen sample was not described. There was apparently no uniform opinion on the effects of storage of the sample. Some early workers did realize that electrophoresis should be performed as soon as possible in view of the labile character of the material. These questions of composition and lability were first studied by filter paper electrophoresis (Shulman and Bronson, 1968). A total of nine components were revealed, component 7 accounting for about 60% of the pattern. When samples were refrigerated at 4°C, the percentage of component 7 declined continuously but that of component 5 steadily rose. These changes with time of storage suggested the presence of proteolysis initiated by a seminal plasma enzyme. It seemed unlikely that both the enzyme and the substrate would be elaborated by the same tissue. Accordingly, several ejaculates were obtained in the form of split fractions. The two fractions of a single donation did contain different electrophoretic components, but even more important, each pattern was more stable on storage. It was concluded that these split fractions could therefore be better starting materials for isolation and purification of the major constituents (Shulman and Bronson, 1968).

D. Composition of Human Seminal Plasma: Antigenic Analysis

The heterogeneity of human seminal plasma has also been studied by means of antigenic analysis. Many of the earliest studies of this sort have been described in detail elsewhere and will not be reviewed here (Shulman, 1974, 1975). This survey showed that many reports have appeared in the old literature on the analysis of human seminal plasma by the use of antisera; the results varied in revealing from 4 to 16 components. However, some of these reports suffered from technical or theoretical defects. It has sometimes been overlooked that not all immunized animals will produce equally full collections of antibody responses, and the use of only one antiserum against each antigenic material has led to inadequate studies. Furthermore, the extent of the antibody response to components of blood serum and to components that are common to other tissues of the body has not always been studied. In addition to these theoretical problems, there have been only limited efforts, in the frequent use of gel diffusion methods, to study variations in concentration of seminal plasma or of antiserum, as well as the geometry, time of incubation, and temperature. In some reports, commercial antisera have been put to use, with no studies of the sensitivity or the degree of specificity of these reagents.

In a study by Shulman and Bronson (1969), rabbit antisera to human seminal plasma gave precipitation with normal human serum and revealed several such lines of reaction, indicating the presence of a number of serum components in the seminal plasma that had been used for immunization. (The preimmunization rabbit sera gave no reactions.) The exact number of apparent cross-reacting components varied with the individual rabbit and with the particular blood sample; in addition, the number of indicated lines varied considerably with the geometry of the arrangement of wells. A total of six lines was distinguished for human serum itself. The number of lines, apart from serum lines, was quite different under varying conditions of geometry and dilution but did suggest a total of 8–11 distinctive components (Shulman and Bronson, 1969).

Immunoelectrophoresis using an antiserum selected for its ability to show many well-separated lines was then applied for clearer resolution. This often revealed as many as 11 or 12 distinctive arcs. The exact number varied from one sample to another, but the analysis of numerous experiments revealed a rather typical pattern of precipitation. A schematic diagram is shown in Figure 6. The major arcs were indicated by the letters A, C, E, and F. The lines for C and E were actually groups of lines with very similar mobilities. The individual components were therefore distinguished as C_1, C_2, C_3, E_1, and E_2. A faint additional pair was frequently seen in the F region, and these were termed F_1 and (fainter) F_2. In addition to these eight components, there were several lines at a much greater distance from the antibody trough; these were located near the fast end and the slow end of the C group of arcs. They have therefore been designated as the B and D groups. Since two members of each of these minor groups were detected, it was concluded that there were a minimum of 12 reproducibly detected components in seminal plasma (Shulman and Bronson, 1969). An immunoelectrophoretic pattern for rabbit seminal plasma was published by Menge and Protzman (1967), and this pattern is rather similar in many details to the pattern obtained for human material. An antigenic analysis of this sort has also been made of guinea pig seminal plasma (Maruta and Moyer, 1967).

The presence of serum albumin in seminal plasma is best proven by an experiment according to the method of Osserman (1960), in which one trough contains, instead of antiserum, the antigen, that is, 0.01% human serum albumin; the parallel trough contains the usual antiserum to human seminal plasma. In one such study, a horizontal line of precipitation was seen between the troughs, resulting from migration of the serum albumin toward its corresponding antibody in the antiserum; the line showed a perfect and complete reaction of fusion with the arc that had been designated component A, in the pattern for seminal plasma components (Shulman and Bronson, 1969).

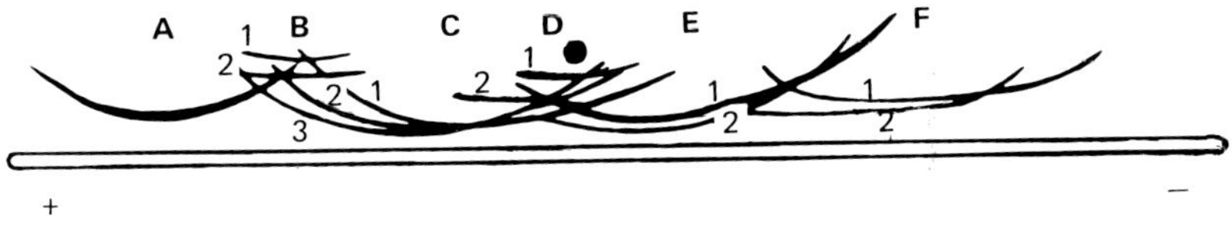

Figure 6. Immunoelectrophoretic sketch, somewhat idealized from a group of individual patterns, of human seminal plasma tested against a rabbit antiserum, according to Shulman and Bronson. (From Shulman and Bronson, 1969.)

This same basic pattern for seminal plasma in immunoelectrophoresis has been presented by other workers, although with different terminology. Thus, Hekman and Rümke (1969b) have presented an immunoelectrophoretic pattern for human seminal plasma that is very similar to that just described. Their study was prompted partly by interest in the spermatozoa-coating antigen (SCA) of Weil. Their pattern is shown in Figure 7, as taken from a more recent report. There are only nine components, but it should be noted that the antiserum used here had been absorbed with human serum. The SCA was definitely shown to be the same as D_1 in our own system (Fig. 6). This SCA fraction and our major fraction, C_2 (see below), are thus of interest for further purification and characterization as possible components of the antigenic stimulus involved in autoantibody formation. Hekman and

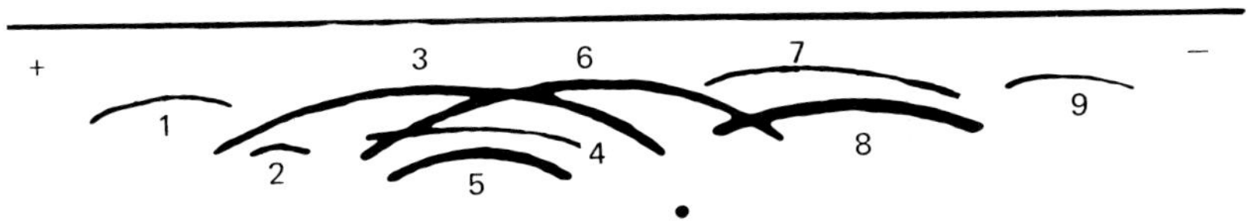

Figure 7. Immunoelectrophoretic sketch, idealized, of human seminal plasma tested against a rabbit antiserum, according to Hekman and Rümke. (From Hekman and Rümke, 1969b.)

Rümke (1969a) showed that seminal vesicle components corresponded to lines 5 and 6 in their pattern, and that three antigens, for lines 3, 7, and 8, came from the prostate gland. The two patterns obtained by these two groups were adjusted photographically, normalizing the lengths, and mounted together. This result is shown in Figure 8. A direct comparison of the patterns can be seen.

Further studies have been made of the purification and properties of the SCA by Weil et al. (Lippiello et al., 1968; Weil and Stetanovic, 1969) and by Boettcher and colleagues (Boettcher, 1969; Roberts and Boettcher, 1969). The latter group showed that the SCA is an iron-binding protein of seminal plasma and that it shares antigenic groups with lactoferrin but not transferrin; they proposed to name it scaferrin (Roberts and Boettcher, 1969), but this name does not seem to be widely used.

Herrmann and Schirren (1961) also described a similar immunoelectrophoretic pattern for human seminal plasma. In later work, a number of organ-specific proteins were described in the seminal plasma, as well as certain blood plasma proteins and other proteins (Herrmann, 1969). A group of eight characteristic proteins have been described in some detail, including two aminopeptidases, both secreted by the prostate gland, which have been studied in terms of antigenic structure, electrophoretic mobility, and molecular weight (Herrmann, 1968). The presence of certain gammaglobulins has been studied by several gel diffusion procedures, and IgG, IgA, and two kinds of molecular fragments of gammaglobulin were detected (Herrmann and Hermann, 1969a). Antigenic studies of seminal plasma have also been reported by Bandhauer (1966) and Zimmermann and Kipping (1967).

Halpern et al. (1967) have shown that human antibodies against constituents of human seminal plasma can occur. This case of antibody formation to such antigens is of special concern because it was a reaginic antibody that caused anaphylactoid reactions in the woman involved, in addition to being detectable by the usual skin-testing procedures. These workers also performed some fractionation studies, and the allergenic activity was associated with a glyco-

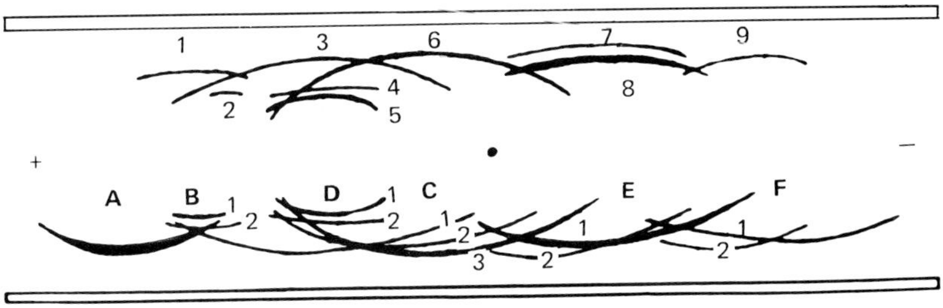

Figure 8. Immunoelectrophoretic sketch, as adjusted photographically and combined, to compare the two patterns for human seminal plasma tested against two rabbit antisera. Bottom half: the pattern presented by Shulman and Bronson. Top half: the pattern presented by Hekman and Rümke. [From Shulman, S. (1971). Antigenicity and autoimmunity in sexual reproduction: A review, *Clin. Exp. Immunol. 9*:267. (1971).]

protein fraction of seminal plasma that was rich in sialic acid and gave a single immunoelectrophoretic line, instead of the six lines seen for whole seminal plasma. Although a precise comparison of the given pattern and that described above is difficult, it seems probable that their allergen is found in our group of E components (Shulman and Bronson, 1969). A reaginic antibody to human seminal plasma has again been described and more thoroughly studied by Levine et al. (1973). Reports by Stevens et al. (1965) have suggested the presence of human autoantibodies to antigens of seminal plasma.

These multitudinous components of human seminal plasma were separated by starch block electrophoresis using preparations from split ejaculates (Shulman et al., 1965b). There was reasonably good resolution into six peaks, arbitrarily designated by numbers. Fraction 3 was the major component, and only this fraction has been further studied in any detail. It was analyzed repeatedly by immunochemical procedures and found to be a much more homogeneous product than the original whole seminal plasma, as judged by filter paper electrophoresis and analytic ultracentrifugation and especially by gel diffusion analysis. The ultracentrifugal result showed a single component with no sign of faster peaks. This single sedimenting peak had a sedimentation coefficient of 1.0S. The immunoelectrophoretic method was also used to confirm the improved homogeneity and to show the identification of this isolated component by the Osserman technique (Osserman, 1960). The single horizontal line of precipitation showed a deviation into an arc that was a component of the C group, probably C_2, of whole seminal plasma. Thus, this major immunoelectrophoretic component has been identified as corresponding to the tallest peak in the zonal electrophoretic pattern (Shulman and Bronson, 1968, 1969). Gel filtration has also been used for fractionation of these antigens (Li and Shulman, 1971; Shulman and Li, 1973; Zappi et al., 1972b). A 1.1S protein was also described by Herrmann, as was a 3.72S protein. This 3.72S component has now been purified, and some of its properties were described by Herrmann and Hermann (1969b).

Isojima et al. (1982) prepared a rat monoclonal antibody and used it for isolation studies. By means of immunoaffinity chromatography, they purified an antigen of human seminal plasma that they termed antigen 7. The purified antigen obtained by rechromatography gave a single band on SDS-PAGE in a position corresponding to a molecular weight of 15,000. The purified antigen 7 contained iron but was different from lactoferrin and transferrin. It did not show any enzymatic activities, such as those of acid phosphatase, lactate dehydrogenase (LDH), or trypsin inhibitor, but it shared antigenicity with human milk protein. It was present in seminal plasma as a molecule with a higher molecular weight but seemed to be cleaved to a monomer of 15,000 during the purification procedures. This antigen is present on spermatozoa as a sperm-coating antigen, and the corresponding antibody, with complement, can immobilize spermatozoa.

Subsequently, this antigen 7 was called Ferrisplan, and its distribution in male genital organs, spermatozoa, and body fluids was studied (Koyama et al., 1983). The amount of Ferrisplan in body fluids was determined by radioimmunoassay. Large amounts were detected in seminal plasma and milk, trace amounts in saliva, and none in the serum and urine. The concentration of Ferrisplan was highest in the seminal plasma of azoospermic patients and gradually decreased from oligospermia to normospermia. Using an immunofluorescent method with anti-Ferrisplan monoclonal antibody, strong staining was observed on the epithelial layers of human seminal vesicles, whereas there was no staining on testes and there was bright staining on the postnuclear cap and midpiece segment of spermatozoa. These results indicate that Ferrisplan is excreted mainly from the seminal vesicle and adheres to the postnuclear cap and midpiece of the spermatozoa as a sperm-coating antigen.

The components of rabbit seminal plasma were fractionated (Shulman, 1975). Gel diffusion on Sephadex G-100 was applied, and four main fractions were eluted, fractions A, B, C, and D. Although fraction D seemed to be mostly nucleic acidlike material, the other three fractions contained protein and they were, respectively, 9.1S, 6.5S, and 2.1S components. Other properties of these fractions, especially various antigenic properties, were also described.

In another report, human seminal plasma and one of its major fractions were studied as ultracentrifugal components (Shulman and Li, 1974). The pattern of the original seminal plasma showed three peaks. The main peak (peak II) was 6.2S components; the other two components had sedimentation coefficients of 12.6S and 1.0S. A previously isolated fraction, identified as the E_1 antigen (Li and Beling, 1973; Li and Shulman, 1971; Shulman and Li, 1973), was also studied. This fraction showed a single homogeneous peak with a sedimentation coefficient of 2.3S, corresponding to a molecular weight of about 31,000, as had been earlier estimated by other means (Li and Beling, 1973). The effects of its antibodies have also been studied (Li and Beling, 1974). This field of investigation has also been reviewed by Li (1974).

A final point should be made concerning the antigenic components of seminal plasma and their specificity characteristics. It is generally assumed that the specific components of seminal plasma are surely components that occur only in the male animal and are absent from the female animal. As a matter of fact, this may not really be true, at least not for all the constituents of interest. For example, a very interesting report was made by De Fazio and Ketchel (1972), who examined this question in the human species. They studied various extracts and secretions from women by means of immunoelectrophoresis using an antiserum against human seminal plasma. They claimed that they could detect a total of 23 antigens of the seminal plasma. Of these antigens, 7 were to be found in blood serum; another 10 antigens were found in other female tissues and secretions. It was found that milk contained 1 of the nonserum components, and that saliva, urine, vagina, and ovary each contained 2. In addition, cervical mucus and the kidney were each found to have 3, the nasal secretion, cervix, endometrium, and Fallopian tube each had 4, and finally gastric fluid had 5 of these antigens. They also presented the hypothesis that women escape sensitization to the antigens of seminal plasma, in general, because these proteins are actually present (and produced) in the female reproductive tract. Finally, we can add the semantic argument that if these findings can be accepted, then the antibodies that women do form against components of semen might well be defined as autoantibodies, instead of isoantibodies, after all.

REFERENCES

Ablin, R. J., and Soanes, W. A. (1972). Experimental production of autoimmune aspermatogenic orchitis in the rabbit in consequences of in situ freezing of the testis. *Eur. Surg. Res. 4*:98.

Ahmed, U., and Shulman, S. (1972). Fractionation of the antigens of canine prostatic fluid. *J. Immunol. 108*:432.

Ahmed, U., and Shulman, S. (1974). Further characterization of the antigens of canine prostatic fluid. *Immunology 26*:1207.

Allhoff, E. P., Proppe, K. H., Chapman, C. M., Lin, C. W., and Prout, G. R., Jr. (1983). Evaluation of prostate specific acid phosphatase and prostate specific antigen in identification of prostatic cancer. *J. Urol. 129*:315.

Aumüller, G., Krause, W., Bischof, W., and Seitz, J. (1983). Carcinoembryonic antigen-like substance is a marker of prostatic secretory function. *Andrologia 15*:159.

Bandhauer, K. (1966). Zum Problem der Antigeneigenschaften des menschlichen Samenplasmas. *Wien. Med. Wochenschr. 116*:318.

Barnes, G., Soanes, W. A., Mamrod, L., Gonder, M. J., and Shulman, S. (1963). Immunologic properties of human prostatic fluid. *J. Lab. Clin. Med. 61*:578.

Barnes, G., Shulman, S., Gonder, M. J., and Soanes, W. A. (1965). Further studies of the immunological properties of human prostatic fluid. *J. Lab. Clin. Med. 66*:741.

Bishop, D. W., Narbaitz, R., and Lessof, M. (1961). Induced aspermatogenesis in adult guinea pig injected with testicular antigen and adjuvant in neonatal stages. *Dev. Biol. 3*:444.

Boehme, D. (1965). Response of reticuloendothelial system of experimental allergic orchitis in a genetically susceptible and resistant mouse genotype. *Proc. Soc. Exp. Biol. Med. 118*:374.

Boettcher, B. (1969). Blood group antigens in seminal plasma, and the nature of human sperm-coating antigen. In *Immunology and Reproduction* R. G. Edwards, ed.), International Planned Parenthood Federation, London, p. 148.

Boursnell, J. C., Johnson, P., and Zamora, J. (1962). An electrophoretic and ultracentrifugal study of boar seminal plasma. *Biochim. Biophys. Acta 63*:374.

Camba, R. (1957). Contributo all'interpretazione del diagramma electroferetico dello sperma umano. *Minerva Medicoleg. 77*:43.

Choe, B. K., Pontes, E. J., Rose, N. R., and Henderson, M. D. (1978). Expression of human prostatic acid phosphatase in a pancreatic islet cell carcinoma. *Invest. Urol. 15*:312.

De Almeida, M., Lefroit-Jolly, M., and Voisin, G. A. (1981). Studies on human spermatozoa autoantigens. I. Fractionation of sperm membrane antigens: Evidence of three antigenic systems. *Clin. Exp. Immunol. 44*:359.

De Fazio, S. R., and Ketchel, M. M. (1972). The occurrence of seminal plasma antigens in the tissues of women. *J. Reprod. Fertil. 30*:125.

Dondero, F., and Isidori, A. (1972). Anti-testicular autoimmunity in man. *Ann. Endocrinol. 33*:417.

Dostal, J., and Matoušek, J. (1973). Isolation and some chemical properties of aspermatogenic substance from bull seminal vesicle fluid. *J. Reprod. Fertil.* *33*:263.

Dufour, D., Gagnon, P. M., Tremblay, A., Proulx, J., and Lemieux, S. (1965a). Charactérisation des relations antigeniques et enzymatiques entre la prostate et l'urine humaine. *Laval. Med.* *36*:643.

Dufour, D., Lafontaine, A., and Lille, S. (1965b). Polymorphisme d'une urophosphatase humaine. *Rev. Immunol.* (*Paris*) *29*:411.

Dufour, D., Tremblay, A., and Lemieux, S. (1966). Différence de spécificité immunologique entre la phosphatase urinaire humaine male et femelle. *Rev. Fr. Etud. Clin. Biol.* *11*:89.

Ekbom, K., and Wetterdal, B. (1961). Paper-electrophoretic studies on human semen with special interest in the distribution of administered Zn^{65}. *Scand. J. Clin. Lab. Invest.* *13*:396.

Eyquem, A., and Krieg, H. (1965). Experimental autosensitization of the testis. *Ann. N.Y. Acad. Sci.* *124*:270.

Feuchter, F. A., Vernon, R. B., and Eddy, E. M. (1981). Analysis of the sperm surface with monoclonal antibodies: Topographically restricted antigens appearing in the epididymis. *Biol. Reprod.* *24*:1099.

Freund, J., Lipton, M. M., and Thompson, G. E. (1954). Impairment of spermatogenesis in the rat after cutaneous injection of testicular suspension with complete adjuvant. *Proc. Soc. Exp. Biol. Med.* *87*:408.

Freund, J., Lipton, M. M., and Thompson, G. E. (1963). Aspermatogenesis in the guinea pig induced by testicular tissue and adjuvants. *J. Exp. Med.* *97*:711.

Gaunt, S. J., (1982). A 28K-Dalton cell surface autoantigen of spermatogenesis: Characterization using a monoclonal antibody. *Dev. Biol.* *89*:92.

Gaunt, S. J., Brown, C. R., and Jones, R. (1983). Identification of mobile and fixed antigens on the plasma membrane of rat spermatozoa using monoclonal antibodies. *Exp. Cell Res.* *144*:275.

Gray, S., and Huggins, C. (1942). Electrophoretic analysis of human semen. *Proc. Soc. Exp. Biol. Med.* *50*:351.

Hagopian, A., Jackson, J. J., Carlo, D. J., Limjuco, G. A., and Eylar, E. H. (1975). Experimental allergic aspermatogenic orchitis. III. Isolation of spermatozoal glycoproteins and their role in allergic aspermatogenic orchitis. *J. Immunol.* *115*:1731.

Hagopian, A., Limjuco, G., Jackson, J. J., Carlo, D., and Eylar, E. H. (1976). Experimental allergic aspermatogenic orchitis. IV. Chemical properties of sperm glycoproteins isolated from guinea pig testes. *Biochim. Biophys. Acta 434*:354.

Halpern, B. N., Ky, T., and Robert, B. (1967). Clinical and immunological study of an exceptional case of reaginic type sensitization to human seminal fluid. *Immunology 12*:247.

Hargis, B. J., Malkiel, S., and Berkelhammer, J. (1968). Immunologically induced aspermatogenesis in the white mouse. *J. Immunol. 101*:374.

Hekman, A., and Rümke, P. (1969). The antigens of human seminal plasma. *Fertil. Steril. 20*:312.

Hekman, A., and Rümke, P. (1969b). The specificity of the antigens of human seminal plasma with special reference to lactoferrin as spermatozoa-coating antigen. In *Immunology of Spermatozoa and Fertilization, Proceedings of the International Symposium, Varna, Bulgaria, 1967* (K. Bratanov, ed.), Bulgarian Academy of Sciences Press, Sofia, p. 107.

Hendry, W. F., Parslow, J. M., and Stedronska, J. (1983). Exploratory scrototomy in 168 azoospermic males. *Br. J. Urol. 55*:785.

Hermann, G. (1960). Le plasma séminal. In *Analyse Immuno-Electrophorétique (P. Grabar and* P. Burtin, eds.), Masson et Cie, Paris, p. 271.

Herr, J. C., and Eddy, E. M. (1980). Detection of mouse sperm antigens by a surface labeling and immunoprecipitation approach. *Biol. Reprod. 22*:1263.

Hermann, W. P. (1968). Immunologische Charakterisierung der Aminopeptidasen in menschlichen Spermaplasma. *Arch. Klin. Exp. Dermatol. 233*:249.

Herrmann, W. P. (1969). Immunologische Charakterisierung menschlischer Spermaplasmaprotein. *Andrologie 1*:11.

Herrmann, W. P., and Hermann, G. (1969a). Immunoelectrophoretic and chromatographic demonstration of IgG, IgA, and fragments of γ-globulin in the human seminal fluid. *Int. J. Fertil. 14*:211.

Herrmann, W. P., nad Hermann, G. (1969b). Purification of the specific seminal fluid 3.72 S protein. *Fertil. Steril. 20*:521.

Herrmann, W. P., and Schirren, C. (1961). Immunoelektrophoretische Untersuchungen des menschlichen Spermaplasma. *Z. Hautkr. 34*:134.

Huggins, C., and Sommer, J. L. (1963). Quantitative studies of prostatic secretion. III. Simultaneous measurement of size and secretion of the canine prostate and the interaction of androgenic and estrogenic substances thereon. *J. Exp. Med. 97*:663.

Isidori, A., Dondero, F., and Lombardo, D. (1970). Antitesticular immunity. Role of the basement membrane. *Experientia 26*:1375.

Isojima, S., Koyama, K., and Fujiwara, N. (1982). Purification of human seminal plasma No. 7 antigen by immunoaffinity chromatography on bound monoclonal antibody. *Clin. Exp. Immunol. 49*:449.

Jackson, J. J., Hagopian, A., Carlo, D. J., Limjuco, G. A., and Eylar, E. H. (1975). Experimental allergic aspermatogenic orchitis. I. Isolation of spermatozoal protein (AP1) which induces allergic aspermatogenic orchitis. *J. Biol. Chem. 250*:6141.

Jackson, J. J., Hagopian, A., Carlo, D., and Eylar, E. H. (1976). Experimental allergic aspermatogenic orchitis. II. Some chemical properties of the AP1 protein of the sperm acrosome. *Biochim. Biophys. Acta 427*:251.

Jagodzinski, R. V., Yantorno, C., and Shulman, S. (1967). An experimental system for the production of antibodies in response to cryo-surgical procedures. *Cryobiology 3*:456.

Kantor, G. L., and Dixon, F. J. (1972). Transfer of experimental allergic orchitis with peritoneal exudate cells. *J. Immunol. 108*:329.

Katsh, S. (1964). Adjuvants and aspermatogenesis in the guinea pig. *Int. Arch. Allergy 24*:319.

Katsh, S., and Aguirre, A. (1968). Biochemical responses in organs of guinea pigs immunized with aspermatogenic antigen. *Int. Arch. Allergy 33*:141.

Katsh, S., and Bishop, D. (1958). The effects of homologous testicular and brain and heterologous testicular homogenates combined with adjuvant upon the testes of guinea pig. *J. Embryol. Exp. Morphol. 6*:94.

Klopstock, A., Haas, R., and Rimon, A. (1963). Immunoelectrophoretic analysis of seminal plasma. *Fertil. Steril. 14*:530.

Kolk, A. H. J., Samuel, T., and Rümke, P. (1974). Autoantigens of human spermatozoa. I. Solubilization of a new autoantigen detected on swollen sperm heads. *Clin. Exp. Immunol. 16*:63.

Koyama, K., Takada, Y., Takemura, T., and Isojima, S. (1983). Localization of human seminal plasma No. 7 antigen (Ferrisplan) in accessory glands of male genital tract and spermatozoa. *J. Reprod. Immunol.* *5*:135.

Larson, B. L., and Salisbury, G. W. (1954). The proteins of bovine seminal plasma. I. Preliminary and electrophoretic studies. *J. Biol. Chem.* *206*:741.

Larson, B. L., Gray, R. S., and Salisbury, G. W. (1954). The proteins of bovine seminal plasma. II. Ultracentrifugal and immunological studies and comparison with blood and milk serum. *J. Biol. Chem.* *211*:43.

Laurence, K. A., and Perlbachs, M. (1962). Studies on the relationship of delayed hypersensitivity to experimental aspermatogenesis in rats. *Bacteriol. Proc.* *88*:88.

Laurence, K. A., Carpuk, O., and Perlbachs, M. (1965). Transfer of testicular lesions by leukocytes from testis-immunized rats. *Int. J. Fertil.* *10*:13.

Lee, C. G., Huang, Y. S., Huang, C. H., Hu, P. C., and Menge, A. C. (1982). Monoclonal antibodies to human sperm antigens. *J. Reprod. Immunol.* *4*:173.

Levine, B. B., Siraganian, R. P., and Schenkein, I. (1973). Allergy to human seminal plasma. *N. Engl. J. Med.* *288*:894.

Li, T. S. (1974). Sperm immunology, infertility and fertility control. *Obstet. Gynecol.* *44*:607.

Li, T. S., and Beling, C. G., (1973). Isolation and characterization of two specific antigens of human seminal plasma. *Fertil. Steril.* *24*:134.

Li, T. S., and Beling, C. G. (1974). The effect of antibodies to two human seminal plasma-specific antigens on human sperm. *Fertil. Steril.* *25*:851.

Li, T. S., and Shulman, S. (1971). Immunoelectrophoretic analysis of human seminal plasma fractions after fractionation by various methods. *Int. J. Fertil.* *16*:87.

Lippiello, L. A., El-Rubaye, F., and Weil, A. J. (1968). Human spermatozoa-coating antigen. Studies on purification. *Fertil. Steril.* *19*:991.

Losos, G. J., Winter, A. J., and McEntree, K. (1968). Induction of testicular degeneration in bulls by isoimmunization. *Am. J. Vet. Res.* *29*:2295.

Macalalag, E. V., Jr., and Prout, G. R., Jr. (1967). Anti-canine prostatic fluid serum and prostatic degeneration. *Invest. Urol. 4*:321.

Mancini, R. E., Andrada, J. A., Saraceni, D., Bachmann, A. E., Lavierei, J. C., and Nemirovsky, M. (1965). Immunological and testicular response in man sensitized with human testicular homogenate. *J. Clin. Endocrinol. Metab. 25*:859.

Mancini, R. E., Huidobro, H., Collazo, E. F., and Monastirsky, R. (1966). Detection of a kinin substance in the testis of guinea pig after induced allergic orchitis. *Proc. Soc. Exp. Biol. Med. 123*:227.

Maruta, H., and Moyer, D. L. (1967). Immunologic studies of the antigens of guinea pig semen. *Fertil. Steril. 18*:649.

Mason, M. M., Keefe, F., and Boria, T. (1961). Specialized surgery of the canine bladder and prostate fluid. *J. Am. Vet. Med. 139*:1007.

Matoušek, J. (1973). Antiembryonic effect of bull seminal vesicle fluid in mice. *J. Reprod. Fertil. 32*:175.

Matoušek, J., Pavlok, A., Dostál, J., and Grozdanovič, J. (1973). Some biological properties of bull seminal vesicle aspermatogenic substance and its effect on mice. *J. Reprod. Fertil. 34*:9.

Menge, A. C., and Christian, J. J., Jr. (1971). Effects of auto- and iso-immunization of bulls with semen and testis. *Int. J. Fertil. 16*:130.

Menge, A. C., and Protzman, W. P. (1967). Origin of the antigens in rabbit semen which induce antifertility antibody. *J. Reprod. Fertil. 13*:31.

Mettler, L., and Gradl. T. (1975). Solubilization of human spermatozoa and antigen isolation responsible for agglutination. *Res. Exp. Med. 165*:169.

Mettler, L., and Skrabei, H. (1979). Isolation of human spermatozoa membrane antigens binding spermimmobilizing and spermagglutinating antibodies. *Int. J. Fertil. 24*:44.

Mischler, T. W., and Reineke, E. P. (1966). Some electrophoretic and immunological properties of human semen. *J. Reprod. Fertil. 12*:125.

Moncure, C. W., and Prout, G. R., Jr. (1970). Antigenicity of human prostatic acid phosphatase. *Cancer 25*:463.

Myles, D. G., Primakoff, P., and Bellvé, A. R. (1981). Surface domains of the guinea pig sperm defined with monoclonal antibodies. *Cell 23*:433.

Nadji, M., Tabei, S. Z., Castro, A., Chu, T. M., Murphy, G. P., Wang, M. C., and Morales, A. R. (1981). Prostatic specific antigen. An immunohistologic marker for prostatic neoplasms. *Cancer 48:*1229.

Oliphant, G., and Singhas, C. A., (1979). Iodination of rabbit sperm plasma membrane: Relationship of specific surface proteins to epididymal function and sperm capacitation. *Biol. Reprod. 21*:937.

O'Rand, M. G., and Porter, J. P. (1982). Purification of rabbit sperm autoantigens by preparative SDS gel electrophoresis: Amino acid and carbohydrate content of RSA-1. *Biol. Reprod. 27*:713.

Orsini, F., and Shulman, S. (1971). The antigen and autoantigens of the seminal vesicle. I. Immunochemical studies on guinea pig vesicular fluid. *J. Exp. Med. 134*:120.

Osserman, E. F. (1960). A modified technique of immunoelectrophoresis facilitating the identification of specific precipitin arcs. *J. Immunol. 84*:93.

Paolella, A. (1957). Electroforesi su carta di liquido seminale umano normale e patologico. *Minerva Medicoleg. 77*:48.

Papsidero, L. D., Kuriyama, M., Wang, M. C., Horoszewicz, J., Leong, S. S., Valenzuela, L., Murphy, G. P., and Chu, T. M. (1981). Prostate antigen: A marker for human prostate epithelial cells. *JNCI 66*:37.

Peel, S. (1968). An immunologic study of dog prostate and the effects of injecting antidog prostate serum. *Invest. Urol. 5*:427.

Pfeiffer, L., Ablin, R. J., Gonder, M. J., and Soanes, W. A. (1970). Antibodies to human prostatic acid phosphatase. *Fertil. Steril. 21*:344.

Pokorná, Z., Vojtíšková, M., Rycliková, M., and Chutná, J. (1963). An isologous model of experimental autoimmune aspermatogenesis in mice. *Folia Biol. (Praha) 9*:203.

Pontes, J. E., Choe, B., Rose, N., and Pierce, J. M., Jr. (1977). Indirect immunofluorescence for identification of prostatic epithelial cells. *J. Urol. 117*:459.

Pontes, J. E., Rose, N. R., Ercole, C., and Pierce, J. M., Jr. (1981). Immunofluorescence for prostatic acid phosphatase: Clinical applications. *J. Urol. 126*:187.

Poulsen, F. (1983). The nature of an iso-antigen of the human sperm membrane. *J. Reprod. Immunol. 5*:49.

Poulsen, F., and Hjort, T. (1981). Identification of auto-antigens of the human sperm membrane. *J. Clin. Lab. Immunol. 6*:69.

Raboch, J. (1961). Electrophoresis of seminal plasma proteins. *Int. J. Fertil. 6*:31.

Raitsina, S. S., and Nilovsky, M. N. (1967). Posttraumatic aspermatogenesis. Resemblance of pathogenesis of autoallergic and posttraumatic orchitis. *Folia Biol. (Praha) 13*:450.

Riera, C., Yantorno, C., and Shulman, S. (1967). Antigenic specificity of seminal plasma and the formation of autoantibodies. *Fed. Proc. 26*:532.

Riera, C. M., Brandt, E. J., and Shulman, S. (1968). Studies in cryo-immunology. IV. Antibody development in rabbits after iso-immunization followed by freezing. *Immunology 15*:779.

Roberts, T. K., and Boettcher, B. (1969). Identification of human sperm-coating antigen. *J. Reprod. Fertil. 18*:347.

Ross, V., Moore, D. H., and Miller, E. G., Jr. (1942). Proteins of human seminal plasma. *J. Biol. Chem. 144*:667.

Ross, V., Miller, E. G., Jr., Moore, D. H., and Sikorski, H. (1943). Electrophoretic patterns of seminal plasma from some "abnormal" human semens. *Proc. Soc. Exp. Biol. Med. 54*:179.

Rozin, S., Graff, E., and Shafrir, E. (1963). Electrophoretic resolution and characterization of human seminal plasma proteins. *Int. J. Fertil. 8*:523.

Schmell, E. D., Yuan, L. C., Gulyas, B. J., and August, J. T. (1982). Identification of mammalian sperm surface antigens. I. Production of monoclonal antimouse sperm antibodies. *Fertil. Steril. 37*:249.

Searcy, R. L., Craig, R. G., and Bergquist, L. M. (1964). Immunochemical properties of normal and pathological plasma. *Fertil. Steril. 15*:1.

Shulman, S. (1968). Cryo-immunology: The production of antibodies by the freezing of tissue. In *Cryosurgery* (R. W. Rand, A. P. Rinfret, and H. von Leden, eds.), Charles C. Thomas, Springfield, Illinois, p. 78.

Shulman, S. (1969). Experimental cryosurgery and antibody response. *J. Cryosurg. 2*:90.
Shulman, S. (1970). Les auto-antigènes de la vesicule seminale. *Ann. Inst. Pasteur (Paris) 118*:529.
Shulman, S. (1974). The reproductive system. In *Tissue Specificity and Autoimmunity* (S. Shulman, ed.), Springer-Verlag, Berlin, p. 71.
Shulman, S. (1975). *Reproduction and Antibody Response*, CRC Press, Cleveland.
Shulman, S., and Ahmed, U. (1971). Prostate antigens and antibodies. *Proc. Soc. Exp. Biol. Med. 137*:97.
Shulman, S., and Bronson, P. (1968). Immunochemical studies on human seminal plasma. I. Changes in composition during storage, as demonstrated by electrophoresis. *Fertil. Steril. 19*:549.
Shulman, S., and Bronson, P. (1969). Immunochemical studies on human seminal plasma. II. The major antigens and their fractionation. *J. Reprod. Fertil. 18*:481.
Shulman, S., and Ferber, J. (1966). Multiple forms of prostatic acid phosphatase. *J. Reprod. Fertil. 11*:295.
Shulman, S., and Keane, T. (1981). Human soluble antigens and their use in sperm antibody testing. *Am. J. Reprod. Immunol. 1*:69.
Shulman, S., and Li, T. S. (1973). The analysis of the antigens of human seminal plasma. In *Immunology of Reproduction, Proceedings of the Second International Symposium, Varna, Bulgaria, 1971* (K. Bratanov, ed.), Bulgarian Academy of Sciences Press, Sofia, p. 133.
Shulman, S., and Li, T. S. (1974). Immunochemical studies on human seminal plasma. III. Ultracentrifugal studies on human seminal plasma and a purified fraction. *Int. J. Fertil. 19*:19.
Shulman, S., and Orsini, F. (1970). The antigens of seminal vesicle and seminal plasma. *Fertil. Steril. 21*: 794.
Shulman, S., and Orsini, F. (1975). The antigens and autoantigens of the seminal vesicle. II. Immunochemical studies on rabbit vesicular fluid. *J. Immunol. 115*:545.
Shulman, S., and Yantorno, C. (1971). Postnatal development of tissue-specific antigens of the male reproductive accessory glands. In *Protides of the Biological Fluids, Brugge, 18th Colloquium, 1970* (H. Peeters, ed.), Pergamon, Oxford, p. 153.

Shulman, S., and Zappi, E. (1972). Cryo-immunology: An aspect of cryobiology, In *Cryogenics in Surgery* (H. von Leden and W. Cahan, eds.), Medical Examination Publishing Co., Flushing, New York, p. 42.

Shulman, S., and Zappi, E. (1973). Cryo-immunization and the reproductive system: Aspermatogenesis, orchitis and epididymitis. In *Immunology of Reproduction, Proceedin gs of the Second International Symposium, Varna, Bulgaria, 1971* (K. Bratanov, ed.), Bulgarian Academy of Sciences Press, Sofia, p. 75.

Shulman, S., Mamrod, L., Gonder, M. J., and Soanes, W. A. (1964). The detection of prostatic acid phosphatase by antibody reactions in gel diffusion. *J. Immunol. 93*:474.

Shulman, S., Mamrod, L., Lang, R., Gonder, M. J., and Soanes, W. A. (1965a). Measurement of prostatic acid phosphatase by gel diffusion methods. *J. Reprod. Fertil. 10*:55.

Shulman, S., Yantorno, C., Barnes, G. W., Gonder, M. J., Soanes, W. A., and Witebsky, E. (1965b). Studies on autosensitization to prostatic tissue and related tissue. *Ann. N.Y. Acad. Sci. 124*:279.

Shulman, S., Brandt, E. J., and Yantorno, C. (1968a). Studies in cyro-immunology. II. Tissue specificity of the antibody response and comparison to isoimmunization. *Immunology 14*:149.

Shulman, S., Bronson, P., Gonder, M. J., and Soanes, W. A. (1968b). Ultracentrifugal constituents of human canine prostatic fluid. *Nature 197*:58.

Shulman, S., Bronson, P., Riera, C., Brandt, E. J., and Yantorno, C. (1968c). Studies in cryo-immunology. III. The immunoglobulin nature of the antibody response. *Immunology 14*:541.

Shulman, S., Riera, C., and Yantorno, C. (1968d). Studies on organ specificity. XIX. Antigenic specificity of seminal plasma and the formation of autoantibodies. *J. Immunol. 100*:682.

Soanes, W. A., Shulman, S., Mamrod, L., Barnes, G. W., and Gonder, M. J. (1963). Electrophoretic analysis of prostatic fluid. Classification according to agar gel electrophoresis. *Invest. Urol. 1*:269.

Stevens, K. M., Fost, C. A., and Balows, A. (1965). Circulating antibodies to human seminal plasma in man. *J. Reprod. Fertil. 10*:137.

Teuscher, C., Wild, G. C., and Tung, K. S. K. (1983). Acrosomal autoantigens of guinea pig sperm. I. The purification of an aspermatogenic protein, AP2. *J. Immunol. 130*:317.

Tung, K. S. K., Unanue, E. R., and Dixon, F. J., (1971). Pathogenesis of experimental allergic orchitis. I. Transfer with immune lymph node cells. *J. Immunol. 106*:1453.

Voisin, G. A., and Toullet, F. (1968). Étude sur l'orchite aspermatogénétique autoimmune et les auto-antigènes des spermatozoides chez le cobaye. *Ann. Inst. Pasteur (Paris) 114*:727.

Voisin, G. A., and Toullet, F. (1969). Relation between hypersensitivity responses to autoantigens and tissue damage in the male reproductive tract. In *Immunology and Reproduction* (R. G. Edwards, ed.), International Planned Parenthood Federation, London, p. 93.

Voisin, G. A., Delaunay, A., and Barber, M. (1951). Sur des lésions testiculaires provoquées chez le cobaye par iso- et auto-sensibilisation. *Ann. Inst. Pasteur (Paris) 81*:48.

Vottero-Cima, E., Vides, M. A., and Yantorno, C. (1973). Humoral autoimmune response against rabbit accessory glands elicited by untreated and chemically modified rabbit seminal plasma. *Ann. Immunol. (Inst. Pasteur) 124C*:273.

Wang, M. C., Valenzuela, L. A., Murphy, G. P., and Chu, T. M. (1979). Purification of a human prostate specific antigen. *Invest. Urol. 17*:159.

Wang, M. C., Papsidero, L. D., Kuriyama, M., Valenzuela, L. A., Murphy, G. P., and Chu, T. M. (1981). Prostate antigen: A new potential marker for prostatic cancer. Prostate *2*:89.

Weil, A. J. (1960). Immunological differentiation of epididymal and seminal spermatozoa of the rabbit. *Science 131*:1040.

Weil, A. J. (1961). Antigens of the adnexal glands of the male genital tract. *Fertil. Steril. 12*:538.

Weil, A. J., and Finkler, A. E. (1958). Antigens of rabbit semen. *Proc. Soc. Exp. Biol. Med. 98*:794.

Weil, A. J., and Finkler, A. E. (1959). Isoantigenicity of rabbit semen. *Proc. Soc. Exp. Biol. Med. 102*:624.

Weil, A. J., and Rodenburg, J. M. (1960). Immunological differentiation of human testicular (spermatocele) and seminal spermatozoa. *Proc. Soc. Exp. Biol. Med. 105*:43.

Weil, A. J., and Rodenburg, J. M. (1962). The seminal vesicle as the source of the spermatozoa-coating antigen of seminal plasma. *Proc. Soc. Exp. Biol. Med. 109*:567.

Weil, A, J., and Stefanovic, D. (1969). Spermatozoa-coating antigen (SCA): Its persistence in the genital tract of female rabbits. *Fertil. Steril. 20*:689.

Weil, A. J., Kotsevalov, O., and Wilson, L. (1956). Antigens of human seminal plasma. *Proc. Soc. Exp. Biol. Med. 92*:606.

Weil, A. J., Herman, R. R., Goldberg, A. S., and Rodenburg, J. M. (1961). Immunological and chemical studies of spermatocele fluid. *J. Urol. 85*:665.

Wentworth, B. C., and Mellen, W. J. (1964). Active immunity induced in spermatogenesis suppressed by testicular antigen in the male Japanese quail (Coturnix coturnix japonica). *J. Reprod. Fertil. 8*:215.

Yantorno, C., Shulman, S., Gonder, M. J., Soanes, W. A., and Witebsky, E. (1966). Studies on organ specificity. XVIII. Immunological and biphysical characterization of canine prostatic fluid. *J. Immunol. 96*:1035.

Yantorno, C., Shulman, S., Gonder, M. J., and Soanes, W. A. (1967). Studies in cryo-immunology. I. The production of antibodies to urogenital tissue in consequence of freezing treatment. *Immunology 12*:395.

Yantorno, C., Debanne, M. T., and Vottero-Cima, E. (1971). Autoimmune orchitis induced by autoimmunization with seminal plasma in the rabbit. *J. Reprod. Fertil. 27*:311.

Yantorno, C., Vottero-Cima, E., and Galmarini, M. (1973). Experimental autoimmune damage to rabbit male accessory glands. *Invest. Urol. 10*:397.

Young, L. G., and Goodman, S. A. (1980). Characterization of human sperm cell surface components. *Biol Reprod. 23*:826.

Zappi, E., and Shulman, S. (1971). Cryo-immunization. The cold propagation in the target tissue and the resulting volume of the lesion. *Cryobiology 8*:235.

Zappi, E., and Shulman, S. (1972). Cryo-immunology, Antibody response to epididymis freezing in the rabbit. *Invest. Urol. 10*:226.

Zappi, E., and Shulman, S. (1974). Early histological changes in experimental contralateral epididymo-orchitis in the rabbit. *J. Reprod. Fertil. 36*:23.
Zappi, E., Orsini, F., and Shulman, S. (1972a). Cryo-immunoization. Antibody responses after selective and repeated cryostimulations of the coagulating gland and the seminal vesicle of the male rabbit. *Invest. Urol. 10*:171.
Zappi, E., Smith, D. J., and Shulman, S. (1972b). Preparative separation of rabbit seminal plasma and immunochemical study of the resulting fractions. *Int. J. Fertil. 17*:145.
Zimmermann, H., and Kipping, D. (1967). Erfahrungen mit der Immunoelektrophorese des Spermatoplasmas bei der Fertilitätsdiagnostik des Mannes. *Dermatol. Wochenschr. 153*:945.

2
Detection of Antisperm Antibodies

TAGE HJORT

Institute of Medical Microbiology
University of Aarhus
Aarhus, Denmark

I. GENERAL PROBLEMS IN TESTING FOR ANTISPERM ANTIBODIES AND INTERPRETATION OF THE FINDINGS

To describe and discuss how to detect antisperm antibodies could easily become an odyssey through immunologic techniques in general, since a multitude of different test systems, often with minor modifications by individual investigators, have been or are being used. Many techniques for a given purpose often signify that none of them are really good. Furthermore, the most commonly used techniques might to most immunologists appear rather old-fashioned. This could explain why antisperm antibody techniques are sometimes met with a certain skepticism by colleagues from other fields. One of the aims of this review is to try to show that such a general skepticism is not justified. Antisperm antibody testing may still be at a relatively primitive stage, but provided the tests are carried out with the proper materials (in particular, optimal sperm samples) and proper controls are included, the results with the most common techniques seem as reliable as results of testing for antibodies to most other autoantigens. Nevertheless, there are certain special problems and difficulties related to testing for antisperm antibodies that should be kept in mind.

The large number of techniques is to some extent explained by the fact that spermatozoa contain an extraordinarily large number of sperm-specific components, which can induce immune responses in the male and female organism (i.e., auto- and isoimmune responses), and different techniques are required for different groups of antigens. For evaluation of the pathogenic significance of the immune responses, a distinction is usually made between antigens expressed on the surface of the spermatozoa and those hidden within the cell. To the former group belong various integral membrane proteins, such as the glycoprotein RSA-1 in rabbit spermatozoa (1), apparently at least three different proteins, including two glycoproteins, in human sperm (2,3), and the T antigen, a lipoprotein in guinea pig spermatozoa. (2). The latter group contains protamines from the sperm nucleus (4), the sperm-specific lactate dehydrogenase LDH-C4, which is predominantly found within the cell but is also detectable in the plasma membrane in the postacrosomal region and tail (5,6), various acrosomal enzymes, such as acrosin and hyaluronidase, which are released at the acrosomal reaction (7,8), and a number of poorly characterized antigens detectable by immunohistological techniques (in the acrosome, equatorial segment, and tail) (9). The distinction between surface antigens, accessible for reaction with antibodies in the intact cell, and hidden antigens is equally relevant when techniques are being discussed. Since only a few sperm antigens have been purified (protamines and LDH-C4), most antibodies have to be detected by using whole spermatozoa as antigen. Consequently, different procedures are required for the two categories of antigens: detection of antibodies to membrane antigens is usually done with fresh untreated or washed spermatozoa, whereas for demonstration of antibodies to subsurface antigens pretreatment of the cells is needed to make the antigens accessible for reaction.

The use of whole spermatozoa (in most of the tests for antibodies to membrane antigens, even motile spermatozoa from fresh ejaculates) means that the first requirement for any immunologic test system, i.e., a well-defined antigen, which can be kept constant from one day to another, cannot be fully met but merely approached. It is therefore essential to select sperm donors with semen samples of good quality [$\geq 70 \times 10^6$ spermatozoa per milliliter with at least 70% motile cells and only a few leukocytes (10)]. But even when adjusted sperm suspensions from such samples are used, day-to-day variations are inevitable. The dilution of semen, the percentage of immotile cells, the degree of motility, and the admixture of leukocytes will vary. For test systems in which only small volumes of sperm suspension are needed, the effect of some of these variations can be reduced by using only motile cells harvested from the semen samples as described by Hellema and Rümke (11). Usually, small volumes of the fresh semen sample (0.1–0.2 ml) are carefully layered under a similar volume of buffer in small test tubes. After incubation at 37°C for 30–60 min, a sperm suspension with nearly 100% motile cells and freed of other cells and most of the seminal plasma proteins can be harvested in the buffer. With good sperm donors the sensivitity of the various test systems can usually be kept fairly constant; i.e., the negative control serum will give a completely negative reaction and strongly positive sera will give the expected titer ± 1 titer step. However, every now and then the sensitivity will not meet these requirements, so the whole batch will have to be discarded. In tests with motile cells a loss of motility is the most common complication, leading to a reduced sensitivity in, for instance, agglutination tests (in our laboratory, where we use semen samples from a small group of selected donors, roughly 5% of the batches have to be disregarded owing to this complication, but the next semem sample from the same donor may turn out to be fully acceptable).

The immunologic findings should be properly interpreted. Apparently it is often expected that a test for antisperm antibodies should tell whether a person is infertile owing to the presence of these antibodies. Most investigators working with antisperm antibodies have been told about patients with such antibodies, maybe even in high concentrations, who appeared not to be infertile, and the conclusion from the case history is often that testing for antisperm antibodies is of little value. Such a general conclusion is not justified, but several other factors should be taken into account.

First, the occurrence of antisperm antibodies should always be considered together with other findings in the infertile couple, particularly with the quality of semen. Whether antibodies to membrane antigens are produced in the male partner and bound in vivo to the sperm membrane or formed in the female partner and reach cervical mucus, one of the main effects seems to be that the antibody molecules link the spermatozoa to the glycoprotein micelles of the mucus, thereby impairing sperm penetration (12). To what extent the penetration will be impaired therefore depends not only upon the number of antibody molecules attached to the spermatozoa, but also upon the motility of the spermatozoa—the better the motility, the lesser the effect of a given amount of antibody.

There is now evidence that antibody molecules of the IgA class prevent sperm migration through cervical mucus more effectively than IgG antibodies (13). Consequently, not only the amount of antibody, but also the immunoglobulin class should be taken into consideration.

There is no constant relation between antibody levels in serum and genital secretions. Therefore, determination of antisperm antibodies in seminal plasma, on the spermatozoa, or in cervical mucus provides better guidance for evaluation of fertility than antibody titers in serum. In women, antisperm antibodies seem rather often to occur in cervical mucus without being detectable in serum (14). In men antibodies are very rarely found in seminal plasma without also being present in serum, but the contribution of locally produced IgA antibodies in seminal plasma may vary considerably (15).

Finally, it should be remembered that only antibodies to antigens accessible in the living cell may play a potential role in infertility, i.e., antibodies to antigens expressed on the sperm surface, and in females possibly also antibodies to sperm-specific enzymes released at the acrosome reaction.

The ideal test for antisperm antibodies should thus provide information about the antigen against which the antibodies are directed, the immunoglobulin class of the antibodies, and the amount of antibody, particularly in the genital secretions or–in males–even better on the spermatozoa. With such information the test should offer valuable guidance for the evaluation of fertility, but even so the results should be interpreted with caution. Generally speaking, the demonstration of antibodies to the relevant sperm antigens can provide evidence for a higher or lower degree of fertility reduction, depending upon the strength of the immune response and various other factors (sperm motility). Only in the strongest cases, and particularly in cases with a strong local immunity, is conception so unlikely that the patient can be considered infertile. In cases with more moderate responses conception might occur, but it could take years (16).

II. METHODS USED FOR THE DETECTION OF ANTISPERM ANTIBODIES

In males there are two different ways of demonstrating autoantibodies to spermatozoa: detection of antibodies bound in vivo to the target cell or determination of (unbound) antibodies in serum or seminal plasma. In the female only the latter principle is applicable by determining antibodies in serum or cervical mucus. The advantages and disadvantages of each of the two procedures will be discussed in more detail in the following sections; it is sufficient to stress here that the great advantage of the former procedure is that that the antibodies bound to the patient's spermatozoa are obviously those that may exert a pathogenic effect and cause subfertility or infertility.

The antisperm antibody techniques to be discussed are listed in Table 1. This chapter is not intended to give a full technical description, but merely to evaluate the techniques in more general terms. More technical reviews have been given by Rose et al. (10), Mettler et al. (17), and Linnet and Suominen (18).

Table 1 Methods for Detection of Antisperm Antibodies

I. Antibodies bound in vivo to spermatozoa

Direct MAR test Immunobead-binding technique "Panning" procedure[a]	applied on patients spermatozoa reveal Ig class of antibodies

II. Antibodies in serum and secretions

Test	Suitable for testing: Male sera	Seminal plasma	Female sera	Cervical mucus[b]
Gelatin agglutination test (Kibrick test)	+	+		
Tray agglutination test (Friberg test)	+	+	+	+
Tube-slide agglutination test (Franklin-Dukes test)			(+)	(+)
Sperm immobilization and spermocytotoxicity test	+	(+)[c]	+	(+)[c]
Radioimmunoassays[a]	+	+	+	+
ELISA technique[a]	+?	+?	+?	+?
Indirect MAR test and immunobead-binding test	(+)	+	(+)	+
Passive hemagglutination[a]	+	+	+	
Indirect immunofluorescence				
methanol-fixed sperm	+		+	
swollen sperm heads	+		+	

[a]Experience limited, further studies needed for final evaluation.
[b]Liquefied cervical mucus or extracts of cervical mucus.
[c]Does not detect locally produced IgA antibodies.

A. Detection of Antibodies Bound In Vivo to the Sperm Surface

1. Direct MAR Test (Mixed Antiglobulin Reaction)

This test is carried out in the most simple way. On a slide one volume (5 or 10 μl) of the patient's fresh semen is mixed with a similar volume of a suspension of erythrocytes with human IgG or IgA attached to the surface, and finally the same volume of anti-IgG or anti-IgA, respectively, is added. After mixing again, the mixture is covered with a coverslip, and the reaction is observed under the microscope. If the spermatozoa carry immunoglobulins on the surface, the erythrocytes carrying the same immunoglobulin class on their surface will in the presence of the corresponding antiserum adhere to the surface of the spermatozoa (Fig. 1), and owing to the motility of the sperm cells this phenomenon is very easy to observe. A positive reaction for IgG antibodies can usually be noted immediately after mixing and is completed within 15 min. In a strongly positive reaction, spermatozoa will hardly be visible at that time, since they are often fully covered by erythrocytes, and one can merely observe agglutinates of erythrocytes showing motility. The reaction for IgA antibodies usually takes a bit longer to develop. Attachment of erythrocytes may be seen after 10–15 min, but the reaction will not be fully developed until after about 30 min incubation at 37°C.

This test was described in 1971 (19), although as an indirect procedure in which the binding of antibodies to the sperm membrane was performed in vitro. But it was not until the direct MAR test, i.e., the test carried out directly on the patient's ejaculate, was described by Jager and co-workers, first for IgG antibodies (20) and later for IgA antibodies (21), that the technique attracted attention. During the last years it has been widely used not only with erythrocytes but also with latex particles as carriers of immunoglobulin (13,22), and most investigators seem to agree that it is a simple and reliable test for detection of clinically significant cases of autoimmunity to sperm. Of particular importance is that the test provides information not merely about the presence of antisperm antibodies but also about their Ig class.

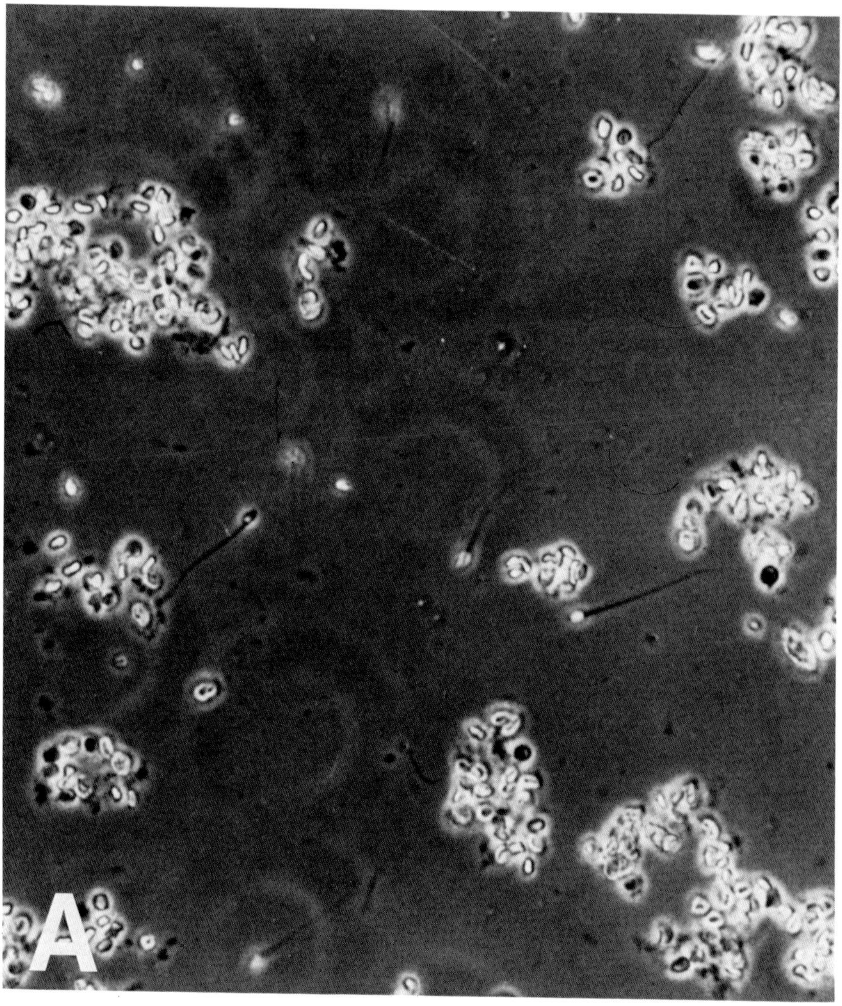

Figure 1. Direct MAR test. (A) Negative reaction, erythrocytes agglutinated, spermatozoa move freely between agglutinates without sticking to them. (B) Positive reaction, early phase, i.e., a few minutes after mixing the reagents, when the erythrocytes are beginning to agglutinate and adhere to the spermatozoa, in this case to the head and distal part of the tail. At a later stage the spermatozoa were fully covered with erythrocytes and hardly visible in the shaking agglutinates.

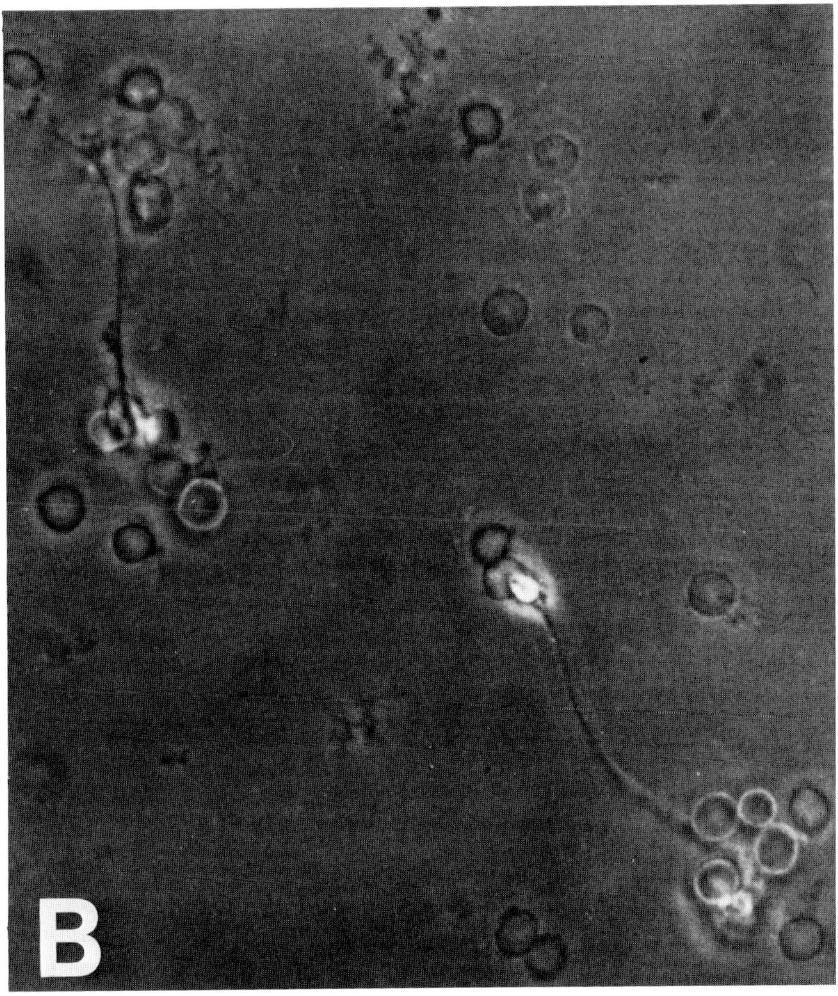

Figure 1 (Continued).

Yet the technique is not without its problems. It can only be performed if there are a sufficient number of motile spermatozoa in the ejaculate (>1–2 million motile cells per milliliter). This means that ejaculates usually cannot be sent to other laboratories for testing but have to be examined in the infertility clinic. The preparation of erythrocytes covered with immunoglobulin, particularly with IgA, requires some immunologic experience. For the IgG test, most laboratories use group O, Rh D-positive human erythrocytes, sensitized with incomplete human anti-D antibody as originally described by Jager et al. (20), and it is then necessary to prepare sensitized cells regularly. The same procedure may be used for the IgA test if an anti-D antiserum of the IgA class is available (13). But such sera are rare, and most laboratories will therefore have to isolate IgA from colostrum or serum and use this for coating erythrocytes. Jager et al. (21) absorbed the IgA to human blood group O, Rh-negative erythrocytes after pretreatment of the cells with formalin and tannic acid. In our laboratory we prefer to use glutaraldehyde-fixed sheep erythrocytes to which purified fractions of IgG and IgA, prepared by ion-exchange chromatography and immunoaffinity chromatography, respectively, can be absorbed without further treatment (23). The purity of the IgG and IgA preparations is not crucial, since the monospecific anti-immunoglobulins (anti-IgG and anti-IgA) will guarantee the specificity of the reactions. Stored in a glycerol-buffer mixture, the coated cells have a shelf life of more than 1 year. We have preferred this procedure mainly because the reactivity of the coated cells remains constant over a long period and the optimal dilutions of the antisera need therefore only be determined once. However, daily preparation of the cells is also easier, since they need only be washed to remove the glycerol.

The erythrocytes should form agglutinates before the MAR test result can be evaluated. This is a built-in control to ensure that the erythrocytes are properly covered with immunoglobulin and that the amount of anti-immunoglobulin antibody is sufficient. From a theoretical point of view, the test system is far from optimal, since the semen contains free immunoglobulins, which could be expected to interfere with the reaction by neutralizing the anti-immunoglobulin. However, the experience in our laboratory has been that nothing is gained by using harvested motile or washed spermatozoa in order to remove (most of) the seminal plasma components. When using harvested motile cells the sperm density was often close to the lower limit for reading the test, and when using washed spermatozoa the motility was usually somewhat reduced. Thus, the original procedure with untreated semen was generally easier to read than the more complicated procedures, and the results were very much the same. In the few cases in which the erythrocytes do not agglutinate, the test should be repeated with a higher concentration of anti-immunoglobulin.

Usually, the reaction is considered negative if less than 10% of the motile spermatozoa are involved in mixed agglutinates, but in most negative reactions only 1–2% of the motile spermatozoa may have a single erythrocyte attached to the surface. In contrast, most positive reactions are strongly positive, with the majority of motile cells (>80%) incorporated into mixed agglutinates, usually with several erythrocytes attached to the surface. This makes reading the tests very easy but on the other hand indicates that the direct MAR test is essentially qualitative. Different patterns of attachment of erythrocytes to the spermatozoa can be observed. Most commonly, attachment starts at the tail tip. In some cases it remains restricted to the tail tip, but usually other areas of the cell (entire tail, neck, and head) are gradually involved in the agglutinates. Strangely, these patterns are poorly correlated with the various modes of agglutination observed in microscopic agglutination tests, and it is still unknown whether the different patterns of attachment are of different clinical significance.

2. Immunobead-Binding Technique

The immunobead-binding technique is basically similar to the direct MAR test, as the presence of immunoglobulins is also demonstrated here by attachment of particles by means of an anti-immunoglobulin antibody. However, polyacrylamide beads are used instead of erythrocytes, and the purified anti-immunoglobulin antibody (anti-IgG, anti-IgM, or anti-IgA) is covalently bound to the beads. Thus, the reaction is carried out simply by mixing spermatozoa and washed, antibody-covered beads on a slide and observing the attachment of beads to the sperm surface (24,25). The main advantage of this technique, compared with the direct MAR test, is that the anti-immunoglobulin-covered beads are commercially available (Immunobeads, Bio-Rad, Richmond, California) and that the particles are smaller than erythrocytes, thereby allowing a more precise recording of the regional binding of immunoglobulin on spermatozoa. The occurrence of antibodies of the IgM class has also been investigated with this technique, but only a few weak reactions were observed in the semen (24,26). Bronson et al. (27) observed that antibodies of the IgG and IgM class directed primarily against the sperm head could in the presence of complement reduce sperm penetration into zona-free hamster eggs.

The drawback of this technique is that free immunoglobulins from seminal plasma can neutralize the immunobeads and thus block their reaction with the antibody-covered spermatozoa. Therefore, it is necessary to wash the spermatozoa carefully before mixing them with the suspension of immunobeads, and the repeated centrifuging of the sperm will unavoidably affect their motility, thereby making the reading of the tests more difficult. The technique has not yet been widely used, and it seems too early to evaluate whether it should be preferred over the MAR test. Clarke et al. (25) compared the two tests and found generally good agreement.

3. "Panning" Procedure

Recently, a third and somewhat different technique for the demonstration of antibody-coated spermatozoa has been described, i.e., the "panning" procedure by Hancock and Faruki (28). The test is carried out in wells in plastic trays, coated with anti-immunoglobulin. The suspension of sperm to be tested is added to such a well and left for an hour at room temperature. If the spermatozoa carry antibodies on their surface they will stick to the bottom of the well and remain there after washing the tray. In principle it is thus a very easy test. However, to obtain effective binding of the sperm the coating of the wells should be performed with a purified anti-immunoglobulin preparation. Therefore, it is necessary to isolate the anti-immunoglobulin antibodies from the antiserum by immunoaffinity chromatography or even to use a monoclonal antibody for the coating. Another and perhaps easier procedure is to coat the wells with immunoglobulins of a given immunoglobulin class (IgG or IgA) and after washing add the monospecific anti-immunoglobulin (anti-IgG or anti-IgA) so that the immunoaffinity chromatography takes place in the wells. As in the immunobead binding technique, the spermatozoa have to be washed carefully to remove immunoglobulins from seminal plasma since they might otherwise block the binding of spermatozoa. The washing causes no problem here, since the main advantage of this technique is that it can be performed regardless of the motility of the sperm.

So far the procedure has been worked out only for IgG, and the sensitivity of the test system, compared to the previously mentioned techniques, has not yet been studied. If the test finds a place in sperm immunology, it will probably be because it can be applied to ejaculates with poor motility.

B. Dectection of Antisperm Antibodies in Serum, Seminal Plasma, and Cervical Mucus

Antibodies to antigens located on the sperm surface have for a number of years been detected mainly by means of various agglutination and immobilization tests. More recently, the anti-immunoglobulin techniques described above have been modified for the testing of serum and secretions; i.e., the antisperm antibodies are allowed to bind to normal spermatozoa in vitro and then are detected as already described. These latter, essentially qualitative tests have mainly been used to study the immunoglobulin classes of antisperm antibodies. During the last years more modern immunologic techniques, i.e., radioimmunoassays, enzyme-linked immunosorbent assays (ELISA), and immunoblotting techniques, have been introduced. These tests are still at the experimental stage, and more experience is needed before they can replace the conventional antisperm antibody tests for clinical purposes. The main advantage of such tests would be that they do not require motile sperm, and it may be possible to use spermatozoa from the same ejaculate for longer periods and thus have a constant and carefully tested antigen preparation. That these techniques may be expected to show a higher sensitivity than conventional techniques would, on the other hand, be less important, since several of the tests now available are so sensitive that weak reactions are considered of little clinical interest.

1. Gelatin Agglutination Test (Kibrick Test)

This test was originally designed for studies of rabbit antisera to mammalian spermatozoa (29) but was shortly afterward (in 1954) applied to the detection of human autoantibodies by Rümke (30). Fresh semen, adjusted to a sperm density of 20 million per milliliter in a gelatin solution, is mixed with an equal volume of dilutions of serum or seminal plasma (usually starting with a dilution of 1:4). The mixtures are transferred to narrow test tubes (internal diameter, 2–3 mm), incubated at 37°C for 2 hr, and then read macroscopically (10). Negative reactions appear as a homogeneous, grey, hardly transparent suspension, whereas positive reactions show clearing of the suspending medium with small white floccules (Fig. 2). Carried out with high-quality semen samples from selected sperm donors and with proper positive and negative control sera, the test is very reliable and reproducible, as shown in a comparative methodological study in which several laboratories tested the same sera (31,32). The main disadvantage of the gelatin agglutination test is that relatively large volumes of semen are needed—for each test tube 0.15 ml of the sperm suspension with 20 million sperm per milliliter. In order to be able to test a suitable number of samples, it is therefore important to select sperm donors with high sperm counts, and the higher dilution of the semen will at the same time facilitate reading the tests. Another disadvantage is that the part of the spermatozoa involved in the agglutination cannot be observed and the motility of the spermatozoa in the

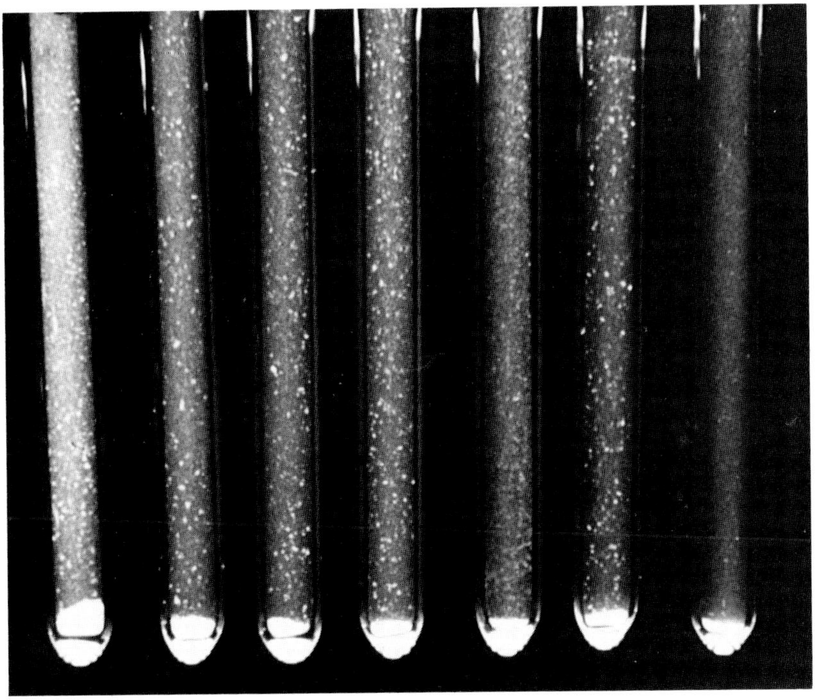

Figure 2 Gelatin agglutination test. Tubes 1–5 represent dilutions of seminal plasma (1:4–1:64); tubes 6 and 7 are examples from the positive and negative control sera, respectively. Although mixtures with seminal plasma appear more opaque than mixtures with serum (tube 6), the agglutinates can easily be seen (titer 32).

test mixture cannot be controlled. It is usually claimed that false-positive reactions may occur, e.g., caused by various microorganisms. However, with properly handled and stored samples false-positive reactions must obviously be very rare, at least in seminal plasma, since in a study of seminal plasma from more than 400 men not a single positive agglutination reaction was observed unless the direct MAR test with the patient's spermatozoa was also positive (23), and the use of anti-immunoglobulin in the latter test system should guarantee the immunologic specificity of the reactions. Although ABO blood group antigens have been demonstrated on spermatozoa (33), ABO antibodies do not influence the results.

The gelatin agglutination test has been widely used for testing male sera and seminal plasma (34–37). Investigations from different laboratories have been in good agreement, showing that in serum weak reactions were of little interest, whereas titers ⩾ 32 were extremely rare among fertile men but occurred in about 4% or more of the infertile men and in about 10% of the men from couples with "unexplained" infertility. In a recent prospective study of men with antisperm antibodies and normal semen samples with good motility, serum titers seemed of little value, but patients with detectable antibodies in seminal plasma had a lower fertility rate than patients with negative seminal plasma reactions (38).

In the study of female infertility, the gelatin agglutination test has, on the other hand, turned out to be of little value. Owing to the relatively large volumes required it is not suitable for testing liquefied cervical mucus, and with female sera most investigators have found only few and weak reactions, i.e., practically no reactions among fertile women and from 0 to 6% positive reactions (titer of 4 or more) among women from infertile couples (31,39). However, for female sera there is not the good agreement among different laboratories as for male sera. Thus, Shulman has recorded positive reactions in the gelatin agglutination test in about 20% of women from couples with unexplained infertility (40,41). The explanation for the weak reactions with female sera in this technique is apparently that sperm agglutinins in female sera in most cases cause the formation of small head-to-head agglutinates, which cannot be observed macroscopically. In contrast, male sera most commonly produce large tail-to-tail agglutinates, which are easily visible (32).

In the search for techniques requiring smaller amounts of semen, and not necessarily motile spermatozoa, a macroscopic agglutination test in capillary tubes has been developed (42), but it has found only limited use (43), probably because the tray agglutination test, using even less semen, appeared shortly afterward.

2. Tray Agglutination Test (Friberg Technique)

This technique, introduced by Friberg in 1974 (44), was based on the technology that had just been developed for tissue typing of lymphocytes, in which the reactions were carried out in drops under liquid paraffin. It was designed to overcome the drawbacks of the gelatin agglutination test; i.e., smaller volumes were used, and the mode of agglutination could be recorded.

The test is performed in trays (e.g., Møller-coates, Moss, Norway, with 3 × 6 microchambers) filled with liquid paraffin. By means of a microsyringe, 5-μl dilutions of serum, seminal plasma, or liquefied cervical mucus are deposited in the microchambers under the liquid paraffin, and 1 μl of a freshly prepared sperm suspension with 40 million sperm per milliliter is added. Serum or secretions are diluted in phosphate-buffered saline (pH 7.4), usually starting with a 1:4 dilution of serum. Some laboratories add normal human serum or bovine serum albumin to the buffer in order to preserve a better sperm motility. When preparing the sperm suspension, leukocytes and cellular debris should as far as possible be removed from the ejaculate in order to avoid nonspecific agglutinates around cellular debris. Friberg therefore kept small portions of the ejaculate in narrow test tubes for about an hour and omitted the bottom layer when preparing the sperm suspension. An even better procedure, now used in most laboratories, is to harvest motile cells in buffer as previously described.

The agglutination reactions are recorded under an inverted microscope after 4 hr at room temperature or 2 hr at 37°C (45). The degree of agglutination is evaluated at low magnification (×40) and the mode of agglutination at a higher magnification (×400). In the original description no coverslip was used, but some laboratories let a coverslip of proper size for the tray sink slowly into the liquid paraffin, thereby flattening the drop and providing much better conditions for microscopy. Reading the test and determining a titer may require some experience. Nevertheless, when different laboratories tested the same sera, the results were generally in good agreement (31). Usually three main modes of agglutination are distinguished: head-to-head, tail-to-tail, and mixed agglutination (10). In recording the reactions only agglutinates with motile spermatozoa should be taken into consideration. Head-to-head agglutinates are rather small (with 10 or fewer spermatozoa), and the free tails move vigorously. Often such agglutinates are seen rotating, always counterclockwise as a result of the structure of the axoneme (46). In strong reactions larger aggregates of the small agglutinates are formed, as the tail tips from one agglutinate are linked to the heads of another agglutinate (Fig. 3), indicating that the antibodies bind not only to the head but also to the tail tip (the same distribution is seen in the indirect MAR test with head-to-head agglutinating sera). Tail-to-tail agglutinates usually appear as large, solid agglutinates, from which the sperm heads stick out (Fig. 3). The involvement of only the tails is best seen in weak reactions (high dilutions) in which the smaller agglutinates look like tied bouquets of spermatozoa. A special tail tip-to-tail tip agglutination can be distinguished in the early phase of the formation of agglutinates, but as the agglutinates grow larger this mode of agglutination can hardly be distinguished from the common tail-to-tail agglutination. In mixed agglutination both heads and tails are involved in the formation of agglutinates.

The meaning of the various modes of agglutination remains a mystery. One might assume that a special antigen was involved in each mode of agglutination, but this seems to be true only for tail tip agglutination. There is now evidence that at least two different glycoproteins may be involved in both head-to-head and tail-to-tail agglutination. In titration of sera a shift in agglutination patterns, e.g., from predominantly head-to-head over mixed to tail-to-tail agglutination, may be seen with increasing dilution. Similarly, a switch may occur during the immune response as observed in vasectomized men (47). Soon after vasectomy, the various modes of agglutination were about equally common, but later nearly all sera revealed tail-to-tail agglutination. Finally, in absorption experiments with labeled glycoprotein fractions from solubilized spermatozoa, it was found that sera reacting with the same antigen(s) showed different modes of agglutination (48).

The tray agglutination test is more sensitive for detecting head-to-head agglutination than the gelatin agglutination test, whereas the two tests have very much the same sensitivity for the other modes of agglutination (31,32,45). However, if harvested "100% motile" spermatozoa are used, the sensitivity of the tray agglutination test is somewhat reduced for tail agglutination (49). Since head-to-head agglutination is the predominant mode of agglutination with female sera, the tray agglutination test is more suitable for testing female sera than the gelatin agglutination test. Thus, Friberg recorded positive reactions (i.e., titers $\geqslant$ 8) in 17% of women from couples with unexplained infertility, and studies from other centers have revealed incidences from 6 to 22% (50–52).

With female sera, head-to-head agglutination may be caused not only by antibodies, but also by a nonimmunoglobulin factor, often referred to as β-spermagglutinin, because it migrates with β-globulin in electrophoresis (39,53). The head-to-head agglutinates formed by the β-spermagglutinin are small, involving only two to five spermatozoa, and visible only at high magnification, whereas the antibody-dependent head-to-head agglutinates are usually larger, often with formation of aggregates as described above. The β-spermagglutinin, but not agglutinating antibodies, can be absorbed by means of a cell-free eluate from spermatozoa, and absorption experiments have revealed β-spermagglutinin in 3–4% of women from infertile couples as well as from various control groups. These reactions were usually weak, and the highest titer observed was 16 (54).

In testing male sera, the β-spermagglutinin does not play any role as a cause of false-positive reactions (55). With male sera, the tray agglutination test yields essentially the same results as the gelatin agglutination test. Strongly positive reactions (titers $\geqslant$ 64) have been recorded in 13–16% of men from infertile couples, but not in fertile males (44,56).

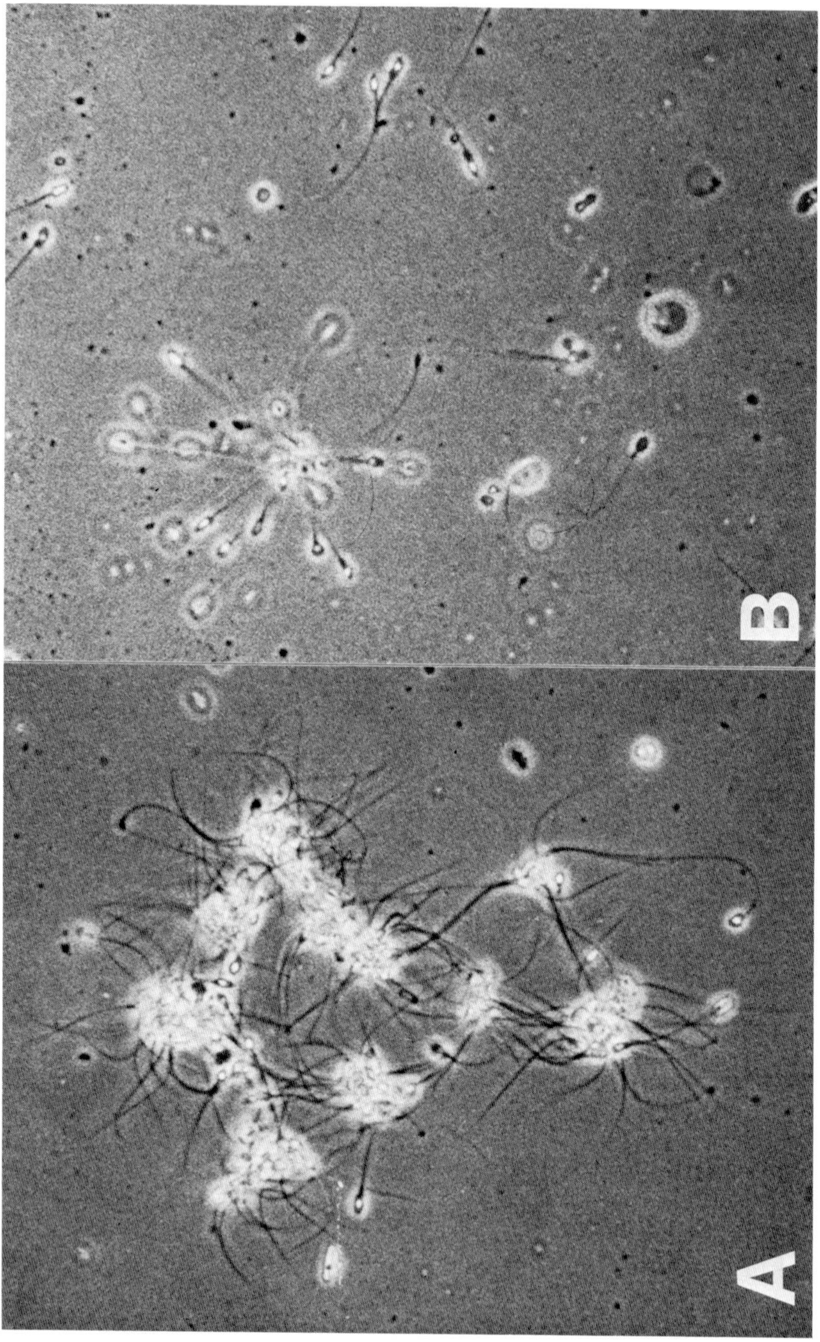
A
B

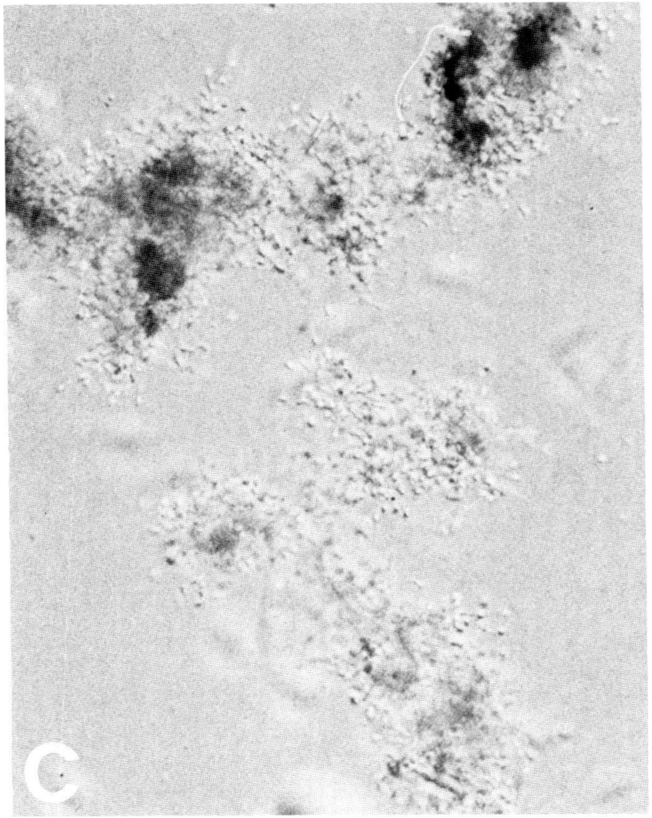

Figure 3. Tray agglutination test. (A) Head-to-head agglutination; strong reaction with formation of a large agglutinate by aggregation of several small agglutinates. (B) Small tail-to-tail agglutinate as seen in weakly reacting dilutions. (C) Large tail-to-tail agglutinate.

3. Tube-Slide Agglutination Test

This test, based on the early studies by Franklin and Dukes (57), has been used in various modifications (10,58,59). Usually, 10 volumes of inactivated serum (undiluted or diluted 1:4) are mixed in a test tube with 1 volume of a sperm suspension (50 million spermatozoa per milliliter) and incubated at 37°C. After 1 hr and again after 2 or 4 hr, 1 drop of the mixture is transferred to a slide and covered with a coverslip. The motile cells are immediately observed in the microscope, and the number of cells involved in agglutinates is recorded in relation to the total number of motile cells. The test has been considered positive if more than 10% of the motile cells were agglutinated (59).

The very simple, although rather time-consuming technique was for a number of years used for many studies of female sera, whereas it has been little applied to male sera. The results from different laboratories have been rather divergent and often confusing, with high incidences of positive reactions (up to 70%) not only in infertile women, but also in various control groups, particularly pregnant women and oral contraceptive users (for reviews, Refs. see 39, 41, 50, 51, and 60). There are good explanations for these findings: (1) nearly exclusively head-to-head agglutinates can be detected, since tail-to-tail agglutinates are apparently disrupted by pipetting onto the microscope slide; (2) the high serum-sperm ratio makes the test very sensitive for detection of the β-spermagglutinin, which can frequently be found in sera from pregnant women and oral contraceptive users; (3) it is difficult to quantitate the reactions; (4) in a comparative methodological study, the results with the tube-slide agglutination test did not show the high degree of concordance among laboratories as observed in the gelatin and tray agglutination test (31); and (5) even within the individual laboratory the test may reveal poor reproducibility (51,61).

For these reasons the test is not much used any longer. It would hardly be justified to use it as the only test, but it might be used in combination with one of the tests already discussed, e.g., the gelatin agglutination test (41).

4. Sperm-Immobilization and Spermocytotoxicity Tests

Antibodies reacting with cell membrane antigens may activate complement and thereby induce a cytotoxic effect on the cell. This will occur if the antibody is of the IgM class or of the IgG class (strictly only IgG1, IgG2, and IgG3) and present on the cell surface in such density that the first component of complement is able to react with two IgG molecules. This reaction lends itself to the detection of antisperm antibodies to surface components since the sperm-cytotoxic effect can be observed directly through immobilization of the sperm cell.

The immobilizing activity of antisperm antibodies in the presence of complement was demonstrated in an early study by Rümke (30), and later sperm-immobilization tests were described by Fjällbrant (62) and Isojima and co-workers (63). In the latter procedure, which has been widely used, 10 volumes of inactivated test serum were incubated at 32°C for 1 hr with 2 volumes of guinea pig complement and 1 volume of a fresh sperm suspension with good motility (60 million spermatozoa per milliliter). The percentage of motile cells (T) was then counted by examining a drop of the mixture under the microscope. At the same time, the percentage of motile cells (C) in a similarly treated control mixture with normal human serum was determined, and the sperm-immobilization value SIV = C/T was calculated. However, this value is suitable only for quantitating relatively weak reactions, since when nearly all spermatozoa have been immobilized the SIV approaches infinity. Therefore, many laboratories have preferred to titrate serum and determine the titer as the reciprocal of the highest dilution in which at least half the initially motile cells have been immobilized. A procedure to determine the dilution at which exactly 50% of the motile cells are immobilized has also been developed (10).

As described here, the immobilization test is simple and very reliable, with good agreement among different laboratories testing the same sera (31). Various control reactions have to be included (10), among these testing of the patient's serum with inactivated complement in order to show that the immobilizing activity is complement dependent and thus a true immunologic reaction. The only technical problem is that guinea pig sera may be sperm cytotoxic, so samples from animals without a sperm-cytotoxic effect have to be selected. If necessary, the toxic activity may be removed by absorption with packed spermatozoa (11). The optimal dilution of complement should be determined as in other complement-dependent test systems (e.g., twice the amount necessary to immobilize all spermatozoa in the presence of a strong antiserum).

The main disadvantage of the technique is that antibodies of the IgA class cannot be detected. Even though positive reactions have been recorded in both seminal plasma (64) and cervical mucus (14,65), the test is not optimal for testing secretions, since the locally produced IgA antibodies—probably the most important—will be missed. A minor disadvantage is the low sensitivity compared with agglutination tests. This is due to the fact that the antisperm antibodies in serum are usually of the IgG class and a certain density of antibody molecules on the sperm membrane is therefore required. In rare cases with IgM antibodies, the titers obtained in immobilization may be of the same order as those seen in gelatin or tray agglutination. It has for years been discussed whether the antibodies detected by immobilization are the same as those demonstrated by agglutination. As technical standards have gradually been improved, more and more investigators seem to agree that the same antibodies are detected in the two test systems (31). This means that if a serum can immobilize spermatozoa it will also cause agglutination (in our laboratory we have never observed exceptions from this rule). However, there is no fixed ratio between titers in the two systems, and sera with pure tail tip-to-tail tip agglutinins of the IgG class in high titers have been unable to immobilize spermatozoa (31). On the other hand, in the immunobead-binding technique, a high degree of immobilization was found only when IgG binding occurred on the distal two-fifths to three-fifths of the main tail piece or when IgM bound to the tail end-piece (66).

Microtechniques, in which the reaction takes place in a drop under liquid paraffin, have been also been developed for immobilization

(11,51,67,68). However, it is difficult to obtain the same high ratio between serum and sperm in microchambers as in the test tube technique, and the sensitivity of the microtechniques is therefore generally lower. These techniques offer an advantage when little material is available for testing (e.g., cervical mucus), but are now often used also for other purposes because they are less time consuming. They are now commonly carried out with "100% motile" cells, which facilitates the readings (11).

The spermocytotoxicity test is essentially an extension of the immobilization tests. Instead of counting the immotile cells after incubation with serum and complement, a dye, usually trypan blue, is added and incubation is prolonged, usually for an hour. The dye will penetrate into the dead cells, and the number of dead cells is therefore determined, either on an air-dried smear of the sediment or in a drop under a coverslip. Hamerlynck and Rümke (69) quantitated the reactions by calculating a spermocytotoxic index (STI) expressing the percentage of unstained cells in a control mixture with normal human serum that had become stained (and thus had been killed) in the mixture with the patient's serum. Several modifications of the original technique (69) have been described, e.g., the use of a microtechnique (67), the use of eosin Y instead of trypan blue (70), the use of harvested 100% motile spermatozoa (71), and the use of formalin for fixation of the spermatozoa (10). Also, a microcytotoxicity test with double-fluorescent staining of the cells has been developed (72). Living cells were stained with diacetylfluorescein and dead cells with ethidium bromide, so that they appeared apple-green and orange-red, respectively. A more advanced modification involves the use of tritiated actinomycin D, which can penetrate damaged cells and bind tightly to nuclear DNA. After incubation with labeled actinomycin D, the spermatozoa can therefore be carefully washed and the spermocytotoxic activity of serum can be quantitated by determining the radioactivity in a liquid scintillation counter (73). A new principle for measuring spermocytotoxicity on the basis of biochemical changes was introduced with the ATP release test. A decrease in ATP release from spermatozoa incubated with test serum and complement, compared with the release from spermatozoa in normal human serum, forms an objective measure for spermocytotoxic activity (74).

The various spermocytotoxicity techniques have not been widely used. The reason is obviously that they are more complicated than the immobilization test, and the results are nearly identical, although generally with a tendency for the spermocytotoxicity tests to be a bit less sensitive than the immobilization test (18,31, 67). Only the microcytotoxicity test with double-fluorescent staining (72) has revealed an exceptionally high percentage of positive reactions in infertile males, but these results are difficult to evaluate, since the technique has apparently not yet been compared to any of the classic tests.

5. Radioimmunoassays

Radioimmunoassays have been scarcely used in sperm immunology. Young (75) developed a solid-phase microradioimmunoassay in which washed spermatozoa were affixed by drying onto the bottom surface of wells in microtiter plates. These cells were then incubated with serum dilutions and, after washing, with ^{125}I-labeled antihuman immunoglobulin. The results were closely correlated with immobilization results, whereas most of the sera with sperm agglutinins and no immobilizing activity (i.e., generally sera with low agglutination titers) were negative. Thus, the sensitivity of the test seemed a bit lower than that of agglutination tests.

Haas et al. (76) used an essentially similar test but kept the fresh washed spermatozoa in suspension. Therefore, repeated washings were required after incubation with undiluted plasma and ^{131}I-labeled rabbit anti-IgG, respectively. In a study of 275 men and 276 women from infertile couples, 21 men (7.6%) and 42 women (15.2%) revealed increased deposition of labeled anti-IgG onto the sperm (compared with a group of fertile controls). Even though undiluted plasma was used, the incidences of positive reactions were thus of the same order as with some of the conventional tests. Comparison with gelatin agglutination reactions revealed a close correlation. That some sera were positive only in the radioimmunoassay is not surprising, since the gelatin agglutination test has a low sensitivity for the head-to-head agglutinins commonly found in female sera. Recently, the same group has also developed a solid-phase radioimmunoassay (77), but it has not yet been clinically tested.

The conclusions from these studies are thus that these radioimmunoassays detect the same antibodies as the conventional tests and with nearly the same sensitivity. Their main advantages are that an objective measure is obtained and that motile spermatozoa may not be needed; their disadvantages are that more equipment is required and they seem more laborious (particularly in that repeated washings must be performed with meticulous care in order to avoid the loss of spermatozoa).

In contrast to these results, radioimmunoassays with sera from animals immunized with sperm have shown a high sensitivity both to human sperm (78) and to guinea pig testicular cells and spermatozoa (79).

Recently also, a solid-phase radioimmunoassay with methanol-fixed spermatozoa in microtiter plates has been described (80). IgG antibodies bound to the spermatozoa were here detected by means of ^{125}I-labeled protein A. The results of this technique were not correlated with agglutination or immobilization reactions, probably because of antigenic changes in the sperm membrane due to the methanol fixation.

6. Enzyme-Linked Immunosorbent Assay (ELISA)

The ELISA test is carried out essentially as a solid-phase radioimmunoassay, i.e., with spermatozoa attached to the bottom of wells in microtiter plates, which are subsequently incubated with dilutions of the test sample and anti-immunoglobulin. But instead of using an isotope-labeled anti-immunoglobulin, the anti-IgG, anti-IgA, or anti-IgM is here labeled with an enzyme (e.g., alkaline phosphatase). After washing away unbound enzyme-conjugate a substrate is added, which will be turned into a colored substance by the enzyme so that the reaction can be quantitated in the spectrophotometer.

An ELISA test would seem most suitable for the detection of antisperm antibodies: it is generally a sensitive and relatively inexpensive technique, suitable for large-scale testing and giving an objective measure; only small amounts of semen and test samples are needed; the test does not require motile spermatozoa, so the same sperm preparation might be used for several days; the antibody class of the antisperm antibodies can be determined; and in using whole spermatozoa, antibodies to all accessible sperm antigens would probably be detected. Furthermore, the test could be used for the detection of antibodies bound in vivo to the patient's spermatozoa (81). This explains why several laboratories have recently tried to develop ELISA techniques with whole sperm (77,81–85), but the results have not been as clear-cut as one might have expected, and they are at this stage difficult to evaluate.

First, the various ELISA tests cannot be directly compared, since the procedures used have not been identical. It seems that fresh and frozen spermatozoa give similar results (77), but the number of cells added to each well is important (optimally, 0.5–1 million cells per well) (77,83). The spermatozoa have been affixed to the wells in different ways; air-dried cells were as good as glutaraldehyde-fixed cells, whereas fixation with methanol revealed slightly lower values for optical density (84). Second, only few of the studies allow evaluation of the significance of the test in clinical studies. Alexander and Bearwood (84) examined sera with and without antibodies detectable in gelatin agglutination and immobilization tests and recorded a significantly higher mean in the antibody-positive group than in the control group, but the ranges for the ELISA reading indicate some overlapping between the two groups. Zanchetta et al. (82) tested sera from 46 infertile patients with both ELISA and gelatin agglutination, recording 8 and 9 positive reactions, respectively. They state that only 3 of the sera were positive in both test systems (but a table indicates 4) and conclude that the ELISA was an easier but less sensitive method than the gelatin agglutination test. Finally, Brandeis et al. (85) found no agreement between ELISA and sperm immobilization, but unfortunately details about the technique were not given. The latter results are in line with experiences from our own laboratory. Although positive reactions in ELISA (carried out with harvested 100%

motile cells from group O sperm donors, affixed in the wells with glutaraldehyde) were more common among infertile patients than among fertile persons, there was no correlation with results from gelatin agglutination, tray agglutination, or immobilization tests (whereas the latter three tests closely correlated), and personal information from certain other laboratories indicate that we are not the only laboratory faced with such confusing results.*

The conclusion at this stage is therefore that ELISA with whole sperm is a difficult test system and more work is needed before it can replace conventional tests. The reasons for the difficulties with the test might be (1) treatment of the spermatozoa might expose new antigens (that frozen cells gave the same reactions as fresh cells supports such an explanation); (2) the presence of Fc receptors for IgG on the spermatozoa causes a high nonspecific binding; and (3) that an exceptionally large amount of spermatozoa is needed to absorb agglutinating or immobilizing antibodies from serum indicates that the relevant antigens may be present in only minute amounts and that the specific antibody binding is therefore low.

ELISA with purified sperm antigen fractions may hold more promise. Rajgopal and Rao (87) used a sperm extract prepared by repeated freezing and thawing of spermatozoa followed by ultrasonication and found an incidence of positive ELISA reactions higher than with sperm immobilization but lower than with agglutination, and Alexander and Bearwood (84) obtained with a lithium-diiodosalicylate (LIS) extract from washed spermatozoa results that were quite closely correlated with agglutination and immobilization reactions.

7. Other Anti-immunoglobulin Tests

Under this heading are various tests in which antisperm antibodies are allowed to react with donor spermatozoa, and the antibodies are then detected on the sperm surface by means of an unlabled anti-immunoglobulin. Examples are the indirect MAR test and the immunobead-binding technique. Apart from a first step with incu-

*Confirmed by multi-center study: L. Mettler et al., *J. Reprod. Immunol. 8*: 301 (1985).

bation of test samples with donor spermatozoa, the indirect immunobead-binding test is carried out as already described. When the indirect MAR test is carried out with serum, it is necessary to remove unbound immunoglobulins by washing the spermatozoa before they are mixed with the immunoglobulin-covered erythrocytes and the anti-immunoglobulin. For the detection of antibodies in serum, these techniques seem rather complicated, but they are useful for analyzing the immunoglobulin classes of antisperm antibodies. Jager et al. (88) also used the indirect MAR test for characterization of immunoglobulin classes of antisperm antibodies in cervical mucus in selected patients known to possess such antibodies. It is difficult to understand why this technique has apparently not been used as a routine test for cervical mucus, since it seems most suitable for this purpose.* Because of the low concentration of immunoglobulins in cervical mucus, washing the spermatozoa after incubation with liquefied cervical mucus is not needed. In our laboratory we have used this test for some time, and the preliminary results indicate that it is an easy and reliable method, more sensitive than the tray agglutination test.

8. Passive Hemagglutination

Previous attempts to use this very sensitive technique for the detection of antisperm antibodies in human sera have been unsuccessful (10), but more recently it has been introduced again, now with a high incidence of positive reactions in both males and females from infertile couples (89). Seminal plasma or sperm extracts prepared by ultrasonication were coated onto human blood group O erythrocytes, and these cells were used in passive hemagglutination tests with serum and seminal plasma and in a modified Coombs test with anti-IgG, anti-IgA, and anti-IgM. Of particular interest is that reactions appear to have been rather similar whether sperm extract or seminal plasma was used for coating the cells and that a cross-reactivity between the sperm-seminal plasma antigen(s) involved in the hemagglutination test and T lymphocytes could be

*Just after finishing this review such a study, with the immunobead-binding test, was published by G. N. Clark [*Am. J. Reprod. Immunol.* 6:195 (1984)].

shown to exist (90). Such reactivities have not been found with antibodies detectable in the conventional agglutination test; i.e., no reduction of titers in gelatin or tray agglutination has been observed after absorption with seminal plasma (31), and selected sera with high levels of sperm-agglutinating and sperm-immobilizing antibodies (of the IgG class) revealed no cytotoxic activity on either T or B lymphocytes (Kissmeyer-Nielsen, unpublished results). It therefore seems likely that antigens are involved in the passive hemagglutination test other than those in the conventional tests.*

9. Indirect Immunofluorescence Technique (IFT)

The indirect IFT is apparently not a suitable technique for the detection of antibodies to sperm membrane antigens. With unfixed spermatozoa, Feltkamp et al. (91) recorded some correlation between agglutination and immunofluorescence staining, but although agglutination did in most cases involve the sperm tails, the fluorescence was mainly on the sperm heads. Other studies have suggested that sperm-agglutinating sera may particularly stain the postnuclear cap area (15,92). The immunoperoxidase technique seems a better way than IFT to depict the localization of antibodies bound to the membrane (93,94).

Most immunofluorescent studies on spermatozoa have been carried out with methanol-fixed spermatozoa because characteristic staining patterns can be recorded, i.e., staining of the acrosome, the equatorial segment, the main tail piece, and the tail end-piece (Fig. 4) (92,95). Acrosome staining may be homogeneous or speckled (96). Subjective evaluation of the fluorescence staining require some experience, because nonspecific background staining is unavoidable in low dilutions of serum. This problem was reflected in a comparative study in which relatively poor agreement was seen when different laboratories tested the same sera (31). Therefore, only dilutions of serum (1:10 or more) should be tested.

It is still a question whether testing for antibodies reacting with methanol-fixed spermatozoa is of more than academic interest. With unfixed spermatozoa only a few cells (depending upon the

*This assumption has now been confirmed: R. Bronson et al., *J. Reprod. Immunol.* *8*:279 (1985).

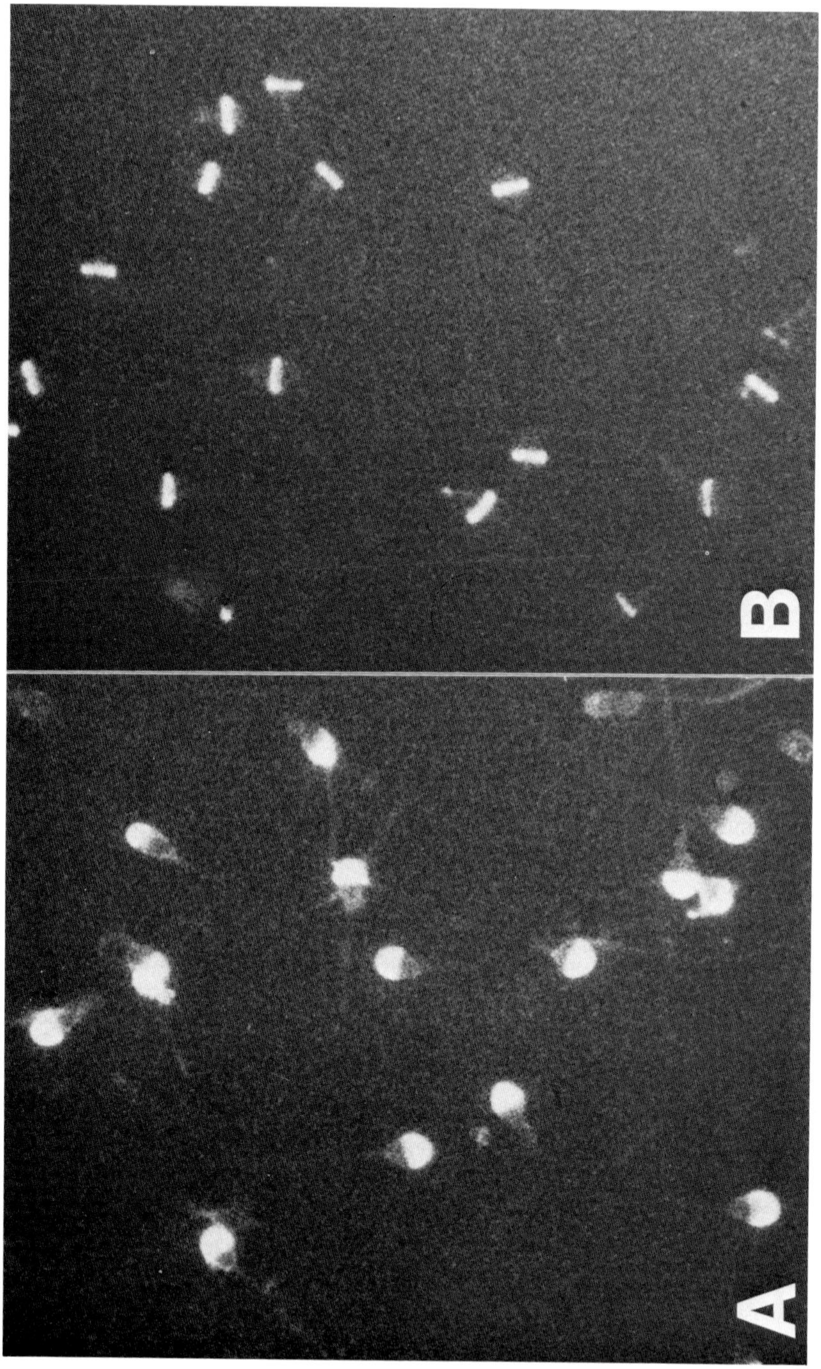
A
B

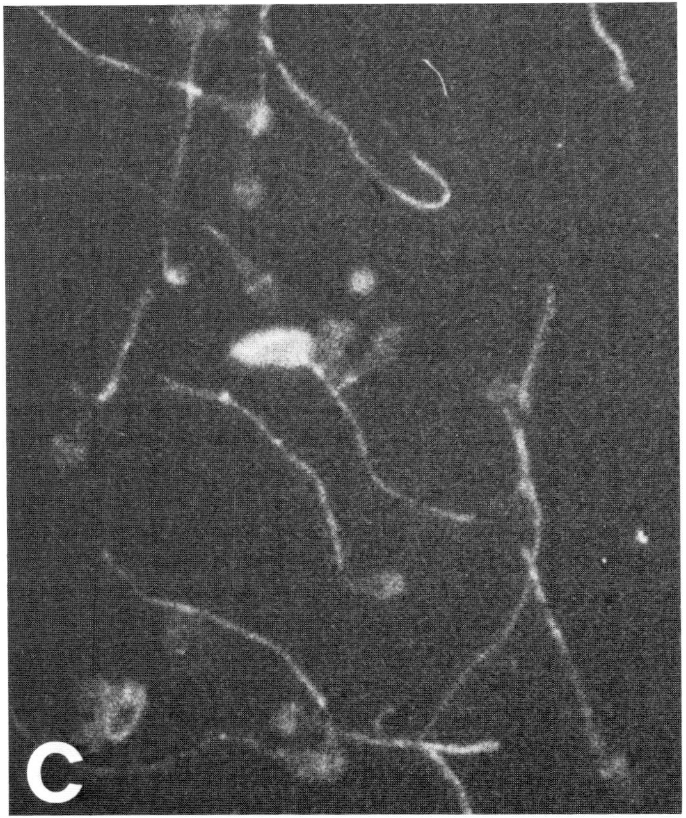

Figure 4. Indirect immunofluorescence technique for detection of antisperm antibodies. (A) Staining of the acrosome. (B) Staining of the equatorial segment. (C) Staining of the main tail piece.

quality of the sperm sample, and therefore apparently only dead cells) are stained by sera known to contain antibodies. Thus, the antigens seem inaccessible for reaction in the ejaculated sperm, and the antibodies could therefore hardly play any role in immune infertility (at least in males). This point of view fits with the fact that the various IF antibodies are common in fertile persons (including children) as well as in infertile patients. Only reactions in titers $\geqslant$ 16 have been recorded more frequently among women from couples with unexplained infertility than in other groups (95). Antibodies to the homogeneous acrosome antigen and to the antigen in the equatorial segment are the most common, and these antigens seem to cross-react with antigens in various ubiquitous microorganisms (97). This explains why the antibody-incidence is age related, with the highest incidence in children (97). Only antibodies to the acrosomal antigen, giving speckled fluorescence, formed an exception to this pattern, being rare in the younger groups and increasing in incidence with age as most true autoantibodies do. However, the production of IF antibodies is not solely caused by cross-reacting antigens in microorganisms, since the incidence of antibodies to the various antigens have been found to increase after vasectomy, although in varying degrees in different studies (97,98). For some years the IFT on fixed spermatozoa has not been much used in human studies, whereas it has been useful in animal experiments (99) and it is now also used for studies of monoclonal antibodies (100).

By using sperm heads artificially swollen by treatment with dithiothreitol and trypsin, Kolk et al. (101) detected hidden antigens also in the sperm nucleus, which were subsequently shown to be protamine 1 and 2 (102). The true autoimmunogenicity of these antigens was demonstrated in studies of vasectomized men and monkeys (103). Within 2 years after vasectomy, about 30% of the patients developed antibodies to protamine. Rather surprisingly, the antiprotamine antibodies occur practically exclusively in sera that at the same time contain sperm agglutinins in high titers and therefore very rarely in female sera (31,104). Owing to the pretreatment of the spermatozoa, nonspecific fluorescence does not cause problems as with methanol-fixed spermatozoa, and the testing for antibodies to swollen sperm heads has therefore revealed nearly identical results in different laboratories (31,104).

III. CONCLUSIONS

Technical development continues, and new techniques are continuously being described, for instance the blot-immunobinding technique (105), which may turn out to be useful for the detailed analysis of both antisperm antibodies and sperm antigens. There are, as has been illustrated, several options for studying immunity to sperm.

For the clinician mainly interested in the antifertility effects of antisperm antibodies, a sensible testing programme might be the following.

1. In males, the direct MAR test would be the first choice. If this is negative no further tests are needed. If the direct MAR test is positive—or if it cannot be performed owing to poor sperm motility—the classic agglutination tests (gelatin and tray agglutination tests), carried out on serum and seminal plasma, still seem to be the most reliable and clinically valid.
2. In females, the tray agglutination test, carried out on serum and liquefied cervical mucus, seems the optimal test, but it might also turn out to be useful to include the indirect MAR test on cervical mucus in the testing program.

For the basic scientist interested in all aspects of immunity to sperm there are more choices; particularly the modern tests, such as radioimmunoassays and ELISA with purified antigens and blot-immunobinding techniques, might be attractive. As indicated in this review, there are still many unsolved problems with these techniques.

REFERENCES

1. M. G. O'Rand, in *Immunological Aspects of Infertility and Fertility Regulation* (D. S. Dhindsa and G. F. B. Schumacher, eds.), Elsevier/North-Holland, New York, 1980.
2. G. A. Voisin, in *Immunological Factors in Human Reproduction, Serono Symposia,* Vol. 45 (S. Shulman, F. Dondero, and M. Nicotra, eds.), Academic Press, London, 1982.
3. T. Hjort, S. P. Ahuja, and F. Poulsen, in *Immunological Factors in Human Reproduction, Serono Symposia,* Vol. 45 (S. Shulman, F. Dondero, and M. Nicotra, eds.), Academic Press, London, 1982.
4. A. H. J. Kolk and T. Samuel, *Biochim. Biophys. Acta 393*:307 (1975).
5. M. Hintz and E. Goldberg, *Devl. Biol. 57*:375 (1977).
6. R. P. Erickson, D. S. Friend, and D. Tennenbaum, *Exp. Cell Res. 91*:1 (1975).
7. H. Fritz, B. Förg-Brey, E. Fink, M. Meier, H. Schiessler, and C. Schirren, *Hoppe-Seylers Z. Physiol. Chem. 353*:1943 (1972).
8. R. P. Erickson and S. R. Martin, *Int. J. Biochem. 9*:145 (1978).
9. K. S. K. Tung, W. D. Cooke, T. A. McCarty, and P. Robitaille, *Clin. Exp. Immunol. 25*:73 (1976).
10. N. R. Rose, T. Hjort, P. Rümke, M. J. K. Harper, and O. Vyazov, *Clin. Exp. Immunol. 23*:175 (1976).
11. H. W. J. Hellema and P. Rümke, *Clin. Exp. Immunol. 31*:1 (1978).
12. J. Kremer, S. Jager, and J. Kuiken, in *Immunological Influence on Human Fertility* (B. Boettcher, ed.), Academic Press, Sidney, 1977.
13. W. F. Hendry, J. Stedronska, and R. A. Lake, *Fertil. Steril. 37*:108 (1982).
14. M. De Almeida and P. Jouannet, in *Immunological Factors in Human Reproduction, Serono Symposia Vol.* 45 (S. Shulman, F. Dondero, and M. Nicotra, eds.), Academic Press, London, 1982.
15. S. Husted and T. Hjort, *Int. J. Fertil. 20*:97 (1975).
16. P. Rümke, N. van Amstel, E. N. Messer, and P. D. Bezemer, *Fertil. Steril. 25*:393 (1974).

17. L. Mettler, D. Shirwani, and T. Gradl, *Am. J. Obstet. Gynecol. 136*:106 (1980).
18. L. Linnet and J. J. O. Suominen, *J. Reprod. Immunol. 4*:133 (1982).
19. R. R. A. Coombs, P. Rümke, and R. G. Edwards, in *Immunology of Reproduction*, Proceedings of the Second International Symposium, Varna (K. Bratanov, ed.), Bulgarian Academy of Sciences Press, Sofia, 1973, p. 354.
20. S. Jager, J. Kremer, and T. van Slochteren-Draaisma, *Int. J. Fertil. 23*:12 (1978).
21. S. Jager, J. Kremer, and T. van Slochteren-Draaisma, *Int. J. Androl. 3*:1 (1980).
22. L. Vermeulen, I. Comhaire, and F. Comhaire, *Contraception-Fertilite-Sexualite 11*(Suppl.):381 (1983).
23. H. M. Jensen and T. Hjort, *Ugeskr. Laeger* 147:2654 (1985).
24. R. A. Bronson, G. W. Cooper, and D. L. Rosenfeld, *Fertil. Steril. 41*:609 (1984).
25. G. N. Clarke, A. Stojanoff, and M. N. Cauchi, in *Immunology of Reproduction*, Proceedings of the Fifth International Symposium, Varna (K. Bratanov, ed.), Bulgarian Academy of Sciences Press, Sofia, 1982, p. 482.
26. G. N. Clarke and H. W. G. Baker, in *Immunology of Reproduction*, Proceedings of the Fifth International Symposium, Varna (K. Bratanov, ed.), Bulgarian Academy of Sciences Press, Sofia, 1982, p. 337.
27. R. A. Bronson, G. W. Cooper, and D. L. Rosenfeld, *Fertil. Steril. 40*:91 (1983).
28. R. J. T. Hancock and S. Faruki, *J. Immunol. Methods 66*:149 (1984).
29. S. Kibrick, D. L. Belding, and B. Merrill, *Fertil. Steril. 3*:430 (1952).
30. P. Rümke, *Vox Sang. 4*:135 (1954).
31. WHO Reference Bank for Reproductive Immunology, *Acta Pathol. Microbiol. Scand.* [C] Suppl. 258 (1977).
32. WHO Reference Bank for Reproductive Immunology, *Clin. Exp. Immunol. 30*:173 (1977).
33. P. Boettcher, *J. Reprod. Fertil. 16*:49 (1968).
34. P. Rümke and G. Hellinga, *Am. J. Clin. Pathol. 32*:357 (1959).

35. B. Fjällbrant, *Acta Obstet. Gynecol. Scand. 47*:89 (1968).
36. S. Husted *Int. J. Fertil. 20*:113 (1975).
37. W. F. Hendry, H. Morgan, J. Stedronska, G. Scammel, and G. V. P. Chamberlain, in *Spermatozoa, Antibodies and Infertility* (J. Cohen and W. F. Hendry, eds.), Blackwell Scientific, Oxford, 1978.
38. T. Hjort and K. Brogaard Hansen, in *Immunological Factors in Human Contraception* (S. Shulman and F. Dondero, eds.), Field Educational Italia, Acta Medica, Rome, 1983.
39. H. J. Ingerslev, *Acta Obstet. Gynecol. Scand.* Suppl. 100 (1981).
40. S. Shulman, H. Jackson, and M. L. Stone, *Am. J. Obstet. Gynecol. 125*:139 (1975).
41. S. Shulman, in *Spermatozoa, Antibodies and Infertility* (J. Cohen and W. F. Hendry, eds.), Blackwell Scientific, Oxford, 1978.
42. S. Shulman and A. Hekman, *Clin. Exp. Immunol. 9*:137 (1971).
43. M. Nicotra, F. Dondero, and I. M. Coghi, in *Immunological Factors in Human Reproduction*, Serona Symposia, Vol. 45 (S. Shulman, F. Dondero, and M. Nicotra, eds.), Academic Press, London, 1982.
44. J. Friberg, *Acta Obstet. Gynecol. Scand.* Suppl. 36 (1974).
45. H. W. J. Hellema and P. Rümke, *Fertil. Steril. 27*:284 (1976).
46. L. Linnet, *Arch. Androl. 2*:157 (1979).
47. L. Linnet and T. Hjort, *Clin. Exp. Immunol. 30*:413 (1977).
48. F. Poulsen and T. Hjort, *J. Clin. Lab. Immunol. 6*:69 (1981).
49. H. W. J. Hellema and P. Rümke, *Clin. Exp. Immunol. 31*:12 (1978).
50. A. C. Menge, in *Immunological Aspects of Infertility and Fertility Regulation* (D. S. Dhindsa and G. F. B. Schumacher, eds.), Elsevier/North-Holland, New York, 1980.
51. L. Mettler, Immunologie der weiblichen Sterilität (Thesis), *Fortschritte der Fertilitätsforschung IV*, Grosse Verlag, Berlin, 1977.
52. H. J. Ingerslev and M. Ingerslev, *Fertil. Steril. 33*:514 (1980).
53. B. Boettcher and D. J. Kay, Nature *223*:737 (1969).
54. H. J. Ingerslev and T. Hjort, *Fertil. Steril. 31*:496 (1979).
55. T. B. Hargreave and T. Hjort, *Andrologia 15*:90 (1983).

56. T. B. Hargreave, M. Haxton, J. Whitelow, R. Elton, and G. D. Chisholin, *Br. J. Urol. 52*:566 (1980).
57. R. R. Franklin and C. D. Dukes, *Am. J. Obstet. Gynecol. 89*:6 (1964).
58. B. Boettcher, J. Hay, D. J. Kay, B. A. Baldo, and T. K. Roberts, *Int. J. Fertil. 15*:143 (1970).
59. S. Shulman, H. Jackson, and M. L. Stone, *Am. J. Obstet. Gynecol. 123*:139 (1975).
60. W. R. Jones, in *Karolinska Symposia on Research Methods in Reproductive Endocrinology*, Seventh Symposium: Immunological Approaches to Fertility Control (E. Diczfalusy, ed.), Karolinska Institutet, Stockholm, 1974.
61. L. Mettler and T. Gradl, *J. Reprod. Fert. 44*:217 (1975).
62. B. Fjällbrant, *Acta Obstet. Gynecol. Scand. 47*:102 (1968).
63. S. Isojima, T. S. Li, and Y. Ashitaka, *Am. J. Obstet. Gynecol. 101*:677 (1968).
64. S. Husted, *Acta Pathol. Microbiol. Scand.* [C]*83*:338 (1975).
65. A. C. Menge, N. E. Medley, C. M. Mangione, and J. W. Dietrich, *Fertil. Steril. 38*:439 (1982).
66. R. A. Bronson, G. W. Cooper, and D. L. Rosenfeld, *Am. J. Reprod. Immunol. 2*:222 (1982).
67. S. Husted and T. Hjort, *Clin. Exp. Immunol. 22*:256 (1975).
68. S. Isojima and K. Koyama, in *Immunology of Reproduction*, Proceedings of the Third International Symposium, Varna (K. Bratanov, ed.), Bulgarian Academy of Sciences Press, Sofia, 1978, p. 215.
69. J. Hamerlynck and P. Rümke, *J. Reprod. Fertil. 17*:191 (1968).
70. S. Jager, J. Kuiken, and J. Kremer, *Fertil. Steril. 41*:294 (1984).
71. M. D'Almeida, M. Lefroit-Joliy, and G. A. Voisin, *Clin. Exp. Immunol. 44*:359 (1981).
72. S. Mathur, H. O. Williamson, F. C. Dirrick, P. R. Madyastha, J. T. Melchers, G. L. Holtz, E. R. Baker, C. L. Smith, and H. H. Fudenberg, *J. Immunol. 126*:905 (1981).
73. J. S. Sung, H. Shizuya, D. D. Black, and D. M. Mumford, *Clin. Exp. Immunol. 27*:469 (1977).
74. J. J. O. Suominen, S. Multamäki, and B. M. Djupsund, *Arch. Androl. 4*:257 (1980).

75. L. G. Young, *J. Cell Biol. 79*:256a (1978).
76. G. G. Haas, D. B. Cines, and A. D. Schreiber, *N. Engl. J. Med. 303*:722 (1980).
77. D. P. Wolf, D. T. Rowlands, and G. G. Haas, *Biol. Reprod. 26*:140 (1982).
78. L. A. Hill and J. K. Hampton, *Fertil. Steril. 33*:308 (1980).
79. L.-P. B. Han and K. S. K. Tung, *Biol. Reprod. 21*:99 (1979).
80. A. B. Czuppon and L. Mettler, *J. Clin. Chem. Clin. Biochem. 21*:357 (1983).
81. S. S. Witkin, G. Zelikovsky, R. A. Good, and N. Day, *Clin. Exp. Immunol. 44*:368 (1981).
82. R. Zanchetta, F. Busolo, and I. Mastrogiacomo, *Fertil. Steril. 38*:730 (1982).
83. S. Paul, V. Baukloh, and L. Mettler, *J. Immunol. Methods 56*:193 (1983).
84. N. J. Alexander and D. Bearwood, *Fertil. Steril. 41*:270 (1984).
85. V. T. Brandeis, R. Shelden, and E. Kemmann, *Fertil. Steril. 41*:995 (1984).
86. K. K. Sethy and H. Brandis, *Eur. J. Immunol. 10*:964 (1980).
87. R. Rajgopal and S. S. Rao, *Indian J. Med. Res. 70*:440 (1979).
88. S. Jager, J. Kremer, J. Kuiken, and T. van Slochteren-Draaisma, in *Immunological Influence on Human Fertility* (B. Boettcher, ed.), Academic Press, Sydney, 1977
89. S. Mathur, H. O. Williamson, S. C. Landgrebe, C. L. Smith, and H. H. Fudenberg, *J. Immunol. Methods 30*:381 (1979).
90. S. Mathur, J. M. Goust, H. O. Williamson, and H. H. Fudenberg, *Am. J. Reprod. Immunol. 1*:113 (1981).
91. T. E. W. Feltkamp, K. Kruyff, N. C. J. J. Ladiger, and P. Rümke, *Ann. N.Y. Acad. Sci. 124*:702 (1965).
92. W. L. Johnson and A. C. Menge, *Fertil. Steril. 26*:721 (1975).
93. T. Hjort, in *Development of Vaccines for Fertility Regulation* (WHO, ed.), Scriptor, Copenhagen, 1976.
94. M. D'Almeida, S. Righenzi, and G. A. Voisin, Abstracts, Fourth International Congress Immunology, Paris (J. L. Preud'Homme and V. A. L. Hawken, eds.) Abstract No. 16.1.06.
95. T. Hjort and K. B. Hansen, *Clin. Exp. Immunol. 8*:9 (1971).
96. K. S. K. Tung, *Clin. Exp. Immunol 20*:93 (1975).

97. K. S. K. Tung, W. D. Cooke, T. A. McCarty, and P. Robitaille, *Clin. Exp. Immunol. 25*:73 (1976).
98. P. Crewe, L. Dawson, R. D. Barnes, E. Tidmash, I. Chanarin, T. Hjort, and J. Ingerslev, *Int. J. Fertil. 22*:104 (1977).
99. N. J. Alexander and D. J. Anderson, *Fertil. Steril. 32*:253 (1979).
100. M. Isahakia and N. J. Alexander, *Am. J. Reprod. Immunol. 5*:117 (1984).
101. A. H. J. Kolk, T. Samuel, and P. Rümke, *Clin. Exp. Immunol. 16*:63 (1974).
102. A. H. J. Kolk and T. Samuel, *Biochim. Biophys. Acta 393*:307 (1975).
103. T. Samuel, L. Linnet, and P. Rümke, *Clin. Exp. Immunol. 33*:261 (1978).
104. T. Samuel, Antigenicity of protamines and autoimmunity after vasectomy. Thesis, Rodopi , Amsterdam, 1978.
105. C.-Y. G. Lee, Y.-S. Huang, P.-C. Hu, V. Gomel, and A. C. Menge, *Anal. Biochem. 123*:14 (1982).

3

Immunologic Regulation of Fertility with Spermatozoal Antigens

L. METTLER and A. B. CZUPPON

Christian Albrecht's University
Kiel, Federal Republic of Germany

The union of the genetically dissimilar sperm and egg in the female reproductive tract and the ensuing pregnancy has a profound but as yet poorly characterized immunologic background. Following demonstration of the antigenic potential of the gametes and the embryo, it became evident that internal fertilization in vivo and viviparity in mammals in dependent upon specialized mechanisms that permit sperms, oocytes, and the embryo to evade destruction by humoral and cell-mediated transplantation reactivity in the female host. Indeed, there is some evidence that an antipaternal immunologic response in the female may even facilitate fertilization and pregnancy. On the other hand, certain cases of infertility may be due to autoimmune and alloimmune reactions against the gametes, block of fertilization, or early embryonic development. In the context of the present monograph we shall discuss only spermatozoal antigens as well as spermatozoal isoantibodies or autoantibodies. Although the presence of antispermatozoal antibodies in the male and female have been correlated with sterility in various studies, the corresponding antigens on the spermatozoa have not yet been positively identified in spite of recent advances in this field (Shulman, 1972; Mettler, 1977; Fjällbrant, 1968). Recently, a sialoglycoprotein antigen was purified from human spermatozoa that reacts with naturally occurring iso-/and autoantibodies in sterile patients (Czuppon et al., 1981). This molecule is thought to be broken down by acrosin or acrosomal enzymes during autolysis, resulting in the release of antigenic peptides from the spermatozoa. The latter peptides are of sufficiently low molecular weight to allow chemical synthesis and to study the induction of immunologic infertility. Up to now, efforts have been made to develop synthetic vaccines using peptide immunogens of human chorionic gonadotropin (Stevens et al., 1981) and antigenic peptide fragments of the spermatozoal enzyme LDH-X (Goldberg et al., 1981a). However, no clear-cut specificity has been established for either in cross-reactions with FSH and in the latter cases possibly with other LDH subunits. From this point of view, the possibility that the LDH-X subunit (i.e., substrate binding sites, allosteric regulation sites, or coenzyme binding) might share common sequences with other LDH enzymes from the various tissues has not been fully investigated.

In this chapter an alternative approach is presented in order to develop a synthetic vaccine for immunoregulation of fertility or as a therapeutic agent to block circulating antibodies and enhance natural fertilization in the female. A peptide antigen with an amino acid sequence of Asp-Pro-Trp-Trp-Cys-Phe-Asp-Lys-Phe-Glu was purified by immunoaffinity chromatography from a mixture of solubilized spermatozoal peptides. Following synthesis of this peptide by the Merrifield solid-phase method and testing with a solid-phase radioimmunoassay and enzyme-linked immunosorbent assay (ELISA), the peptide was shown to react with rabbit anti-human spermatozoal antibodies, with naturally occurring iso- and autoantibodies in steril patients, and with a monoclonal antibody that was generated against whole spermatozoa. Testing for tissue specificity indicated that the synthetic peptide is confined to the spermatozoal surface and eventually to the seminal plasma. Whether the latter is a result of shedding of antigens or the antigen itself is a coating antigen cannot be determined at present. Since the synthetic peptide clearly cross-reacts with primate spermatozoal peptide analogs, an investigation in that direction using a primate animal model has recently been initiated in our laboratory.

I. SPERMATOZOAL AND SEMINAL PLASMA ANTIGENS

Available evidence indicates that spermatozoal possess a complex membrane composed of a variety of proteinic and glycoproteinic antigens. There has been some controversy in regard to expression of HLA antigens on spermatozoa (Goldberg et al., 1970; Kerek and Afzelius, 1972; Law and Bodmer, 1978). However, recent studies employing well-defined monoclonal antibodies (Prabhu- and Hedge, 1982), indicate the presence of HLA-A, B, and C antigens on about 60% of sperm, and it was suggested that the density of expression of these antigens was variable. The haploid expression of HLA antigens (Fellous and Dausset, 1970) has been suggested on the basis that when one particular HLA specificity was tested, 50% of sperm were killed in a cytotoxicity assay, whereas with two HLA specificites, 80% sperm killing was obtained. The HLA-DR locus, antigens that initiate the provocation of a cell-mediated immune response, are expressed on about 50% of human spermatozoa (Prabhu and Hedge, 1982). Functional evidence for the presence of the DR locus on spermatozoa was provided by Halim and Festenstein (1978), who found that human spermatozoa stimulated DNA synthesis in lymphocytes from unrelated donors. The expression of an isoenzyme of lactate dehydrogenase (LDH-X) on the sperm membrane and its sperm specificity are well documented (Goldberg, 1975).

LDH-C_4 was first observed in human spermatozoa and testes (Goldberg, 1963; Blanco and Zinkham, 1963), and its presence has been confirmed in every mammalian species examined (summarized in Wheat and Goldberg, 1975; Goldberg, 1976). This isozyme has never been detected in any tissue of females, and its association with the male reproductive system has been rigoruosly established. The synthesis of LDH-C_4 is linked to active spermatogenesis as demonstrated both by the onset of this process in normal development and by a variety of pathological disturbances (Wheat and Goldberg, 1983). LDH-C_4 is first synthesized in the primary spermatocyte (Hintz and Goldberg, 1977; Wheat et al., 1977). The concentration of this enzyme increases as spermatogenesis proceeds (Hintz and Goldberg, 1976; Meistrich et al., 1977), and LDH-C_4 is the major, probably sole, LDH isozyme of spermatozoa. The absolute restriction of LDH-C_4 to male gametes is well suited to its use in the development of an immunocontraceptive.

Purification of LDH-C_4 from mouse testes was achieved by appropriate combination of salt fractionation, ion-exchange chromatography, and crystallization (Goldberg, 1972). Recent advances in affinity chromatography have greatly simplifed the isolation of this enzyme such that batches of a few hundred milligrams can be routinely prepared (Wheat and Goldberg, 1977; Lee et al., 1982). This technology has also facilitated the preparation of small amounts of rabbit and human LDH-C_4 (Wheat and Goldberg, 1977; Bachmann and Lee, 1976).

The availability of pure LDH-C_4 has permitted its biochemical characterization. A variety of enzymological studies confirm that the primary role of this protein is the interconversion of pyruvate and lactate. LDH-C_4, however, differs from the other LDH isozymes in the details of its kinetic properties and specificity (Goldberg, 1976; Wheat and Goldberg, 1983). These enzymic properties are presumably well adapted to the metabolic requirements of spermatozoa, but no satisfactory model of this physiological rationale has yet been established (Wheat and Goldber, 1983).

The structure of mouse LDH-C_4 has been determined. Examination of the crystalline enzyme bu x-ray diffraction reveals that the overall fold of the polypeptide chain is essentially identical to that of the other LDH isozymes (Musick and Rossmann, 1979). Some parts of the structure, particularly near the amino terminal and the carboxyl terminal, are different, and, at least in crystals, the coenzyme binding loop is in a closed conformation (Musick and Rossmann, 1979). The primary structures of both mouse and rat

LDH-C4 have been determined by classic chemical methods (Pan et al., 1983). The amino acid sequences reveal numerous differences in structure from the other LDH isozymes, but the homologies aming this family of proteins are readily apparent (Li et al., 1983a, b). Although the LDH isozymes have extensive common structural features, they are immunologically distinct.

The availability of highly purified and biochemically well-characterized LDH-C4 makes the analysis of immunologic properties possible. The antibody response to LDH-C4 is T dependent, and a delayed-type hypersensitivity response indicates cellular recognition of the antigen (Kille et al., 1978). Immunization of male and female rabbits, mice, and baboons with mouse LDH-C4 elicits circulating antibodies (Goldberg, 1971; Goldberg et al., 1981b; Lerum and Goldberg, 1974). These immunoglobulins both precipitate and inhibit the enzyme activity of LDH-C4. Rabbit antimouse LDH-C4 reacts with LDH-C4 from all species tested, but no cross-reactivity with LDH isozymes composed of A and B subunits can be detected (Goldberg, 1971). Quantitative differences in the degree of immunologic cross-reactivity among LDH-C4 isozymes of various species can be discerned with microcomplement fixation or with monoclonal antibodies (Goldberg and Wheat, 1976; Goldman-Leikin and Goldberg, 1983).

The immunogenicity of LDH-C4 in mice facilitates the analysis of the genetic control of the immune response. Comparisons of different mouse strains reveal that separate genes control the magnitude and the kinetics of the immune response (Kille et al., 1978). The regulation of the rate at which the immune response to LDH-C4 develops in mice is an X-linked trait (Marsh et al., 1977, 1981).

These data confirm the suitability of LDH-C4 as a test antigen for immunocontraception. This protein only occurs in male reproductive cells and is a potent, highly specific antigen. It is well established that the immune response to LDH-C4 significantly impairs fertility. Active immunization of female mice with mouse LDH-C4 reduces the number of offspring compared with parallel controls (Lerum and Goldberg, 1974). The same effect, with an even greater reduction in fertility, was observed in female rabbits (Goldberg, 1973, 1974). Similarly, immunized male rabbits sired fewer offspring (Goldberg and Wheat, 1976). The most recent test of the immunocontraceptive potential of LDH-C4 was conducted in nonhuman primates (Goldberg et al., 1981b). About 80% fewer pregnancies were observed in female baboons immunized with mouse LDH-C4 than in control baboons. Conceptions were restricted to baboons with a poorly developed immune response. In addition, some animals that had remained infertile over several matings subsequently conceived when they were rested from booster immunizations (Goldberg et al., 1981b). This trial in a small group of nonhuman primates conclusively demonstrates that immunization with LDH-C4 can suppress fertility.

The properties of LDH-C4 are consistent with the requirement for an immunocontraceptive antigen. This protein is absolutely restricted to spermatozoa. Significant immunosuppression of fertility has been clearly demonstrated in three species. However, the amount of LDH-C4 that can be isolated from natural sources is incompatible with a widely used contraceptive. Small, synthetic peptides that could be substituted for the natural product because they represent antigenic domains of LDH-C4 have now been identified (Gonzales-Prevatt et al., 1982; Wheat and Goldberg, 1981, 1984; Wheat et al., 1986). Such peptides provoke an immune response to the native enzyme (Gonzales-Prevatt et al., 1982; Wheat et al., 1984). They can be readily synthesized in any desired quantity and provide great flexibility in the design of an antigen for immunocontraception. The development of such peptides has proceeded by identifying peptide fragments that react with antibody to LDH-C4 (Gonzales-Prevatt et al., 1982; Wheat and Goldberg, 1981, 1986).

Rabbit antimouse LDH-C4 binds to the mixture of peptides in a tryptic digest of LDH-C4 (Gonzales-Prevatt et al., 1982). Purification of these peptides by either cation-exchange chromatography or by high-performance liquid chromatography separates fragments that bind antibody from those that do not. Amino acid sequencing with Edman degradation was used to identify these peptides in the overall structure of LDH-C4. A total of 13 peptides representing antigenic domains was identified in this way (Gonzales-Prevatt et al., 1982; Wheat and Goldberg, 1981). An additional domain was recognized with monoclonal antibodies (Goldman-Leikin and Goldberg, 1983). Examination of these antibody combining sites in the three-dimensional structure suggests that virtually every residue on the surface of LDH-C4 can be in one or more antigenic domains (Wheat and Goldberg, 1981). This model provides a wealth of potential synthetic antigens that can be manufactured as linear fragments or as surface simulation peptides (Atassi, 1979).

Peptides representing four of these domains have been synthesized and tested as immunogens (Gonzales-Prevatt et al., 1982). These peptides, ranging in size from 8 to 12 residues, were conjugated to macromolecular carriers and used to immunize rabbits. The injections elicited an immune response that, in every case, included antibodies that bound specifically to native LDH-C4 (Gonzales-Prevatt et al., 1982). The antibody titer increased with booster immunizations, and there were differences in the magnitude of the response among the peptides (Wheat et al., 1984). A peptide-carrier conjugate has now been shown to elicit anti-LDH-C4 immunoglobulins in both mice and baboons (unpublished). These data identify some candidates for synthetic antigens for immunocontraception and confirm the utility of this strategy for replacing the natural product antigen. There is no evidence at present to suggest that the best peptide or combination of peptides has been identified, but the data certainly warrant a more detailed survey of this class of antigens.

Having established a strategy for replacing natural product LDH-C4 in a contraceptive vaccine, it is appropriate to consider the mechanism of the immunosuppression of fertility so that the immunization protocol can be modified. Although anti-LDH-C4 inhibits enzyme activity and could thereby derange sperm metabolism, it is likely that these antibodies inhibit fertilization by their direct action at the sperm membrane.

The surface of the spermatozoon displays numerous binding sites for anti-LDH-C_4 (Goldberg, 1976). In vitro tests demonstrate that rabbit antimouse LDH-C_4 agglutinates mouse spermatozoa, and antibody-mediated complement-dependent lysis is readily observed (Goldberg et al., 1981a). These specific immunoglobulins inhibit in vitro fertilization of mouse sperm (Beyler and Goldberg, unpublished). Antibodies to LDH-C_4 have been detected in oviductal fluid (Kille and Goldberg, 1979). Further, the transport of sperm is virtually eliminated in the oviducts of rabbit simmunized with LDH-C_4 (Kille and Goldberg, 1980). Therefore, fertilization can be prevented by a high concentration of anti-LDH-C_4 in the female reproductive tract. This can be accomplished by local immunization to stimulate the secretory immune system.

The local immune response involves the secretion of IgA specific for the immunogen by cells residing in the mucosal lining. This response can be elicited by direct immunization of the local area. Stimulation of a local secretory response to LDH-C_4 would ensure the high antibody levels in the reproductive tract necessary for complete abrogation of fertility. In addition, since the local response is short-lived, it may be readily reversible. Female mice, immunized with LDH-C_4 directly into the reproductive tract, exhibit elevated levels of LDH-C_4-specific IgA in their uterine fluids. A larger response is observed in animals that received a systemic immunization with LDH-C_4 7–10 days prior to intrauterine inoculation (Shelton and Goldberg, unpublished, 1983). These results suggest that manipulation of the secretory immune system of the female reproductive tract could enhance the immunocontraceptive effects of LDH-C_4.

Specific stimulation of local humoral immunity can be accomplished without cumbersome injection procedures. The female tract can be directly immunized with antigen-releasing devices, such as vaginal rings or suppositories. In addition, indirect immunization of any mucosal site results in antibody secretion at all other mucosal sites (Montgomery et al., 1980; Weisz-Carrington et al., 1979). Oral or nasal immunization of this common secretory immune system would elicit anti-LDH-C_4 in the female reproductive tract. These alternative routes of immunization would be convenient and widely acceptable.

The carbohydrate ABO antigens are also present on sperms, due to either haploid expression or passive adsorption (Erikson, 1977). The acrosomal enzymes (hyaluronidase and acrosin) necessary for penetration of the cumulus mass and zona pellucida investments of the oocyte are antigenic but do not appear to be sperm specific (Jilek and Pavlok, 1975). Similarly, a number of spermatozoal antigens capable of eliciting and reactive with xenogeneic or allogeneic antisera have been described (Isojima and Li, 1968; Rao and Sadri, 1960; Tumbo-Oeri and Kwendo, 1982). Some of these antigens were implied to be sperm specific. Using monoclonal antibodies, we have recently identified an antigenic determinant composed of 10 amino acids and a high-molecular-weight antigen present on spermatozoa and in seminal plasma (Figs. 1 and 2) that does not appear to be present on somatic tissues (Czuppon and Mettler, 1982; Paul et al., 1983). A synthetic decapeptide was established after careful structural analysis of sperm membrane antigen amino acid composition. The preparation of the synthetic decapeptide antigen has been described previously (Czuppon and Mettler, 1982). Solid-phase radioimmunoassay with the synthetic peptide antigen was carried out as described by Czuppon and Mettler (1983). In our tests, 50 ng of the purified synthetic peptide was used for coating the microtiter plates. All 239 monoclonal sperm antibodies were tested with the synthetic peptide in one enzyme-linked immunosorbent assay (Paul et al., 1983). In order to test the tissue specificity of our synthetic decapeptide, absorption experiments with acetone powder extracts of tissues of various human organs were carried out. These included brain, kidney, liver, muscle (smooth and nonsmooth), and lung. The monoclonal antibody (Ki-Sp VII/5) was absorbed by increasing amounts of the acetone powder tissue extracts (10, 20, 50, 100, 200, and 500 ng). After each absorption step an ELISA was carried out. The double-antibody sandwich method was used as it was first described by Nakane and Pierce (1967) for immunohistochemical staining.

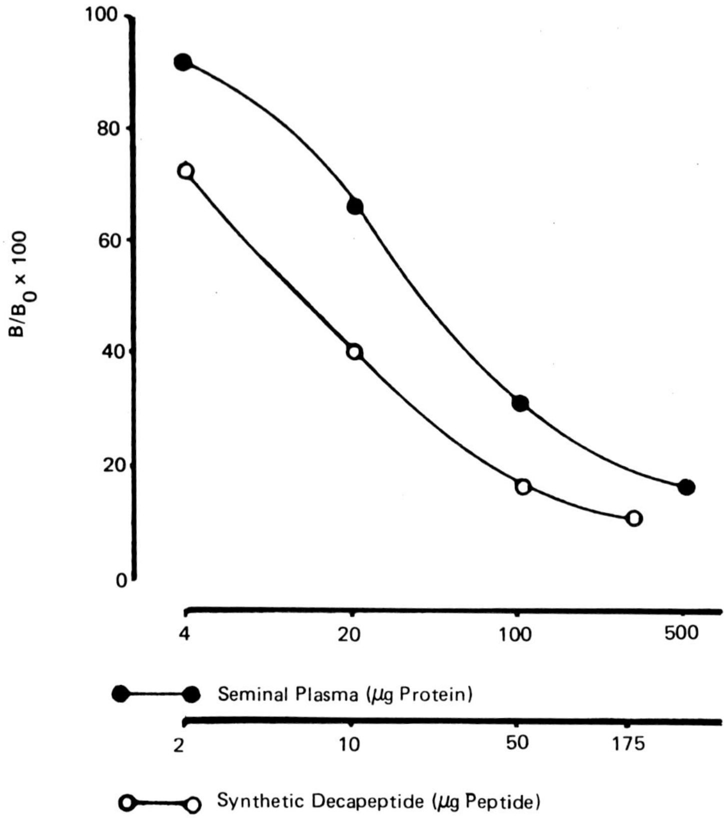

Figure 1. Demonstration of the reactivity of monoclonal antibody VII5 with the synthetic decapeptide in a competitive ELISA test. Various doses of the decapeptide or seminal plasma were allowed to compete with immobilized spermatozoa for binding to the antibody. Values are means of triplicates. (From Paul et al., 1983.)

Cryostate sections of various human tissues were used to investigate the organ specificity of our monoclon antibody (Ki-Sp VII/5). Rabbit antihuman spermatozoal antiserum was purchased from Behring Institute (F.R.G). For the the radioimmunoassay, serial dilutions were used before and after absorption with whole fresh human spermatozoa. Absorption of the naturally occurring anti-spermatozoal antibodies in sera of steril patients was carried out with the synthetic decapeptide. The antispermatozoal antibody titers of clinically defined WHO reference sera were determined as described previously (Hustedt and Hjort, 1974), before and after absorption with the synthetic decapeptide at a concentration of 50 ng peptide per 50 μl serum. The incubation was carried out for 24 hr at 4°C, and the titers were estimated again after the absorption experiment.

Antigenicity of the spermatozoal synthetic decapeptide. Antigenicity has been clearly established by the following reactions.

1. Reactivity with polyvalent rabbit antihuman spermatozoal antiserum in the radioimmunoassay (RIA) is shown in Figure 2. The antigenicity was lost following absorption with fresh human spermatozoa, indicating the spermatozoal origin of the synthetic decapeptide.
2. During the ELISA, the synthetic decapeptide reacted with the monoclonal antibody Ki-Sp VII/5 (Fig. 3).
3. The in vitro absorption of naturally occurring sperm-agglutinating and sperm-immunobilizing antisperm antibodies in sera of infertile patients is shown in Table 1. After absorption of the patient's sera a significant reduction of agglutination occurred ($\chi^2 = 11.44; p < 0.05$) in some cases. It is interesting to note that, although in some cases complete absorption occurred under the experimental conditions, some of the sera did not react at all (i.e., serum 7). The reason for this is not clear at present.

During the ELISA, the reactivity of the synthetic decapeptide with the monoclonal antibody Ki-Sp VII/5 could not be absorbed

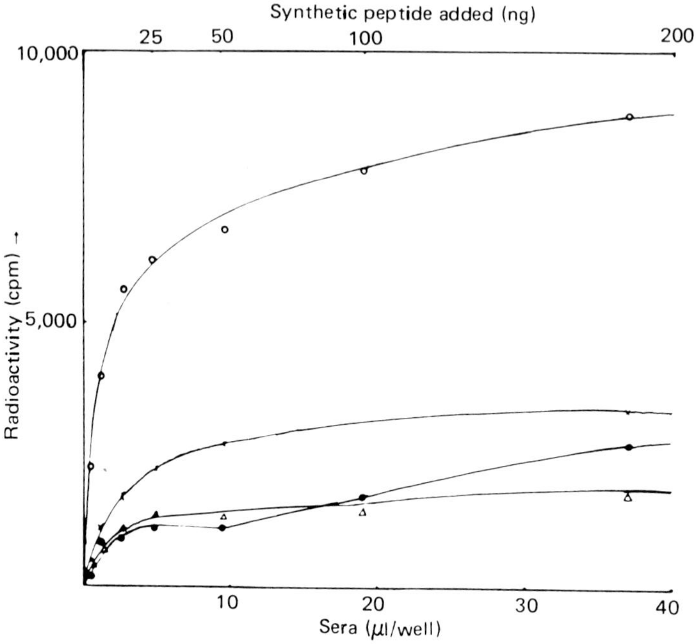

Figure 2 Absorption of the polyvalent rabbit antihuman spermatozoal antiserum with the synthetic human spermatozoal decapeptide. Ordinate = radioactivity (cpm). Abscissa (top) = amount (ng) of synthetic decapeptide added to rabbit antihuman spermatozoal antiserum (X). Abscissa (bottom) = µl rabbit antihuman spermatozoal antiserum per well (○). Preimmune (normal) rabbit serum (△); rabbit antiserum against human spermatozoa preabsorbed on fresh human spermatozoa (●) and rabbit antiserum against human spermatozoa in the presence of the synthetic decapeptide (X).

with any of the organs tested. However, a slight cross-reaction with seminal plasma seems to have occurred. Approximately 10–30% of the monoclonal antibody reactivity against the synthetic decapeptide could be absorbed with pooled human seminal plasma. Whether this represents so-called antigen shedding from the spermatozoal surface into the seminal plasma or whether there

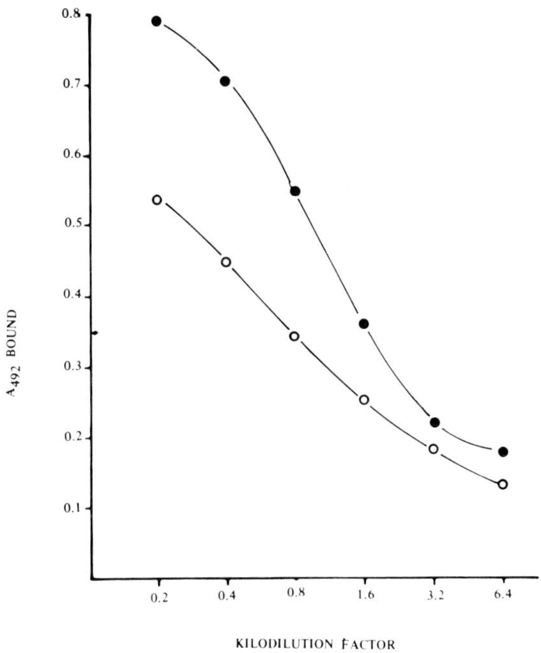

Figure 3 Monoclonal antibody VII-5 dilution curves using the crude solubilized spermatozoal antigens (○) and the synthetic decapeptide (●) as solid phase. Values are means of duplicates.

is a similar antigen present in the seminal plasma cannot be determined from the data. Further studies are being carried out using seminal plasma after vasoligation. Immunohistochemical staining of various tissue sections showed that the monoclonal antibody reacting with the synthetic decapeptide does not react with any of the organs tested.

Apart from intrinsic spermatozoal antigens, seminal plasma contains many antigenic components originating from the testis, accessory glands, and epidydimis. Shigeta et al. (1980) have generated a monoclonal antibody against a seminal plasma antigen that agglutinates and immobilizes spermatozoa. Li and Behrman (1970) could not detect any specific antigens on human sperm but did find three sperm-coating antigens originating from

Table 1 Absorption of Antispermatozoal Antibodies in Sera of Sterile Patients with the Synthetic Decapeptide[a]

Antiserum no.	Titer prior to incubation	Titer following incubation with the synthetic peptide
1	1:64	1:4[a] (1:8)
2	1:2048	0[b] (0)
3	1:128	1:128 (1:128)
4	1:128	1:16[b] (1:32)
5	1:512	1:64
6	1:16	0[b] (1:4)
7	1:64	1:64[b] (1:128)
8	1:1024	1:64[b] (1:32)

[a]Antisera (50 μl) were preincubated with 50 μg synthetic peptide for 24 hr at 4°C and then assayed by the test (for details, see Sec. III). Results for the native peptide are presented in parentheses.
[b]Titer reduction considered significant (χ^2 = 11.44; $p \Leftarrow 0.05$).

seminal plasma. The extent of shared antigenic determinants in sperm and seminal plasma, due either to coating of spermatozoa by the seminal plasma constituents or to shedding of spermatozoal antigens, is reflected by the observation that 91% of all monoclonal antibodies (n = 239) against spermatozoa also

Table 2 Some Characteristics of Monoclonal Antibodies Generated Against Human Spermatozoa

Characteristic	Number
Positive ELISA reactivity with	
sperm or seminal plasma	149
sperm as well as seminal plasma	136
only sperm	7
only seminal plasma	6
Sperm agglutinating	5
Sperm immobilizing	15
Nonreactive with tonsils	19
Nonreactive with spleen homogenate	13
Total hybrids generated	239

reacted with seminal plasma in ELISA tests (Table 2) (Paul et al., 1983). Moore (1981) observed three epidydimal glycoproteins that bind strongly to rabbit spermatozoa; antisera against these glycoproteins caused spermagglutination and blocked fertilization in vivo. A teratocarcinoma antigen secreted by the epidydimis and coupled to sperm has been reported (Fox et al., 1982).

II. EVIDENCE THAT IMMUNOLOGIC REACTIONS INFLUENCE FERTILIZATION

Theoretically, humoral and/or cell-mediated immune responses can influence fertilization through (1) direct effects on the gametes, such as cytotoxicity, interference with maturation, and modification of the biologic events on the sperm membrane or zona pellucida that precede fertilization, (2) block of recognition and penetration of the egg by the sperm, and (3) neutralization of hormones necessary for ovulation.

Inhibition of fertilization and reproductive performance by antibodies against spermatozoa has been demonstrated by experimental alloimmunization and has been inferred in cases of naturally occurring auto- and alloimmunity. Male guinea pigs immunized with epididymal sperm and Freund's complete adjuvant (FCA) show widespread damage to testis and are rendered infertile. This effect is not obtained in the absence of FCA, although high sperm antibody titers are reached. Apparently, a cell-mediated immune reaction provoked in the presence of FCA is necessary for the induction of aspermatogenesis, although sperm antibodies are also involved in the full expression of tissue damage (Brown and Glynn, 1969; Voisin and Toullet, 1968). Local, but not systemic adoptive transfer of T lymphocytes from immunized guinea pigs causes testicular lesions indistinguishable from primary lesions. (Tung, Teuscher and Meng, 1981).

Female hamsters isoimmunized with spermatozoa show decreased fertility (Isojima et al., 1972; Katsh, 1959). Serum from immunized females inhibits fertilization in vivo and in vitro. Purified IgG from vasectomized guinea pigs contains high antisperm activity and inhibits the acrosome reactions, sperm-zona binding, and sperm-ovum fusion in vitro (Huang et al., 1981). Univalent Fab fragments from vasectomized guinea pigs block sperm-zona binding but not sperm-ovum fusion. Female mice immunized with allogeneic spermatozoa without adjuvant exhibit significant but incomplete reduction of in vivo fertilization correlated with circulating titers of agglutinating and immobilizing sperm antibody (Fig. 4) (Seki and Mettler, 1982). Further, two-cell embryos recovered from the immunized mice generate fewer and smaller blastocysts compared with those from the control group. Allogeneic antisera against mouse spermatozoa inhibit mouse in vitro fertilization (Table 3). The two-cell mouse embryos exposed in vitro to antispermatozoal antibody did not exhibit reduced cleavage, but a significant block of hatching of the embryos occurred (Mettler et al., 1982). In the female rat, immunization with a low-molecular-weight spermatozoal peptide conjugated to bovine serum albumin (BSA) and FCA yielded a significant reduction of

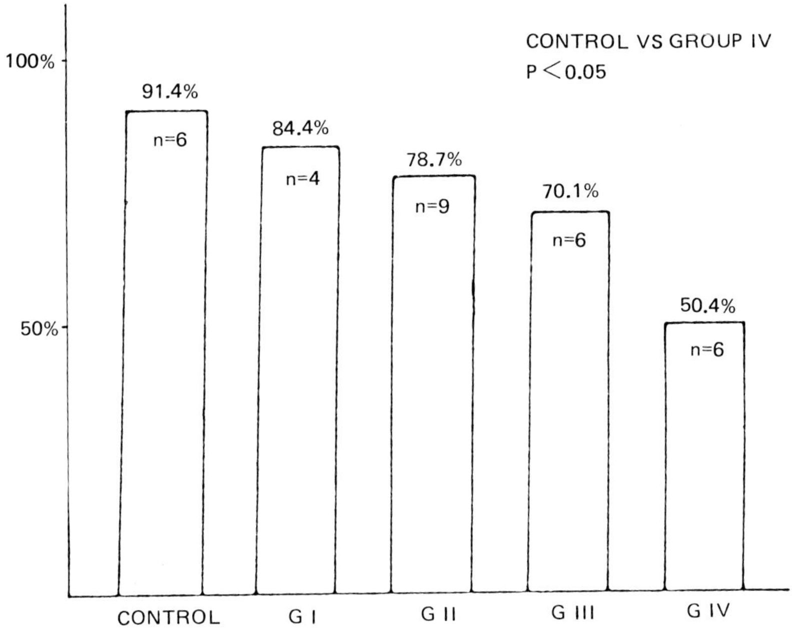

Figure 4 Influence of immunization with spermatozoa on in vivo fertilization in allogeneic mice. The mice were injected twice a week for 2 weeks (GI and GII) or 8 weeks (GIII and GIV) with 4, 8, 12, or 16 million spermatozoa in groups GI, GIII, and GIV, respectively. Following mating, embryos were flushed out and examined for cell stage in vitro. (From Seki and Mettler, 1982.)

fertility; surprisingly, a more dramatic fertility reduction was obtained using the peptide-BSA conjugate in liposomes as adjuvant (Table 4).

With regard to the natural incidence of antisperm antibodies in humans, a number of investigations have attempted to correlate their occurrence with infertility. Using the techniques of sperm agglutination and complement-dependent sperm immobilization, most reports show a higher or slightly higher incidence of sperm antibodies in infertile patient collectives compared with fertile groups (Franklin and Dukes, 1964; Isojima et al., 1972; Mettler, 1977a). Results from our own laboratory are given in Tables 5 and 6. In general, it can be stated that whereas sperm agglutination can also be caused by nonantibody material, such as steroids and bacteria (Boettcher and Kay, 1973), complement-dependent sperm immobilization is probably a more reliable indicator of sperm antibody and fertility status (Isojima et al., 1959; Mettler, 1977b). In our own experience and as also reported by Chen and Jones (1981), some human sera immobilize spermatozoa without utilizing complement. This immobilizing activity is associated with the IgG fraction of these sera. Possibly such antibodies bind and neutralize contractile constituents or molecules involved in the energy generating system and thus immobilize spermatozoa.

Table 3 In Vitro Fertilization of Mouse Oocytes: Influence of Antisera Against Mouse Spermatozoa on the Fertilization Rate

	Oocytes (total)	Fertilization rate (%)
In vitro fertilization (control)	112	49
Adding control sera (non-treated)	51	41
Adding control sera (erythrocyte sensitized)	43	40
Adding antisera against spermatozoa	68	3
Adding gammaglobulin fractions out of antisera	80	1

Sperm antibodies present in the blood may not be a faithful reflection of their presence in the female reproductive tract. Indeed, compared with serum, better correlation of male and female infertility with the incidence of sperm-agglutinating and sperm-immobilizing antibodies in the seminal plasma and cervical mucus, respectively, has been reported (De Almeida and Eyquem, 1978; Jager et al., 1980; Rümke, 1982). Relatively low titers of sperm-agglutination and sperm-immobilizing antibodies antibodies observed in vitro may be physiologically irrelevant owing

Table 4 Inhibition of Fertility in Female Rats by Immunization with a Spermatozoal Liposomal Peptide

Immunogen	Number of pregnancies[a]	Number of newborn/rat	Antibody titer in RIA (cpm)[b]
Controls (liposomes alone)			
before immunization	10	9.9	0
after immunization	8	8.7	110
Purified spermatozoal peptide-liposomes			
before immunization	10	10.2[c]	0
after immunization	3	2.4[c]	2078

[a]Each group had 10 rats.
[b]Performed according to Czuppon and Mettler (1981).
[c]$p < 0.05$.

Table 5 Pregnancy Rate of 130 Sterile Females with Unexplained Sterility for the Preceding 3 Years[a]

Test method		n	Number of pregnancies	
MAT[b]	Negative	91	12	12
	Positive	39		7
MIT[c]	Negative	103		15
	Positive	27		0

[a]Including 45 females with persisting sperm-agglutinating and sperm-immobilizing antibodies (serum dilution, 1:3).
[b]Sperm microagglutination test.
[c]Sperm microimmobilization test.

to incomplete immobilization or agglutination, and this may be the explanation for the fertile status of many individuals exhibiting these activities. In a recent report using vital staining of spermatozoa with the dye fluorescein diacetate, sera, cervical mucus, and seminal plasma samples from infertile individuals had average antibody titers significantly higher than fertile individuals, with 40–40% of the infertile patients exhibiting antibody titers higher than the fertile controls (Mathur et al., 1981).

According to the sperm-agglutination and sperm-immobilization assays, naturally occurring human sperm auto- and isoantibodies are species specific (with the exception of closely related primates) but individually nonspecific; i.e., they are directed against tissue-specific spermatozoal antigens. On the other hand, Mathur et al. (19810, using their passive hemagglutination and vital staining assays, observed that the sperm antibody titers in infertile women were significantly higher when tested with husband's spermatozoa compared with controls; surprisingly, sperm antibody titers in cervical mucus and vaginal secretions were similar with both types of spermatozoa.

A correlation between sperm antibody titers in the sera of the husband and the wife in infertile couples has been described by Mathur et al. (1981); similar results were obtained by Czuppon and Mettler (1981) using a solid-phase radioimmunoassay with [^{125}I]protein A as tracer (Fig. 5). Employing this RIA and a well-validated ELISA for antibody against intact sperm (Paul et al., 1983), clear correlations between agglutination-immobilization

Table 6 Sperm Antibodies in Human Sera of Sterile Males and Females[a]

		Positive cases	
Methods	Number	n	%
Females			
FD test	412	26	6.1
Kibrick test	207	5	2.4
MAT	2.067	206	10.0
Isojima	412	5	1.2
MIT	2.067	73	3.5
Males			
FD test	215	4	1.3
Kibrick test	42	2	5
MAT	1.025	20	2
Isojima	215	3	1.8
MIT	1.025	10	1

[a]Department of Obstetrics and Gynecology, University of Kid, 1971-1981.
FD = Franklin and Dukes, 1964.
MAT = microtray agglutination test.
MIT = microtray immobilization test.

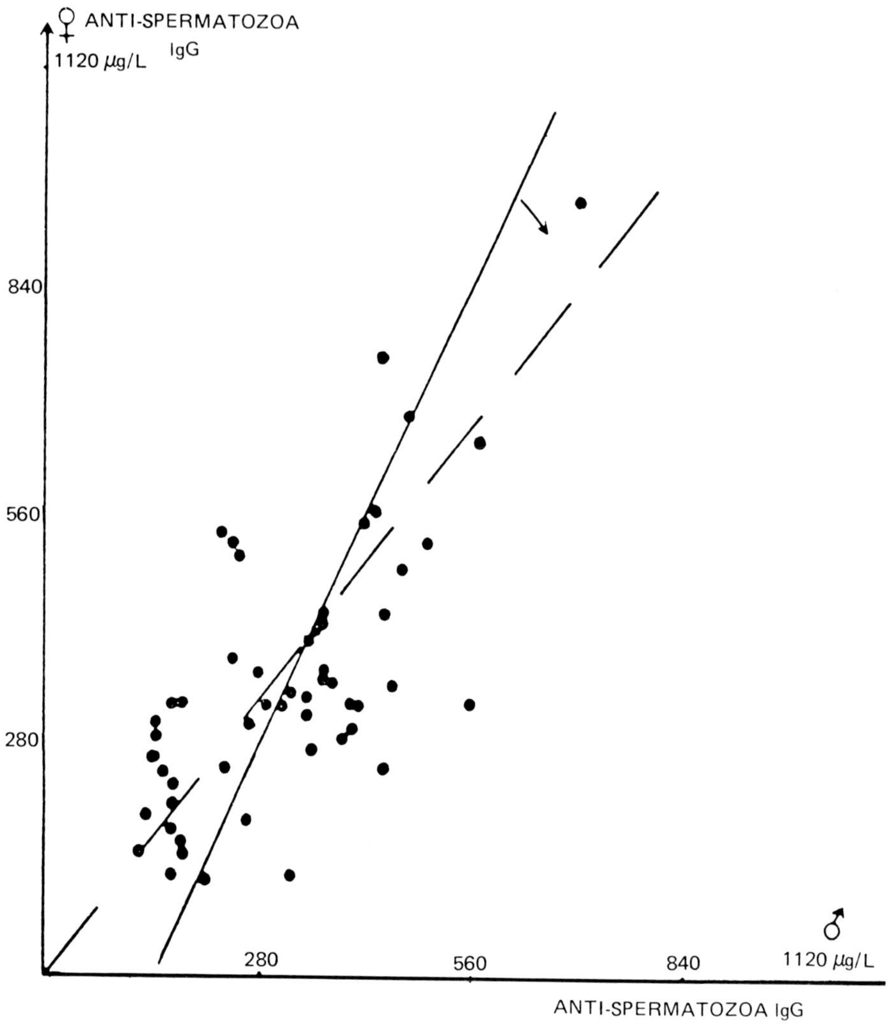

Figure 5 Correlation of antisperm IgG serum levels of sterile married couples. A significant positive correlation (solid line) was observed between the antisperm antibody levels of the wives and their husbands (r = 0.6; n = 52; p 0.01; y = 2.09; x = 27.25). The broken line represents absolute correlation (r = 1).

titers or fertile-infertile status and the RIA and ELISA titers were lacking. In the RIA and ELISA tests, most patient sera showed reactivity greater than control sera that had been absorbed previously with spermatozoa. In view of the demonstration using monoclonal antibodies of cross-reactivity of many spermatozoal antigens with somatic tissues and the high sensitivity of the radioimmune and enzyme-linked probes, the frequent incidence of antisperm antibodies may be explained in terms of reactivity with low concentrations of perhaps physiologically irrelevant autoantibodies that have been postulated to exist under normal, nonpathologic circumstances. Bacteria have also been implicated as the antigeneic stimulus for some of the naturally occurring sperm antibodies (Sarkar, 1974; Tung et al., 1976).

The penetration of zona-free hamster eggs by human spermatozoa has recently been used widely as a model of fertilization. A number of reports demonstrate block of penetration of zona-free hamster eggs by spermatozoa in the presence of human sera or purified IgG possessing antisperm activity (Dor et al., 1981; Haas et al., 1980). This inhibition was not related to the tray agglutination and immobilization titers of the antisperm sera. On the other hand, our group did observe some correlation between the sperm-immobilization and agglutination titers and the inhibition of hamster oocyte penetration by human sperm antibody containing sera. Using the univalent Fab antibody fragment, the ability of the antibody to bind spermatozoa, as well as to inhibit zona-free hamster oocyte penetration by spermatozoa, was retained, whereas sperm-immobilizing and sperm-agglutinating activity was lost (Menge and Black, 1979; Tzartos, 1979). Thus the antifertility effect of the sperm antibodies may occur through steric masking of the sperm receptor for ovum binding sites and/or through interference with the acrosome reaction necessary for fertilization. Studying spermatozoa from a group of infertile donors, a mean hamster oocyte penetration level of 14% was observed, whereas proven fertile donors gave a penetration level of 81% ($p < 0.02$); these penetration levels showed no striking correlation with the survival index of spermatozoa, the sperm count, or the motility of sperm (Guelman et al., 1981; Hall, 1981). Similarly, using penetration of the zona of cryopreserved human ova, statistically significant differences in the penetration capacity of spermatozoa from infertile (12.7%) and fertile (50%) patients is described (Overstreet and Hembree, 1976). It can be speculated that these differences between infertile and fertile patients were due to the greater amount of antibody coated on spermatozoa from the former group (Hancock and Cockett, 1981). On the other hand, one report indicates that spermatozoa coated with antibody, as assayed by RIA, exhibit increased penetration of zona-free hamster oocytes (Bronson et al., 1981). This potentiation of fertilization capacity was hypothesized to occur through activation of acrosomal enzymes by antibody bound on the sperm head. Such results underscore the importance of investigating the heterogeneity of the antibody profile that spermatozoa may provoke. Antibodies directed against the different antigens in the sperm membrane may result in widely disparate biologic consequences.

Further evidence that immunologic mechanisms may participate in the acrosomal reaction comes from a report that complement components bind to spermatozoa during follicular fluid-induced acrosome reaction in capacitated spermatozoa and that the complement binding, acrosome reaction, and fertilization can be blocked by antibody against component C3 of the complement cascade (Cabot and Oliphant, 1978). These blocks were overcome by addition of exogeneous C3.

First, allogeneic mating in the rat is associated with a specific cytolytic T-cell response against paternal strain antigens; this response was enhanced by subsequent intrauterine challenge with allogeneic spermatozoa (Thomas et al., 1982). Allogeneic spermatozoa introduced into the rat uterus produce a local inflammatory reaction, enlargement of the uterine regional lymphnodes, and specific sensitization to subsequent intradermal injection of lymphocytes from the same strain (Beer and Billinghan, 1974). Such sensitization to subsequent reaction apparently enhance, the reproductive efficiency of the sensitized uterine horn compared with the control horn. A facilitating effect of immunologic responses upon reproductive performance may occur through enhancing antibodies, generation of suppressor T lymphocytes, or simply antigen masking.

III. CLINICAL IMPLICATIONS

Prakash and Lang (1980) discovered a seminal plasma constituent that blocks the cell-mediated reactivity of lymphocytes and postulated that the immunosuppressive action of this molecule may possess a role in determining the absence or presence of an antisperm response. Bertling et al. (1982) demonstrated a spermatozoal glycoprotein of molecular weight 40,000 and pH 4.6 that suppressed the one-way mixed lymphocyte culture reactivity of lymphocytes. The development of the cytotoxic T-lymphocyte response against paternal strain cells following mating in rats is a transient phenomenon disappearing 3 days postcoitum (Thomas et al., 1982). The early pregnancy factor (EPF) is alleged to be synthesized by the oocytes 6 hr after fertilization in the mouse and to inhibit T-lymphocyte rosette formation with sheep erythrocytes (Clark et al., 1978; Morton et al., 1974). In culture in vitro of human embryos, EPF was detected 24 hr after fertilization. A great deal of interest has been generated by EPF; unfortunately, assay methods currently employed to detect EPF are not easily reproducible (Cooper and Aitken, 1981).

Knowledge derived from studies of the immunology of fertilization may prove useful both for treatment of infertility as well for achieving immunologic contraception. Female monkeys immunized with the spermatozoal LDH-X isoenzyme show reduced fertility (Goldberg, 1979), as do female rats immunized with a low-molecular-weight spermatozoal peptide-BSA conjugate in liposomes (Czuppon and Mettler, unpublished).

Spermatozoal low-molecular-weight peptides that are reactive with naturally occurring sperm auto- and isoantibodies may be used as active immunogen for contraception or for neutralization of antibodies in the treatment of infertility. The recent availability of monoclonal sperm and seminal plasma antibodies enables the precise identification of potential target antigens on spermatozoa and their tissue specificity. A number of reports state that zona antigens are not shared by somatic tissues and that fertility is reduced after immunization with isolated zona as well as solubilized zona proteins (reviewed by Sacco, 1981). The development of a contraceptive vaccine hinges upon identification of suitable target antigens, selection of a potent adjuvant, and route of immunization resulting in a uniformly individual-independent, long-lasting, but reversible humoral and/or cell-mediated immune response that interferes critically in the reproduction process but does not cross-react with somatic tissues. This is currently an intense area of research.

A. Spermatozoal Antibody Detection by Solid-Phase Radioimmunoassay

Ever since Landsteiner (1899) discovered the antigenic properties of human spermatozoa, there have been numerous tests devised for the diagnosis of immunologically induced infertility. The main difficulties in developing an adequate diagnostic test lie in the methods used for the preparation of the proper antigen (Mettler and Czuppon, 1983) and the detection of the reacting antibodies in the sera of patients with fertility problems.

Most of the tests that are in use require either motile, fresh spermatozoa or fixed intact cells and thus are dependent upon a steady supply of cells. In addition, test results are only as good as the subjective interpretation of the observer. Furthermore, some of these tests are known to be influenced by nonspecific factors (i.e., hormones in the sera) (Boettcher, 1974).

Theoretically, the intact spermatozoal membrane might not al all provide the proper target antigens, since the latter can be masked (Czuppon, 1984) or not expressed on the intact cell membrane surface (Mettler and Czuppon, 1983). In the present study, spermatozoal membranes were first solubilized by the zwitterionic detergent, 3- (3-(cholamidopropyl)dimethylammonoi)propanesulfonate (CHAPS). The solubilized membrane mixture was used as antigen following immobilization on beads. The immune complexes with the naturally occurring antibodies in sera of infertile patients were detected with the aid of [^{125}I]protein A. The assay is simple to perform and requires no vital or intact cells, and large numbers of sera can be processed in a single day (up to 400).

These advantages and the specificity of the reaction suggest that this new immunoassay will be the method of choice for the detection of immunologically induced infertility cases.

1. Material and Methods

The solubilization process was the same as described earlier (Czuppon and Mettler, 1981), except for the presence of 10% w/v CHAPS.

a. Preparation of the Antigen-Coated Beads The plastic beads (3-mm diameter) were incubated with the solubilized mixture (90 mg protein ml^{-1}; 60 beads ml^{-1}), with gentle shaking for 120 min at room temperature. This was followed by overnight incubation at 4°C. After the incubations, the beads were washed with ice-cold 0.05 M phosphate buffer, pH 7.8, dried, and stored at 4°C until use.

b. Solid-Phase Immunoassay Patient sera were diluted 1:100 with the above buffer and 200 μl was incubated with the coated beads in separate RIA tubes for 30 min at 37°C and for 30 min at 25°C. After the incubation, the beads were washed with ice-cold phosphate buffer using a suction pump. Then 200 μl of a I-protein-A solution (60,000 cpm; 7 μl Ci/μg diluted in the above buffer that contained 0.1% w/v BSA) were pipetted to each bead, and these were incubated for another 30 min at 37°C. Following the incubation, the beads were washed again and finally counted separately for 1 min in the gamma counter (Fig. 6).

All assays were carried out in triplicate. In each set of assay a positive control serum, rabbit antihuman sperm antiserum, was also included to maintain quality control.

The bound antispermatozoa IgG concentrations in the sera of patients were calculated according to the equation: ng IgG = average (cpm × BC) × (1268 × SA)$^{-1}$, where BC = binding capacity of I-protein-A in ng, 1268 = constant, and SA = specific activity

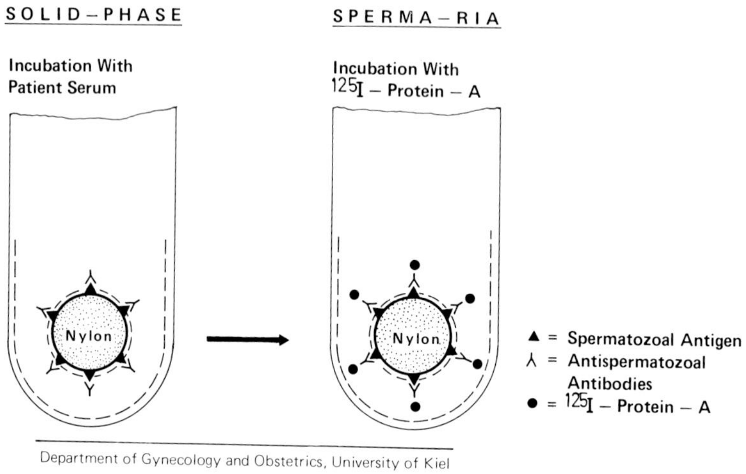

Figure 6 Principle of solid-phase RIA for the detection of spermatozoal antibodies.

of the I-protein-A in nCi/ng. An IgG level of 3.5 ng or greater was considered positive, according to the upper levels of the negative control groups.

Test sera were sent to the laboratory frozen, on dry ice, from the WHO Reference Bank for Reproductive Immunology, Aarhus, Denmark. The double-blind study was coordinated by Hjort under the trial number 77180 and included sera of clinically defined categories as follows:

Females: fertile, postpartum, postmenopausal, primary ammenorrhea, autoimmune ovarian failure, virgin, pregnant, recurrent abortion, unexplained infertility

Males: fertile, congenital absence of vas, aspermatogenesis, vasectomy, and unexplained infertility

In addition there were 24 pairs of duplicates, randomly distributed among the 360 sera.

2. Results

a. Sera of Females There were no positives in the categories of fertile, postpartum, postmenopausal, primary ammenorrhea, autoimmune ovarian failure, or virgins. In the category of unexplained infertiles, however, 6% of the sera showed an elevated antispermatozoal antibody level. All positives were primary sterility cases of 6 years' or more of duration.

b. Sera of Males No positives were found in the catefories of fertile, aspermatogenesis, or congenital absence of vas. In the unexplained infertility group, 3% of the patients showed elevated antispermatozoal IgG levels. In the category of vasectomized men, 8% of the patients were positive. Antibodies in the latter case are known to occur for some time (Fig. 7).

c. Quality Control The intrapair CV was estimated to be around 5%, and the interassay variation was less than 10%. The 23 pairs of duplicate sample that were distributed randomly in the total of 360 sera with coded numbers showed a correlation coefficient of $r = 0.45$ (Spearman correlation). This indicates a significant interpair correlation of the duplicates ($P < 0.05$).

B. Spermatozoal Immunologic Contraception

It has been demonstrated previously that incubation of spermatozoa results in the autolytic release of antigenic peptides from the cell membranes. This process, which can be inhibited by acrosin inhibitors (Czuppon and Mettler, 1981), might conceivably occur under physiological conditions in the female genital tract, where the natural acrosin inhibitors are not present. Autolysis of the spermatozoal membrane results in the release of both high molecular mass ($\geqslant$5000 daltons) and low molecular mass (1.000–2.000 daltons) peptide antigens (Czuppon and Mettler, 1981). It seems reasonable to assume that one or more large antigen molecules are broken down by the sperm proteinase acrosin and the resulting peptides still retain antigenic properties and may still be recognized by antibodies directed against the parent molecule.

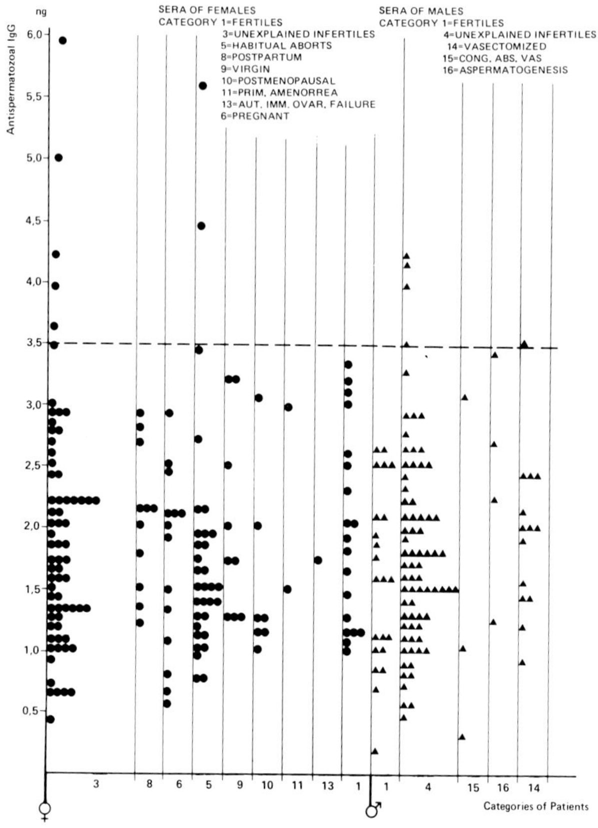

Figure 7 Solid-phase immunoassay of clinically defined (WHO) sera.

The antigenic character of the synthetic peptide is clearly established in the solid-phase radioimmunoassay and ELISA described. In attempting to interpret these absorption experiments, several possibilities can be considered. The two sera that did not react with the synthetic peptide may show nonspecific agglutination in the microsperm agglutination test. Alternatively, it is conceivable that these peptides react only with some of the antispermatozoal antibodies. Considering the polyspecific nature of antispermatozoal antibodies, the results of the abosrption experiments are not entirely unexplected, as only one antigen out of a major number of antigenic peptides generated by autolysis of the sperm proteins was tested. Thus, it is reasonable to assume that testing the mixture of antigenic peptides with a panel of antisera would result in immunoinhibition of all antisera by these different peptides. This phenomenon is the subject of current investigation.

That the synthetic decapeptide exhibits spermatozoal antigen characteristics could pave the way for important future applications in diagnosis and therapy of immunologically based sterility. This is further substantiated by the lack of cross-reactivity with other tissues. In therapy, the synthetic antigen could be applied to block circulating antispermatozoal antibodies in sterile patients in vivo, since it has been shown that even a temporary drop in the antispermatozoal antibody titer can lead to a reversal of immunologically induced sterility (Jones and Ing, 1974). An investigation of this nature using a primate animal model has recently been initiated in our laboratory. Alternatively, the possibility of an immunologic suppression of fertility in the female can be considered by immunization with the synthetic decapeptide, i.e., a sperm immunologic contraception. In an allogeneic rat model we were able to clearly demonstrate the fertility-reducing effect of immunization with out peptide (Mettler et al., 1983).

There is no doubt that, viewed in the light of the escalating appraisals of the long-term safety and acceptability of currently available methods, the principle of a birth control vaccine has several well-defined potential advantages:

1. Use of a nonpharmacologically active agent
2. Ease and convenience of administration making it suitable for distribution by paramedical personnel
3. Long-lasting (at least 12 months) but potentially reversible effect
4. Acceptability of the "vaccine" principle, of particular importance in developing countries

5. Reduced patient failure, since potection is not dependent on constant positive action by the recipient
6. Large-scale synthesis and manufacture of a vaccine at low cost

By far the most advanced approach to birth control vaccine development has involved the principle of immunization against the placental hormone human chorionic gonadotropin (HCG). A great deal of progress is also documented in the role of sperm immunologic contraception and its possible future development as summarized in this monograph.

REFERENCES

Atassi, M. Z. (1979). *CRC Crit. Rev. Biochem. 6*:371.

Bachmann, B. K., and C.-Y. Lee (1976). *Anal. Biochem. 72*:153.

Beer, A. E., and R. E. Billingham (1974). *Reprod. Fertil. 21*:59-88.

Bertling, E., Czuppon, A., and Mettler, L. (1982). Proceedings of the Fifth International Symposium on Immunology of Reproduction, Bulgarian Academy of Medical Sciences Press, Sofia, p. 426.

Blanco, A., and Zinkham, W. H. (1963). *Science 139*:601.

Boettcher, B. (1974). *Reprod. Fertil. (Suppl.) 21*:151-161.

Boettcher, B., and Kay, D. J. (1973). *Andrologie 5*:265-271.

Bronson, R., Cooper, G., and Rosenfeld, M. D. (1981). *Fertil. Steril. 36*:778-783.

Brown, P. C., and Glynn, L. E. (1969). *J. Pathol. 98*:277-282.

Cabot, C. L., and Oliphant, G. (1978). *Biol. Reprod. 19*:666-672.

Chen, C., and Jones, W. R. (1981). *Fertil. Steril. 35*:542-545.

Clark, F. M., Morton, H., and Clunie, G. J. A. (1978). *Clin. Exp. Immunol. 32*:318-323.

Cooper, D. W., and Aitken, R. J. (1981). *Reprod. Fertil. 61*:241-245.

Czuppon, A. B. (1984). *Biochem. Int. 9*:9-19.

Czuppon, A. B., and Mettler, L. (1981). *Am. J. Reprod. Immunol. 1*:303-306.

Czuppon, A. B., and Mettler, L. (1982). *Hoppe-Seylers Z. Physiol. Chem. 363*:1465–1471.
Czuppon, A. B., and Mettler, L. (1983). *J. Clin. Chem. Clin. Biochem. 21*:357–362.
Czuppon, A. B., Mettler, L., Schauer, R., and Pawassarat V., (1981). *Hoppe-Seylers Physiol. Chem. 362*:963–968.
De Almeida, M., and Eyquem, A. (1978). Bulgarian Academy of Sciences Press, Sofia, pp. 432–437.
Dor, J., Rudak, E., and Aitken, R. J. (1981). *Fertil. Steril. 35*:535–541.
Erikson, R. P. (1977). Cambridge University Press, London, pp. 85–107.
Fellous, M., and Dausset, J. (1970). *Nature 225*:191–193.
Fjällbrant, B. (1968). *Acta Obstet. Gynecol. Scand. 47*:102–110.
Fox, N., Damjanov, I., Knowles, B. B., and Solter, D., (1982). *Exp. Cell. Res. 137*:485–488.
Franklin, R. R., and Dukes, C. D. (1964). *Am. J. Obstet. Gynecol. 89*:6–9.
Goldberg, E. (1963). *Science 139*:602.
Goldberg, E. (1971). *Proc. Natl. Acad. Sci. USA 68*:349.
Goldberg, E. (1972). *J. Biol. Chem. 247*:2044.
Goldberg, E. (1973). *Science 181*:458.
Goldberg, E. (1974). Acta Endocrinol. (*Copenh.*) (*Suppl.*) *194*:202.
Goldberg, E. (1975). *Acta Endocrinol (Copenh.) (Suppl.) 194*:202–222.
Goldberg, E. (1976). Alan R. Liss, New York, pp. 133–138.
Goldberg, E. (1979). Elsevier/North-Holland, Amsterdam, pp. 281–290.
Goldberg, E., and Wheat, T. E. (1976). American Elsevier New York, pp. 133-138.
Goldberg, E., Aoki, T., Boyse, E. J., and Bennet, D. (1970). *Nature 225*:191–193.
Goldberg, E., Gonzales-Prevatt, U., and Wheat, T. E. (1981a). In *Human Reproduction* (K. Semm and L. Mettler, eds.) Elsevier/ North-Holland, Amsterdam, pp. 360–364.
Goldberg, E., Wheat, T. E., Powell, J. E., and Stevens, V. C. (1981b). *Fertil. Steril. 35*:214.

Goldman-Leikin, R. E., and Goldberg, E. (1983). *Proc. Natl. Acad. Sci. USA 80*:3774.
Gonzales-Prevatt, V., Wheat T. E., and Goldberg, E. (1982). *Mol. Immunol. 19*:1579.
Guelman, B. Z., Blasco, L., and Wolf, D. P. (1981). *Fertil. Steril. 36*:771–777.
Haas, G. G., Sokoloski, J. E., and Wolf, D. P. (1980). *Am. J. Reprod. Immunol. 1*:40–43.
Halim, A., and Festenstein, H. (1978). *Lancet 2*:937–938.
Hall, J. L. (1981). *Fertil. Steril. 35*:457–463.
Hancock, J., and Cockett, A. T. (1981). *J. Immunol. Methods 43*:103–113.
Hintz, M., and Goldberg, E. (1976). *Dev. Biol. 57*:375.
Hustedt, S., and Hjort, T. (1974). *Clin. Exp. Immunol. 47*:61–69.
Huang, T. T., Tung, S. K., and Yanagimachi, R. (1981). *Science 213*:1267–1269.
Isojima, S., and Li, T. S. (1968). *Fertil. Steril. 19*:999–1008.
Isojima, S., Graham, R. M., and Graham, J. B. (1959). *Science 129*:44.
Isojima, S., Tsuhiya, K., and Koyama, K. (1972). *Am. J. Obstet. Gynecol. 112*:199–207.
Jager, S., Kremer, J., Kuiken, J., and van Slochteren-Craaisma, T. 1977). Academic Press, Sydney, pp. 289–293.
Jager, S., Kremer, J., and Kuiken, J. (1980). *Int. J. Androl. 3*:1–14.
Jilek, A., and Pavlok, A. (1975). *J. Reprod. Fertil. 42*:377–380.
Jones, W. R., and Ing, R. M. Y. (1974). In *Immunology in Obstetrics and Gynaecology* (A. Centaro and N. Caretti, eds.), Elsevier/North-Holland, Amsterdam, pp. 94–99.
Katsh, S. (1959). *Am. J. Obstet. Gynecol. 78*:276–278.
Kerek, G., and Afzelius, B. A. (1972). *Int. J. Fertil. 17*:120–126.
Kille, J. W., and Goldberg, E. (1979). *Biol. Reprod. 20*:863.
Kille, J. W., and Goldberg, E. (1980). *J. Reprod. Immunol. 2*:15.
Kille, J., Wheat, T. E., Mitchell, G., and Goldberg, E., (1978). *J. Exp. Zool. 204*:259.
Landsteiner, K. (1899). *Zentralbl. Bakteriol. Parasitol. 25*:546–549.
Law, H. Y., and Bodmer, W. F. (1978). *Tissue Antigens 12*:249–269.

Lee, C.-Y., Yuan, J. H., and Goldberg, E. (1982). *Methods Enzymol. 89*:351–362.
Lerum, J. E., and Goldberg, E. (1974). *Biol. Reprod. 11*:108.
Li, T., and Behrman, S. J. (1970). *Fertil. Steril. 21*:565–573.
Li, S. S.-L., Feldmann, R. J., Okabe, M., and Pan, Y.-C. E. (1983a). *J. Biol. Chem. 258*:7017.
Li, S. S.-L., Fitch, W. M., Pan, Y.-C. E., and Sharief, F. S. (1983b). *J. Biol. Chem. 258*:7029.
Marsh, J. A., Wheat, T. E., and Goldberg, E. (1977). *J. Immunol. 118*(b):2293.
Marsh, J. A., O'Hern, P., and Goldberg, E. (1981). *J. Immunol. 126*:100.
Mathur, S., Williamson, H. O., and Derrick, F. C. (1981). *J. Immunol. 126*:905–908.
Meistrich, M. L., Trostle, P. K., Frapart, M., and Erickson, R. P. (1977). *Dev. Biol. 60*:428.
Menge, A. C., and Black, C. S. (1979). *Fertil. Steril. 32*:214–218.
Mettler, L. (1977a). Gross Verlag, Berlin,
Mettler, L. (1977b). In Bd. 4 (C. Schirren and K. Semm, eds.), Grosse Verlag, Berlin.
Mettler, L., and Czuppon, A. B. (1983). *Am. J. Reprod. Immunol. 4*:127–132.
Mettler, L., Baukloh, V., and Riedel, H.-H. (1982). In (R. E. Edwards and J. Purdy, eds.), Academic Press, London, pp. 181–189.
Mettler, L., Czuppon, A. B., and Tinneberg, H.-R. (1983). *Andrologia 15*(6):670–675.
Montgomery, P. C., Lemaitre-Coelho, I, M., and Vaer, J. P. (1980). *Immunol. Commun. 9*:705.
Moore, H. D. (1981). *J. Exp. Zool. 215*:77–85.
Morton, H., Hega, V., and Clunie, G. A. (1974). *Nature 249*:459–460.
Musick, W. D. L., and Rossmann, M. G. (1979). *J. Biol. Chem. 254*:7611.
Nakane, P. K., and Pierce, C. B. (1967). *J. Cell. Biol. 33*:307–318.
Overstreet, J. W., and Hembree, W. C. (1976). *Fertil. Steril. 27*:815–831.
Pan, Y. C.-E. Sharief, F. S., Okabe, M., Huang, S., and Li, S. S.-L. (1983). *J. Biol. Chem. 258*:7005.

Paul, S., Baukloh, V., and Mettler, L. (1983). *J. Immunol. Methods* *56*:193–199.
Prahbu, G., and Hedge, U. C. (1982). *Am. J. Reprod. Immunol.* *2*:243–245.
Prakash, C., and Lang, R. W. (1980). *M. Sinai J. Med. (NY.)* *47*:491–510.
Rao, S. S., and Sadri, K. K. (1960). *J. Comp. Pathol. 70*:1–9.
Rümke, P. (1982). In (S. Shulman, F. Donero, and M. Nicotra, eds.), Academic Press, London, pp. 69–76.
Sacco, A. C. (1981). *Obstet. Gynecol. Annu. 10*:1–26.
Sarkar, S. K. (1974). *J. Reprod. Med. 13*:93–99.
Seki, M., and Mettler, L. (1982). *Am. J. Reprod. Immunol. 2*:225–232.
Shigeta, A., Watanabe, T., Maruyama, S., Koyama, K., and Isojima, S. (1980). *Clin. Exp. Immunol. 42*:458–462.
Shulman, S. (1972). *Obstet. Gynecol. Surv. 27*:553–563.
Stevens, V. C., Cinader, B., Powell, J. E., Lee, A. C., Koh, S. W. (1981). *Am. J. Reprod. Immunol. 1*:307–314.
Thomas, I. K., Leeming, G., and McLean, J. M. (1982). *Am. J. Reprod. Immunol. 2*:165.
Tumbo-Oeri, A. G., and Kwendo, J. (1982). *Am. J. Reprod. Immunol. 2*:165–166.
Tung, K. S. K., Cooke, W. D., McCarty, T. A., and Robitaille, P. (1976). *Clin. Exp. Immunol. 25*:73–79.
Tung, S. K., Teuscher, C., and Meng, A. (1981). *Immunol. Rev.* *55*:217–255.
Tzartos, S. K. (1979). *J. Reprod. Fertil. 55*:447–455.
Voisin, G. A., and Toullet, F. (1968). *Ann. Inst. Pasteur 114*:727.
Weisz-Carrington, P., Roux, M., McWilliams, M., Phillips-Quagliata, J., and Lamm, M. (1979). *J. Immunol. 123*:1705.
Wheat, T. E., and Goldberg, E. (1975). *Development Biology*, Academic Press, New York, pp. 325–346.
Wheat, T. E., and Goldberg, E. (1977). In: (B. Boettcher, ed.), Harcourt, Brace, Jovanovich, Australia, pp. 221-227.
Wheat, T. E., and Goldberg, E. (1981). In: (D. H. Rich and E. Gross, eds.), Pierce Chemical Co., Rockford, Illinois, pp. 557–560.
Wheat, T. E., and Goldberg, E. (1983). *Med. REs. 7*:113–130.

Wheat, T. E., and Goldberg, E. (1986). Antigenic Domains of the Sperm Specific Lactate Dehydrogenase C_4 Isozyme. In preparation.

Wheat, T. E., Hintz, M., Goldberg, E., and Margoliash, E. (1977). *Differentiation* 9:37.

Wheat, T. E., Gonzales-Prevatt, Shelton, J. A., and Goldberg, E. (1986). Immune Response to Synthetic Antigen Domains of the Sperm Specific Lactate Dehydrogenase C_4 Isozyme. In preparation.

4

Autoimmune Responses to Testicular Antigens in Male Infertility

FRANCO DONDERO

University of Rome
Rome, Italy

Even though the immune response to sperm antigens was demonstrated independently by Metchnikoff (1) and by Landsteiner (2) as early as 1899, it was only at the beginning of the 1950s that any systematic study of experimental allergic orchitis really began, with the work of Voisin et al. (3) and of Freund et al. (4) and with the observations of Rümke (5) and of Wilson (6), who really came to grips with the problem of autoimmune infertility in men. Now, more thorough diagnostic study and many case histories have allowed us to make some sense out of the problematic relationship between antisperm autoimmunization and infertility, even if there are still numerous and fundamental problems to solve (7-21).

The aim of this chapter is to point out the immunologic problems of infertile men and to discern if the antisperm autoimmune response should be considered (1) a mere epiphenomenon (2) an aggravating factor of a pathological situation already able to cause infertility, or (3) a pathogenetic factor.

A more detailed description of what can happen in experimental immunization can be found in Chapter 8; here, I will only report the data necessary for clinical purposes.

Classic experimental allergic orchitis (EAO) after sensitization with testicular homogenate plus complete Freund's adjuvant histologically determines vacuolation and sloughing of germinal epithelium and diffuse or perivascular infiltrates of monocytes, lymphocytes, and plasma cells; along the basement membrane and in the lumen of efferent ducts of the epididymis and vas deferens, foci of polymorphonuclear leukocytes can be observed. Differences in the temporal evolution of the histological lesions (22–24) are probably due to (1) the diversity in the time and the duration of the period of observation; (2) the process of immunization, and, above all, (3) the antigen employed. In fact, using three different highly purified spermatozoal autoantigens, it has been observed in the guinea pig that the histological lesions, even though indistinguishable at their mature stage from one antigen to another, show differences at an early examination (25).

After immunization, humoral and cell-mediated immune responses can be demonstrated and the expression of the immune response may vary according to the antigens employed for the immunization. The passive transfer of EAO by immune sera is demonstrated even though there is no strict correlation between antisperm antibodies and histological lesions. Also in this case, different results are obtained by using antisera against different nemaspermic antigens (26). Passive EAO may be transferred by local injection of lymphnode cells from immunized guinea pigs or peritoneal cells and purified T lymphocytes from peritoneal exudate (27–29).

For clinical purposes I would like to point out that experimental endogenous sensitization can be obtained by means of testicular thermal injury (30), trauma (9), and cryoimmunization (31).

EAO is not induced by using a homogenate of immature testis as antigen, and sensitization in the postnatal period does not inhibit further spermatogenesis (32). This emphasizes the importance of the ontogenetic appearance of autoantigens in the germinal epithelium. In the guinea pig, autoantigens are not present in diploid germinal cells (spermatogonia and spermatocytes I) but appear in haploid germinal cells (spermatocytes II and spermatids) (33). In the mouse, the temporal appearance of plasma membrane antigens has been demonstrated at late meiotic prophase, coincident with the production of pachytene primary spermatocytes (34).

An antiserum was obtained in rabbits by using as antigen a preparation rich in seminiferous tubule basement membrane from adult rat testis; no cross-reactions were detected with other fractions extracted from the germinal cells (35). When the rats were injected intravenously or under the tunica albuginea with rabbit antiserum against seminiferous tubule basement membrane, multifocal damage of the testis was obtained and a linear deposit of rabbit gammaglobulins was detected by immunohistochemical techniques along the basement membrane of the seminiferous tubules and vessels (36).

It has been noted that the epididymis, although of fundamental importance in the functional maturation of spermatozoa, also plays an important part in the modulation of the immune response against sperm antigens. Particularly noticeable was the presence of lymphocytes and macrophages in the human, both of which have been known to migrate in the interstitial tissue in cases of obstructive azoospermia (37,38).

Many experts have dedicated themselves to a study of the antigenetic structure of the human spermatozoa by means of the indirect immunofluorescence technique (39–41). Thanks to technical progress, significant steps have been made, thus paving the way for such attempts as the isolation and purification of the various surface and internal antigens.

At present, some extremely important, if disputable, observations have been made. These may be of particular use in our clinical studies.

1. Of the blood group antigens (ABO, Rh, MNS, Kell, Duffy, and P), none can be safely said to be linked with immunologic infertility (42–44).
2. The significance of HLA antigens; as far as infertility is concerned, is a cause of some dispute (45–47).

3. The effect of H-Y antigens on fertility has not yet been demonstrated (48).
4. Nuclear proteins are present in the nucleus of the spermatozoa, and, in common with other subsurface antigens present in the acrosome, equatorial segment, postnuclear area, and tail, may be observed by immunofluorescence (39–41,49).
5. Sperm-specific enzymes, such as acrosin (in the acrosome and in the equatorial segment), hyaluronidase (in the acrosome), DNA polymerase (in the nucleus area and in the seminal plasma), and, in particular, the LDH-X enzyme, seem to be of special interest for possible immunologic fertility control (50–52).
6. Membrane antigens are of fundamental importance given that (1) there is an increased incidence of specific antibodies in so-called unexplained infertility (2) the antigens are accessible for antibodies, and (3) specific antibodies can assume a pathogenetic significance for immune infertility (53).
7. Coating antigens are in the seminal plasma and coat the spermatozoa during their transit along the genital tract. The most well known are the isoenzymes of prostatic acid phosphatase and the lactoferrin of vesicular origin. These may act as a defense mechanism during the transit of spermatozoa along the female genital tract, in order to prevent an isoimmune antisperm reaction (54,55). On the other hand, the spermatozoa may be "innocent victims" of an Ag-Ab reaction caused by disease in the adnexal glands.

EAO was also demonstrated in men (56). Selected volunteer patients with prostatic carcinoma showed autologous or homologous sensitization after intradermal injection of testicular homogenate mixed with complete Freund's adjuvant. Histologically, a patchy lesion consisting of congestion, serous edema, and sloughing of germinal cells was observed. Transient low-titer circulating antibodies and a positive delayed-type skin test appeared between 2 and 3 weeks after sensitization. The immunofluorescence technique, using the patients' own sera and testis sections, showed a positive reaction in the germinal cells, presumably spermatids and spermatozoa, and sometimes in the wall of some seminiferous tubules.

Also, vasectomy can be considered, at least in theory, an experimental model of antisperm autoimmunization following a sudden and massive reabsorption of sperm antigens. Recently, a few excellent reviews reported data concerning the relationships between vasectomy and autoimmunity to sperm antigens (57-61). I would like only to emphasize that circulating antisperm antibodies, immune complexes with sperm antigens, and cell-mediated response to sperm antigens have been detected in men, too (see Chap. 5).

The question we can ask ourselves at this moment is, is there also a possibility of an autoimmune orchitis responsible for infertility in human spontaneous pathology?

In 22% of patients with nonobstructive azoospermia, the presence of immunoglobulin deposits was observed, by means of direct immunofluorescence on ultrathin sections of testis from biopsy fragments, with well-differentiated patterns (62-64); positivity that was

1. Localized in the interstitial space
2. Limited to the tubular wall
3. Limited to the germinal epithelium (65)
4. Located simultaneously at tubular wall and germinal epithelial levels.

Histological findings showed maturational arrest, germinal aplasia, and sclerohyalinosis, but no definite relationship could be detected between histology and immunofluorescence patterns. These different patterns, while separately seem to reproduce the various patterns that collectively characterize EAO, may be due to (1) the differences in the inciting antigens, (2) the time of onset and duration of the immune stimulation, (3) the time of observation, correlated with the clinical problem of infertility, and (4) the possible concomitant diseases, both systemic and of the genitourinary tract.

IgG and IgA in the tubular wall and in the cells that sloughed into the tubules were detected in five cases of azoospermia (66). A group of nine patients who had obstructive azoospermia that followed bilateral epididymoorchitis underwent a testicular biopsy. Of these nine cases, six exhibited variable degrees of maturational arrest, mainly at the spermatid stage; disorganization, sloughing of immature cells, and Sertoli cell vacuolization were also found in some speciments. In five cases the germinal cells contained very high concentrations of IgG, and all the control sections for these specimens showed that the stain was specific for immunoglobulins (67). IgG and complement deposits have also been observed in the tubular wall and germinal epithelium in 15 of 20 cases with oligospermia (68).

In 50 cases of male infertility, an immunohistological study of testicular biopsies was carried out. In 10 of the 50 biopsies, immune deposits were observed in various locations. In 6 cases, Ig was discovered in the tubular wall; irregular deposits on both sides of the tunica propria, as well as thin linear deposits on the internal side, were seen. In 1 case all the heads of the spermatozoa were coated with IgM; in another case IgG was found on all germinal cells. In 4 cases IgG and complement were observed under the endothelium of blood vessels, and in 2 cases immune deposits were noted on the Leydig cells (69).

Cryostat-cut sections of biopsies from 212 men of infertile couples were treated with fluorescein-conjugated antibodies to demonstrate tissue-bound IgG, IgA, IgM, IgD, C3, and C4. In 27 cases (12.7%), autoantibodies and/or complement could be detected; in most cases IgG were found bound to walls of seminiferous tubules. In 3 cases, antibodies or complement was found in germinal cells; in 1 case each IgA immunofluorescence was found in spermatids or Leydig cells (70).

Testicular and spermatozoal autoantibodies have been found in chronic alcoholic males with gonadal failure. The hypothesis is that the alcohol produces a primary testicular metabolic and possible cytotoxic injury; therefore, testicular antigens leak from the testes, cross the testicular blood barrier, and induce autoantibody formation (71).

Antibodies reacting with a cytoplasmic component of Sertoli cells were detected in the serum of a 20-year-old man with hypogonadism and azoospermia; testicular biopsy showed Leydig cell hypoplasia and maturational arrest of the germinal epithelium but apparently normal Sertoli cells (72). Similar antibodies have also been found in one case of Sjögren's syndrome (72), in two patients with Addison's disease, in three infertile patients, and in one case of amenorrhea (73). Circulating antibodies directed against testicular basement membranes and germinal cells were demonstrated in an 81-year-old man with multiple primary endocrine gland deficiencies involving thyroid, adrenals, stomach (pernicious anemia), and testes; testicular biopsy revealed focal destruction of seminiferous tubules and interstitial fibrosis (74).

A group of 68 patients with no family history of autoimmune diseases, who had monolateral spermatic cord torsion within the previous 7 years, were examined using frozen sections of human testis. Of these, 9 patients (13.2%) were positive for organ-specific antitestis autoantibodies, 6 patients were positive for autoantibodies against Leydig cells, and another 3 patients were positive for antibodies against germ line cells (75).

Immunofluorescence studies of testicular biopsies were carried out in prepubertal boys and adult males with monolateral or bilateral cryptorchidism. The patterns were negative or nonspecific in all the testicular biopsies, of both the retained and scrotal testes (76).

In summary, these results have led me to the conclusion that an autoimmune orchitis is also possible in spontaneous human pathology. However, the actual clinical frequency of such cases is not yet clear, and we still have to define the precise mechanism able to trigger the autoimmune response.

As far as concerns humoral antisperm immunity, it is now well established that men can produce antibodies against spermatozoa and that these antibodies can negatively interfere with reproduction. Ample information can be found on this subject in a number of excellent reviews (12,13,15,16,20,77). The majority of work has been based on techniques able to detect antibodies against the surface antigens [see reviews (17,78,79) and Chap. 5].

Research has been done with a wide cross section of men of various ages from various countries. From these findings, we can note that 9–10% of men from infertile couples showed positive results for antisperm antibodies compared with 1% in a fertile population (17,80–83).

In cases of comparison between groups, the age of the subjects should always be borne in mind. In fact, using the classic gelatin agglutination test (84) in the group selected without regard to fertility, the incidence of spermagglutinin-positive sera generally increases with age (80). With the capillary tube agglutination test (85), it has been confirmed that, in controls, positive results increase with age, but the percentage of positivity remains stable in infertile patients aged between 20 and 50 years; in the former cases, the positive tests were attributed to increasing sperm reabsorption due to such factors as trauma, inflammatory processes (even though clinically silent), hypertrophy of the prostate, and metabolic disorders, together with the physiologic reduction of the mechanism responsible for the regulation of the autoimmune response (86). A different percentage of positivity between controls and infertile subjects is also observed in seminal plasma.

In general, IgG and IgA are always present in seminal plasma (87–90) in normal men and infertile patients, whereas several investigators did not find IgM. For example, in 168 men of infertile couples, IgM as seen in only 61 (36.3%) (89); in 90 normal control subjects, IgM as absent in 58 cases, present in trace amounts in 23, and ranged between 0.7 and 3.3 mg per 100 ml in 9 cases (90).

By means of the split ejaculated technique to measure the concentration of IgG and IgA, along with albumin, lactoferrin, acid phosphatase, and fructose, it was possible in 1974 to obtain data supporting evidence of the prostatic filtration of serum Ig, but also suggesting the possibility of production by the local immunnocompetent system (88). Further information in this field has been obtained, confirming both the prostatic filtration of serum Ig and IgA and the production of Ig by the local immune system (52).

Although an increase in seminal Ig concentration has not been reported in a study of patients with sperm antibodies (91), in another report the results of Ig tests in 127 sterile patients presenting positive antisperm antibodies showed a statistically significant increase ($P \leqslant 0.001$) for both IgG and IgA in seminal plasma (90).

By using a specific method the enzyme-linked immunosorbent assay (ELISA) recently developed for the determination of the 11S IgA, it has been revealed that antisperm antibodies present in the seminal plasma of infertile patients are of the IgA type (92). A total of 100 samples of semen showing azoospermia, oligozoospermia, or self-agglutination of spermatozoa were examined for evidence of autoimmune disorders. In abnormal samples, secretory IgA (sIgA), IgA, C3, and C4 were present in a greater proportion than in normal samples; IgA content was markedly increased and IgG level slightly increased (93). The presence of sIgA and free secretory piece had already been revealed by means of radial immunodiffusion and the antiglobulin test (94,95) and confirmed employing the immunoprecipitating technique (96). Between 60 and 90% of the IgA present in the seminal plasma is of the secretory type (97); assay of secretory piece revealed an increase parallel to that of total IgA in infertile patients with antisperm antibodies (90).

Besides the difference in the percentage of positivity between controls and infertile subjects, a difference in titers was also observed; this is almost always higher in the latter group. An attempt was made to formulate a clinically significant titer corresponding to 1:32 in the blood serum and to 1:16 in the seminal plasma. This concept has been partially contested, given that, although it has been agreed "the higher the titer the greater the problem," the presence of antisperm antibodies, albeit of a lower titer, is still "of some significance for infertility" (98).

Spermagglutinins can be simultaneously found in both blood serum and seminal plasma or in only one of the two samples. Normally, the titer is higher in the serum than in semen; however, it is possible to observe a higher titer in semen and, even if unlikely, tests for spermagglutinins may be positive only in the seminal plasma.

Sperm-immobilizing and sperm-cytotoxic antibodies are practically absent in control subjects under 40 years of age; the percent positivity therefore rises with increasing age. In contrast to spermagglutinins, in our experience the seminal titer is often the same and in some instances higher than in blood serum.

By means of the immunofluorescence technique, subsurface and internal antigens of the spermatozoa can be studied (39-49). Using regular sperm smears it is possible to reveal antigens in the (1) acrosome (Ac 1 and Ac 2), (2) equatorial region (3) postacrosomal region, (4) main piece of tail and (5) tip of tail. Human spermatozoa pretreated with dithiothreitol and trypsin show two other antigens in the (1) nucleus (protamine) and (2) midpiece of the tail. The immunofluorescence technique is highly useful for experimental purposes but, owing to the (1) possible cross-reaction with bacterial antigens, (2) nonspecific binding of Ig to the sperm membrane, and (3) high percentage of positivity in both prepubertal subjects and fertile control group, cannot effectively be used for clinical purposes (78,79).

To discover antibodies attached to the spermatozoa in the semen, even though specific spermagglutination areas are not present, a very simple and responsive technique is the mixed erythrocyte-spermatozoa antiglobulin reaction test (MAR test) (99,100). This test is beginning to be used in many laboratories and, in addition, is becoming a new standard parameter in routine seminal analysis (101).

Case histories therefore confirm what the experimental data of the antisperm autoimmunization have already shown. Yet there are still those patients in whom the autoimmune response itself represents the only pathological data available, thus assuming a vital role in infertility, independently of any previous illness that might have triggered an immune responses. In these cases we can attribute the infertility to antisperm antibodies. A double check is given by the results gained from therapy aimed exclusively at immune suppression. The various protocols, such as the intermittent high-dose corticosteroid medication method, the continuous low-dose corticosteroid method, and pharmacologically induced azoospermia followed by the administration of corticosteroids, although having met with various degrees of success, are still able to bring about disappearance or significant decrease in antisperm antibodies and to restore fertility (102–108).

In other cases, however, the antisperm autoimmune reaction seems to be a factor aggravating a pathologic situation already able to cause sterility. There are two clinical conclusions that may be drawn from this, which in my opinion are of fundamental importance: (1) in cases of infertility with antisperm antibodies, it is first necessary to deal therapeutically with the basic pathology that has elicited the autoimmune response; and (2) strict control must be kept on the autoimmune response, given that the autoimmunization may well remain and become the primary cause of infertility even after the original illness has completely disappeared—either spontaneously or through therapy.

Normally, there is immunologic unresponsiveness to sperm antigens in spite of their late ontogenetic appearance. In genetically predisposed subjects, a pathologic situation inducing an increased reabsorption of sperm antigens may break this negative immunoregolatory response and lead to the synthesis of antisperm autoantibodies. In point of fact, it has long been noticed that spermagglutinins are present to a high degree in cases of obstructive azoospermia (109,110).

Therapeutically, it has been observed that the surgical removal of an epididymial cyst and of an epididymis with tuberculous inflammation led to the disappearance of spermagglutinins (111). Moreover, after unilateral orchidectomy in a patient with secondary unilateral testicular atrophy and dysspermia, sperm-cytotoxic antibodies in both blood serum and seminal plasma gradually disappeared and the seminal parameters returned to normal (112). More recently, the presence of serum antisperm antibodies has been reported in 26 of 32 (81%) subfertile males with sperm in the ejaculate and unilateral testicular obstruction (113). Serum antisperm antibodies were successively measured in 168 azoospermic males with normal FSH, and the site of obstruction was investigated by means of exploratory scrototomy. Acquired blocks of cauda epididymis (34 cases) and vas (23 cases) were significantly more commonly associated with serum spermagglutinins than congenital bilateral absence of vas (29 cases) or blocks of the caput epididymis. A sperm count of 10 million per milliliter or more was produced in 23 cases after surgical reconstruction, and 11 pregnancies were obtained. Among patients with spermatozoa in the ejaculate after surgery, spermagglutinins were found significantly less often in those whose partners became pregnant compared with those who failed to produce pregnancy (114).

Sperm antibodies were prominent in infertile subjects who had been operated on for inguinal hernia (18). On the contrary, no significant incidence of antisperm antibodies, either in blood serum or in seminal plasma, was observed in 20 infertile subjects with previous cryptorchidism (18) and in 18 monolateral and 6 bilateral adult cryptorchidic males (76).

Also, infective processes in the genital tract could theoretically favor the synthesis of antisperm antibodies. In fact, sperm antigens may extravasate and stimulate the local and/or systemic immunocompetent system, eliciting antisperm antibody production. Even as early as 1968, reports were published suggesting the hypothesis that both genital infections and antisperm antibodies are not only interrelated but are also associated with infertility (115). In the same year, a higher incidence of prostatitis was observed in men with spermagglutinins than in a control group (116). The observation of a 28% positivity for antisperm antibodies in infertile men was attributed to the high incidence of genital tract infections and of urinary schistosomiasis in the cases studied (117). This higher incidence of antisperm antibodies in infertile patients with genital tract infection than in a control group was confirmed by using an enzyme-linked immunosorbent assay (118). Finally, in both blood serum and seminal plasma tests for spermagglutinins, sperm-immobilizing and sperm-cytotoxic antibodies (positivity to at least one test, with a titer of at least 1:4, in at least one of the two biologic samples) were positive in 10.2% of cases in randomly selected infertile patients and in 37.5% of cases in infertile patients with positive sperm culture (119).

In this particular form of infertility with antisperm antibodies, the therapeutic result turned out to be interesting. In 1977, it was observed that in eight cases the treatment of prostatitis was followed by a reduction of the antibody titers, followed in five cases by the pregnancy of the partner (120). Successive experiences confirmed that, in some patients who had recovered from their genital tract infection, tests for antisperm antibodies become negative and the seminal parameters, if pathologic, return to normal (119).

In females, after incubating an antigen preparation from group A streptococci with sera with positive and negative antispermatozoal activity, in most cases a reduction in spermagglutination titers is observed (121). In males, the absorption of positive serum and/or seminal plasma with the streptococcus B α-hemolytic type isolated in the same patient, can lead in some cases to a marked reduction in antibody titers (119).

On the basis of a very high percentage of positivity in tests for antisperm antibodies in patients with genital tract infection and from therapeutic results, the following hypotheses have been advanced: (1) a cross-reaction may exist between sperm antigens and bacterial antigens; (2) bacterial infections may cause a change in the physiological mechanism of enzymatic degradation of sperm antigens in the male genital tract and activation of the immune competent system; this may cause antisperm autoimmunization. Obviously, if the immune response remains even after therapeutic recovery from the infection, antisperm antibodies may become the principle reason for infertility.

Spermagglutinins were observed in 2 of 28 cases with acute mumps orchitis and in 3 of 7 cases with chronic mumps orchitis; indirect immunofluorescence tests on testis biopsies in 5 cases showed positivity at the level of the head and of the perinuclear area of spermatids (122).

In experimental animals, an autoimmune response upon mechanical pressure of the testis is reported (9). In clinical pathology, a high incidence of antisperm antibodies in infertile patients who had suffered anamnestic traumas of the testis has been reported (18,123), whereas an investigation of victims of genital torture did not show any conclusive relationship between testicular trauma and increased production of spermagglutinins (124).

Finally, I would like to mention the possibility of an antisperm immune reaction in homosexuals. Actually, investigations of blood samples obtained from 18 sexually active male homosexuals suggest that intake of spermatozoa, via the alimentary canal, may lead to the development of a humoral immune response to spermatozoa (125). A subsequent investigation of 30 asymptomatic, monogamously homosexual males has also suggested that chronic, repeated exposure to sperm during anal intercourse results in a high frequency of allogeneic immunization and may play a role in the development of acquired immune dysregulation among homosexual males (126).

So far we have seen that numerous factors can trigger an antisperm immune reaction, and this autoimmune state may interfere with reproductive success. What exactly are the possible mechanisms involved in antisperm antibody-mediated infertility?

First, the autoimmune reaction may affect spermatogenesis, thus inhibiting sperm production. Experimental and clinical reports confirm this possibility; nevertheless, in human spontaneous pathology, a strict correlation between antisperm antibodies and lesions of germinal epithelium seems limited to particular conditions and the autoimmune response seems more often than not the consequence rather than the cause of testicular alteration (127 128).

Second, the antisperm antibodies may impair the normal function of the ejaculated spermatozoa. If spermagglutinins are present, seminal fluid only rarely displays oligozoospermia and sperm morphology does not show an increase in abnormal forms, whereas a decrease in progressive motility is almost always present.

The most characteristic finding is the presence of spermagglutination areas. Three types of agglutination may be observed: (1) head-to-head, (2) tail-to-tail, (3) and head-to-tail, with the following features.

1. The spermatozoa are actually agglutinated among themselves, not only crowded around sloughing cells or leukocytes.
2. The agglutinated spermatozoa shake themselves, sometimes very vigorously, and the surrounding spermatozoa maintain progressive and/or nonprogressive motility.
3. During microscopic observation, the spermagglutination areas tend to enlarge and new areas may be observed.

To explain why many spermatozoa are not agglutinated, it has been hypothesized that (1) corresponding surface antigens are not present on all spermatozoa, or are expressed with a variable quantitative degree; (2) nonagglutinating antibodies block the antigenic sites; (3) agglutination may only occur under optimal circunstances of collision (129); and (4) agglutination comes from antibody titer and avidity.

It is interesting that when treatment successfully solves the autoimmune process with the disappearance of spermagglutinins, the spermagglutination areas disappear and motility returns to normal (130).

If sperm-immobilizing antibodies are present, almost 100% of patients show hypomotility and there is a close correlation between the immobilizing titer in the seminal plasma and degree of hypomotility. Sperm-cytotoxic antibodies induce dysspermia with oligozoospermia, hypomotility, and teratozoospermia.

Spermatozoa not agglutinated or immobilized are inhibited in their migration through the female genital tract. In fact, an early report (1954) observed that the spermatozoa of two men with antisperm antibodies did not penetrate the cervical mucus (6). Since then, a statistically significant negative correlation between the spermagglutinating titer in the serum and the degree of sperm penetration of cervical mucus has been demonstrated (131), and an inverse correlation was reported between postcoital test and sperm antibody titer in the male partner (132). Nevertheless, in other reports, no correlation could be observed between postcoital tests and sperm migration tests and antisperm antibodies (133, 134).

In 1976, using a sperm-cervical mucus contact test, it was observed that in ejaculates with partial spermagglutination caused by autoimmunization, the progressively moving spermatozoa show a locally shaking movement (the so-called shaking phenomenon) when they come into contact with cervical mucus and are not able to go on (135). It was hypothesized that the shaking phenomenon is caused by the adherence by the Fc portion of the antisperm antibodies coating the spermatozoa to the glycoprotein micelles in the cervical mucus (136). This shaking phenomenon can be induced by the pretreatment of spermatozoa with sera containing antisperm antibodies (137); in addition, sera with spermagglutinins or the $F(ab)_2$ fragments of IgG obtained from the same sera inhibit sperm migration through cervical mucus in capillary tubes (138).

Recently it has been confirmed that (1) antisperm antibodies can reduce sperm penetration of cervical mucus; (2) sperm motility in the postcoital test is correlated positively with sperm motility in the semen and inversely with sperm-cytotoxic antibodies in the serum and seminal plasma; (3) in couples with an abnormal postcoital test, when male partners exhibited autoimmunity to spermatozoa revealed by means of an immunobead-binding test, the degree of impairment of sperm penetration in cervical mucus is correlated with the proportion of spermatozoa in the ejaculate exhibiting surface-bound immunoglobulins (139–141).

Even if spermatozoa manage to get through the cervical barrier, antibodies binding to antigens on the cell surface may cause phagocytosis of the spermatozoa through opsonic (Fc) immune (C3) adherence, or nonphagocytic extracellular cytotoxicity by killer cells with receptors for Ig Fc.

Another possibility is the inhibition of sperm attachment to and penetration of eggs. In fact, sperm-specific antibodies in the acrosomal region inhibit the binding of human sperm to the human zona pellucida (142). Moreover, antisperm antibodies impair the ability of human spermatozoa to penetrate zone-free hamster eggs (143); this effect is due to immunoglobulins (144). Spermatozoa were incubated with sera that contained IgG, IgA, or IgM directed primarily against the sperm heads, in the presence or absence of complement; IgG and IgM diminished the percentage of eggs penetrated and the number of penetrating sperm per eggs but IgA, which did not fix the first component of complement, did not alter the ability of human sperm to penetrate hamster eggs (145). One of the latest reports is of antibodies to human spermatozoa impeding sperm penetration of hamster eggs. Spermatozoa were of donors with proven fertility and with at lest 50% penetration in the sperm penetration assay. When spermatozoa were exposed to antisperm antibodies, 6 samples totally blocked and another 10 significantly reduced sperm penetration, whereas only 2 samples yielded results comparable with those of controls. The IgG fraction caused a reduction similar to that of whole serum (139).

Finally, there is the possibility of antisperm interference with postfertilization fertility. In women with sperm antibodies, a high incidence of spontaneous abortion in subsequent pregnancies has been reported (146). No similar reports exist for men, but we have found in our experience, which of course needs confirmation, that women who have been fertilized by partners with antisperm antibodies show a high incidence of spontaneous abortion.

Since both humoral and cell-mediated immunity are involved in experimental autoimmune orchitis, it should follow that cellular immunity to sperm may play an important role in human infertility; nonetheless, few reports have as yet appeared in print and even these are sometimes in disagreement.

In 1970, blastoid transformation of lymphocytes was carried out in 31 normal adult males and in 126 patients with nonobstructive azoospermia or severe oligozoospermia, using normal semen homogenate as antigen. The test was negative in the control group, whereas blastoid transformation was observed in 16.6% of patients (147).

Lymphocyte incorporation of tritiated thymidine, using as antigen serial 10-fold dilutions of semen with phosphate-buffered saline, was carried out in 10 male subjects with demonstrated fertility within the preceding 2 years and in 6 patients with antisperm antibodies. Stimulation of the uptake by the cells in culture with semen antigen was observed in 3 of 6 patients with antisperm antibodies , but not in the control group (148).

The macrophage migration inhibition test using as antigen rat testis extract revealed a cell-mediated antisperm immunity in 32% of 22 oligozoospermic infertile patients and in only 6% of 18 healthy men (149).

The reactivity of lymphocytes from men of infertile couples (63 cases) in a lymphocyte transformation test was studied following the application of various sperm antigens (150). The reactivity was at least three times as high in the control culture:

1. In 14% after stimulation with autologous spermatozoa
2. In 11% after stimulation with allogeneic pooled spermatozoa
3. In 24% after stimulation with allogeneic spermatozoa from a single subject

The results of the lymphocyte transformation test (LTT) using washed autologous spermatozoa as antigen were analyzed in relation to sperm count, occurrence of sperm antibodies, and fertile status of the couple. Of men with oligozoospermia, 71% yielded a positive LTT, compared with 30% of men with normozoospermia. All 10 men with high titers of spermagglutinins revealed a positive reaction in the LTT; in contrast, humoral immunity (as demonstrated by immunofluorescence) was not correlated with the LTT response. LTT showed, at least in this series, little clinical significance, because men from infertile couples had negative tests, whereas 1 had a strongly positive reaction of the 5 men who appeared to be fertile during the observation period, (151).

The Clausen test of leukocyte migration inhibition on agarose, using as antigen washed spermatozoa obtained from normal healthy donors, was studied in donors with proven fertility and normal sperm count (18 subjects), in donors with oligozoospermia but proven fertility (11 subjects), and in individuals with selected forms of male infertility (210 patients) (152). The test was always negative in the control groups. A positive response was observed by these authors in

1. Unilateral or bilateral cryptorchidism, 48.5
2. Germinal epithelial disorders, 53.2%
3. Genital tract infections, 38.9%
4. Unilateral left varicocele, 31.2%
5. Idiopathic oligozoospermia, 33.3%

Finally, other investigators have utilized the leukocyte migration inhbition test (LMT), using as antigen a semipurified spermatozoal antigen (153), washed spermatozoa, and seminal plasma. Using washed pooled spermatozoa from normal donors, a very high percentage of positivity to LMT was observed but without a significant difference between the control group and infertile patients (154). It was stressed that spermatozoa are capable, on a dose-dependent basis, of both inhibiting and stimulating normal lymphocyte DNA synthesis, as well as suppressing mitogen-induced responses (155). Using autologous or allogeneic seminal plasma, LMT was positive in all cases, control group and infertile patients. Dialysis of seminal plasma against phosphate-buffered saline did not reduce the inhibiting capacity of leukocyte migration; the seminal plasma of patients with agenesis or obstruction of vas deferens or postvasectomy subjects inhibited leukocyte migration in the same way (154). Actually, a high-molecular-weight fraction prepared from human seminal plasma by gel filtration chromatography can suppress the in vitro lymphocyte activation (156).

Conversely, significantly different results were obtained using a semipurified sperm antigen (157). LMT was constantly negative in the 15 fertile subjects before vasectomy and positive in only 1 of the 25 normal volunteers, but only at the highest concentration of antigen. Infertile patients were incidentally selected because it was expected theoretically that they would present an autoimmune antisperm reaction. All patients were also tested for humoral antisperm immunity (sperm agglutinins and sperm-immobilizing and sperm-cytotoxic antibodies). The results were as follows.

1. LMT was positive in 3 of 16 patients with agenesis or obstruction of vas deferens; in only 2 cases were spermagglutinins detected, with negativity of LMT (all patients presented azoospermia).
2. LMT was positive in 6 of 23 cases with previous orchitis; in only 2 of 6 cases with positive LMT were antibodies detected. Normal seminal parameters were seen in a LMT-positive patients, whereas 2 presented with azoospermia.
3. LMT was positive in 3 of 11 cases with previous testicular injury, without antisperm antibodies. A single LMT-positive patients had normal semen, whereas 2 presented with teratozoospermia or hypomotility.
4. LMT was positive in 6 of 7 cases with previous torsion of the spermatic cord, and antisperm antibodies were observed in 3 of 6 patients with positive LMT. Normal semen was seen in 2 LMT-positive patients, 1 showed oligozoospermia, and 3 were azoospermic.
5. LMT was positive in 3 of 10 patients who remained infertile after successful immune therapy for spermagglutinins (104). LMT positive and LMT negative patients did not show diference in seminal parameters.
6. LMT was positive in 4 of 12 patients with so-called idiopathic infertility but with antisperm antibodies.

Owing to the lack of correlation between humoral and cell-mediated antisperm immunity, it has been hypothesized that the difference in response to the two tests could be attributed to (1) A difference in the antigen employed for the techniques (2) a difference in the mechanism of autoimmunization (3) evolution of the autoimmune disease.

In conclusion, in certain forms of male infertility, not only experimental data but also clinical observations seem to indicate that cell-mediated antisperm immunity can play an important role. Still, it is not yet possible to ascertain if this is of pathogenetic importance or whether it represents a simple, yet significant, marker of a condition that might by itself be responsible for infertility.

As a final point, I would like to emphasize that the specialist faced with solving this problem of infertility should always bear in mind the possibility of an autoimmune antisperm reaction that can prove an important factor in human infertility. It is only by identifying and treating the immune component that we can help the infertile patient succeed in fertilizing his partner.

REFERENCES

1. E. Metchnikoff, *Ann. Inst. Pasteur 13*:737 (1899).
2. K. Landsteiner, *Abt. Bakt. 25*:546 (1899).
3. G. A. Voisin, A. Delaunay, and M. Barber, *Ann. Inst. Pasteur 81*:48 (1951).
4. J. Freund, M. M. Lipton, and G. E. Thompson, *J. Exp. Med. 97*:711 (1953).
5. P. Rümke, *Vox Sang. 4*:135 (1954).
6. L. Wilson, *Proc. Soc. Exp. Biol. Med. 85*:652 (1954).
7. T. S. Li, *Obstet. Gynecol. 44*:607 (1974).
8. S. Shulman, *Reproduction and Antibody Response*, CRC Press, Boca Raton, Florida, 1975.
9. R. E. Mancini, *Immunologic Aspects of Testicular Function*, Springer-Verlag, New York, 1976.
10. J. S. Scott and W. R. Jones, *Immunology of Human Reproduction*, Academic Press and Grune & Stratton, New York, 1976.
11. B. Boettcher, *Immunological Influence of Human Fertility*, Academic Press, New York, 1977.
12. P. Rümke and A. Hekman, *Clin. Obstet. Gynecol. 20*:691 (1977).
13. A. E. Beer and W. B. Neaves, *Fertil. Steril. 29*:3 (1978).
14. J. Cohen and W. F. Hendry, *Spermatozoa Antibodies and Infertility*, Blackwell Scientific, Oxford, 1978.

15. D. M. Mumford, *Invest. Urol. 16*:255 (1979).
16. A. C. Menge, in *Immunological Aspects of Infertility and Fertility Regulation* (D. S. Dhindsa and G. F. B. Schumacher, eds.), Elsevier/North-Holland, Amsterdam, 1980, p. 205.
17. S. Shulman, in *Manual of Clinical Immunology* (N. R. Rose and H. Friedman, eds.), Waverly Press, Baltimore, 1980, p.207.
18. M. De Almeida, A. Soumah, B. Ducot, and P. Jouannet, in *Facteurs de la Fertilité Humaine* (A. Spira and P. Jouannet, eds.) INSERM, Paris, 1981, p. 141.
19. N. Gleicher, *Reproductive Immunology*, Alan R. Liss, New York, 1981.
20. S. Mathur, E. R. Baker, H. O. Williamson, F. C. Derrick, K. J. Teague, and H. H. Fudenberg, *Fertil. Steril. 36*:486 (1981).
21. S. Shulman, F. Dondero, and M. Nicotra, *Immunological Factors in Human Reproduction*, Academic Press, New York, 1982.
22. K. S. K. Tung, E. R. Unanue, and F. J. Dixon, *Am. J. Pathol. 60*:313 (1970).
23. A. L. Kiezszenbaum and R. E. Mancini, *J. Reprod. Fertil. 33*:119 (1973).
24. K. S. K. Tung, in *Immunological Aspects of Infertility and Fertility Regulation* (D. S. Dhindsa and G. F. B. Schumacher, eds.), Elsevier/North-Holland, Amsterdam, 1980, p. 33.
25. G. A. Voisin and F. Toullet, in *Immunological in Obstetrics and Gynaecology* (A. Centaro and N. Carretti, eds.), Excerpta Medica, Amsterdam, 1974, p. 9.
26. F. Toullet and G. A. Voisin, *Clin. Exp. Immunol. 26*:549 (1976).
27. K. S. K. Tung, E. R. Unanue, and F. J. Dixon, *J. Immunol. 106*:1453 (1971).
28. G. L. Kantor and F. J. Dixon, *J. Immunol. 108*:329 (1972).
29. K. S. K. Tung and N. J. Alexander, in *The Testis* (A. D. Johnson and W. R. Gomex, eds.), Academic Press, New York, 1977, p. 491.
30. R. E. Mancini, in *Human Semen and Fertility Regulation in Men* (E. S. E. Hafex, ed.), C. V. Mosby, St. Louis, 1976, p. 287.

31. S. Shulman and E. Zappi, in *Immunology of Reproduction* (K. Bratanow, ed.), Bulgarian Academy of Sciences Press, Sofia, 1973, p. 75.
32. R. E. Mancini, in *Immunology in Obstetrics and Gynaecology* (A. Centaro and N. Carretti, eds.), Excerpta Medica, Amsterdam, 1974, p. 16.
33. I. Radu and G. A. Voisin, *Differentiation 3*:107 (1975).
34. C. F. Millette and A. R. Bellve, *J. Cell Biol. 74*:86 (1977).
35. L. Lustig, B. Denduchis, and R. E. Mancini, *Int. J. Fertil. 22*:16 (1977).
36. L. Lustig, B. Denduchis, N. N. Gonzales, and R. P. Puig, *Arch. Androl. 1*:333 (1978).
37. Y. F. Wang and A. F. Holstein, *Cell Tissue Res. 233*:517 (1983).
38. H. J. Sommer, *Urologe [Ausg. A] 22*:35 (1983).
39. K. B. Hansen and T. Hjort, *Clin. Exp. Immunol. 9*:21 (1971).
40. K. S. K. Tung, W. D. Cooke, T. A. Mc Carty, and P. Robitaille, *Clin. Exp. Immunol. 25*:73 (1976).
41. A. H. J. Kolk, T. Samuel, and P. Rümke, *Clin. Exp. Immunol.* 16:63 (1974).
42. R. G. Edwards, L. C. Ferguson, and R. R. A. Coombs, *J. Reprod. Fertil. 7*:153 (1964).
43. B. Boettcher and J. Kay, *Am. J. Obst. Gynecol. 100*:437 (1968).
44. H. Krieg, A. G. Gathof, P. Netter, and D. Hedrich, in *Immunology of Reproduction* (K. Bratanow, ed.), Bulgarian Academy of Sciences Press, Sofia, 1973, p. 537.
45. K. Halim and H. Festenstein, *Lancet 2*:1255 (1975).
46. R. Hofman, K. H. Ratz, A. Mattheus, and S. Wegener, *Zentralbl. Gynakol 100*:122 (1978).
47. H. Festenstein, K. Halim, and A. Anaiz-Villena, in *Spermatozoa Antibodies and Infertility* (J. Coen and W. F. Hendry, eds.), Blackwell Scientific, Oxford, 1978, p. 11.
48. S. Ohno, Y. Nagai, S. Ciccareses, and H. Iwata, *Recent Prog. Horm. Res. 35*:449 (1979).
49. T. Hjort and K. B. Hansen, *Clin. Exp. Immunol. 8*:9 (1971).
50. E. Goldberg, in *Immunological Approaches to Fertility Control* (E. Diczfalusy, ed.), Bogtrykkeriet Forum, Copenhagen, 1974, p. 202.

51. R. Wellerson, P. Wagstaff, and S. Asculai, *Int. J. Fertil. 19*:65 (1974).
52. B. Boettcher, in *Immunological Factors in Human Reproduction* (S. Shulman, F. Dondero, and M. Nicotra, eds.), Academic Press, New York, 1982, p. 163.
53. T. Hjort, in *Immunological Factors in Human Reproduction* (S. Shulman, F. Dondero, and M. Nicotra, eds.), Academic Press, New York, 1982, p. 77.
54. G. W. Barnes, L. M. Y. Lee, N. Kenny, and M. S. Barnes, *Immunology 35*:589 (1978).
55. L. Veselsky, *Arch. Androl. 7*:1 (1981).
56. R. E. Mancini, J. A. Andrada, D. Saraceni, A. E. Bachmann, J. C. Lavieri, and M. Nemirovsky, *J. Clin. Endocrinol. Metab. 25*:859 (1965).
57. I. H. Lepow and R. Crozier, *Vasectomy: Immunologic and Pathophysiologic Effects in Animals and Man*, Academic Press, New York, 1979.
58. N. J. Alexander and D. J. Anderson, *Fertil. Steril. 32*:253 (1979).
59. T. Samuel and N. R. Rose, *J. Clin. Lab. Immunol. 3*:77 (1980).
60. P. E. Bigazzi, in *Reproductive Immunology* (N. Gleicher, ed.), Alan R. Liss, New York, 1981, p. 461.
61. C. Teuscher, G. C. Wild, E. Johnson, and K. S. K. Tung, *Ric. Clin. Lab. 11*:313 (1981).
62. A. Isidori, F. Dondero, and D. Lombardo, *Experientia 26*:1375 (1970).
63. F. Dondero and A. Isidori, *Ann. Endocrinol.* (*Paris*) *33*:417 (1972).
64. A. Isidori, F. Dondero, and D. Lombardo, in *Immunology of Reproduction* (K. Bratanov, ed.), Bulgarian Academy of Sciences Press, Sofia, 1973, p. 94.
65. G. Le Lorier, J. Salat, and J. Rotman, *Gynecol. Obste. 69*:23 (1970).
66. W. Michalbiewicz, K. Mietkiewski, T. Rucji, and J. B. Warhol, *Folia Histochem. Cytochem.* (*Krakow*) *9*:277 (1971).
67. H. Abdel Aal, A. Abdel Hafiz, O. Kandil, and H. El Tonsy, *J. Reprod. Fertil. 47*:117 (1976).

68. B. S. Rabin, H. R. Nankin, and P. Troen, in *The Testis in Normal and Infertile Men* (P. Troen and H. R. Nankin, eds.), Raven Press, New York, 1977, p. 435.
69. M. Jadot-van de Casseye, G. de Bled, W. Gepts, and R. Schoysman, *Andrologia 12*:122 (1980).
70. H. Donat and J. Morenz, in *Immunology of Reproduction* (K. Bratanov, ed.), Bulgarian Academy of Sciences Press, Sofia, 1982, p. 104.
71. D. H. Van Thiel, J. S. Gavaler, W. I. Smith, and B. S. Rabin, *Clin. Exp. Immunol. 8*:311 (1977).
72. J. R. Wall, J. Stedronska, R. D. David, R. F. Harrison, D. Goriup, and M. Lessof, *Fertil. Steril. 26*:1035 (1975).
73. F. Sotsiu, G. F. Bottazzo, and D. Doniach, *Clin. Exp. Immunol. 39*:97 (1980).
74. G. G. Murthy, N. S. Peress, and S. A. Khan, *J. Clin. Endocrinol. Metab. 42*:637 (1976).
75. R. Zanchetta, I. Mastrogiacomo, P. Graziotti, C. Foresta, and C. Betterle, *Clin. Exp. Immunol. 55*:49 (1984).
76. A. Isidori, F. Dondero, and G. Spera, in *Cryptorchidism* (J. R. Bierich and A. Giarola, eds.), Academic Press, New York, 1979, p. 207.
77. S. Shulman, *Int. J. Fertil. 28*:61 (1983).
78. N. R. Rose, T. Hjort, P. Rümke, M. J. K. Harper, and O. E. Vyazov, *Clin. Exp. Immunol. 23*:175 (1976).
79. B. Boettcher, T. Hjort, P. Rümke, S. Shulman, and O. E. Vyazov, *Acta Pathol. Microbiol. Scand.* Suppl. 258 (1977).
80. B. Fjällbrant, in *Immunology in Obstetrics and Gynaecology* (A. Centaro and N. Carretti, eds.), Excerpta Medica, Amsterdam, 1974, p. 36.
81. T. Hjort and S. Husted, *Proc. Soc. Med. 68*:253 (1975).
82. W. F. Hendry, H. Morgan, and J. Stedronska, *Br. J. Urol. 49*:757, 1977.
83. F. Dondero, V. Bonifacio, and B. Schiavo, *Folia Endocrinol. 27*:650 (1974).
84. S. Kibrick, D. L. Belding, and B. Merril, *Fertil. Steril. 3*:430 (1952).
85. S. Shulman and A. Hekman, *Clin. Exp. Immunol. 9*:137 (1971).

86. F. Dondero, A. Radicioni, F. Mazzilli, P. Giovenco, A. Lenzi, and M. Cerasaro, *Proc. 4th Int. Forum of Andrology*, (A 022), Paris, 1986.
87. W. P. Herrmann, *Andrologia 1*:11 (1969).
88. P. Rümke, *Clin. Exp. Immunol. 17*:769 (1974).
89. H. Donat and S. Schiller, *Andrologia 15*:369 (1983).
90. F. Dondero, A. Radicioni, L. Gandini, and A. Lenzi, *Andrologia 16*:228 (1984).
91. J. Friberg, *Obstet. Gynecol. 136*:671 (1980).
92. S. S. Witkin, G. Zelikousky, R. A. Good, and N. K. Day, *Clin. Exp. Immunol. 3*:368 (1981).
93. H. Sullivan and W. L. G. Quinlivan, *Fertil. Steril. 34*: 465 (1980).
94. D. T. Uehling, *Fertil. Steril. 22*:769 (1971).
95. R. R. A. Coombs, P. Rümke, and R. G. Edwards, in *Immunology of Reproduction* (K. Bratanov, ed.), Bulgarian Academy of Sciences Press,Sofia, 1973, p. 354.
96. H. A. Soliman and H. Olesen, *Clin. Chim. Acta 69*:543 (1976).
97. T. Hjort, in *Immunological Influence on Human Fertility* (B. Boettcher, ed.), Academic Press, New York, 1977, p. 115.
98. S. Shulman, *Contraception-Fertilité Sexualité 10*:507 (1982).
99. R. R. A. Coombs, J. Marks, and D. Bedford, *Br. J. Haematol. 2*:84 (1956).
100. S. Jager, J. Kremer, and T. van Slochteren-Draaisma, *Int. J. Fertil. 23*:12 (1978).
101. J. Stedronska and W. F. Hendy, *Am. J. Reprod. Immunol. 3*:89 (1983).
102. S. Shulman, *Lancet 2*:1243 (1976).
103. M. De Almeida and J. C. Soufir, *Lancet 2*:815 (1977).
104. F. Dondero, A. Isidori, A. Lenzi, M. Cerasaro, F. Mazzilli, P. Giovenco, and C. Conti, *Fertil. Steril. 31*:48 (1979).
105. W. F. Hendry, J. Stedronska, L. Huges, K. M. Cameron, and R. C. B. Pugh, *Lancet 2*:498 (1979).
106. M. Katz and R. Newill, *Lancet 1*:1306 (1980).
107. T. B. Hargreave and R. A. Elton, *Fertil. Steril. 38*:586 (1982).
108. J. F. Shulman and S. Shulman, *Fertil. Steril. 38*:591 (1982).

109. P. Rümke and G. Hellinga, *Am. J. Clin. Pathol.* *32*:357 (1959).
110. A. M. Phadke, *J. Reprod. Fertil.* 7:1 (1964).
111. K. Bandhauer, *Urol. Int.* *21*:247 (1966).
112. F. Dondero, A. Lenzi, A. Isidori, and C. Conti, in *Autoimmune Aspects of Endocrine Disorders* (A. Pinchera, D. Doniach, G. F. Fenzi, and L. Baschieri, eds.), Academic Press, New York, 1980, p. 413.
113. W. F. Hendry, J. M. Parslow, J. Stedronska, and D. M. A. Wallace, *Br. J. Urol.* *54*:774 (1982).
114. W. F. Hendry, J. M. Parslow, and J. Stedronska, *Br. J. Urol.* *55*:785 (1983).
115. E. M. Quesada, C. D. Dukes, G. H. Deen, and R. R. Franklin, *J. Urol.* *99*:106 (1968).
116. B. Fjällbrant and O. Obrant, *Acta Obstet. Gynecol. Scand.* *47*:451 (1968).
117. A. A. Fattah, A. A. Azim, M. Habeib, and M. Rafik, *Fertil. Steril.* *33*:157 (1980).
118. S. S. Witkin and A. Toth, *Fertil. Steril.* *40*:806 (1983).
119. F. Dondero, A. Radicioni, F. Mazzilli, P. Giovenco, A. Lenzi, and M. Cerasaro, *Proc. 4th Int. Forum of Andrology* (A 022), Paris, 1986.
120. B. Fjällbrant and S. Nillson, *Int. J. Fertil.* *22*:255 (1977).
121. H. R. Tinneberg and B. Boettche, *Proc. 10th World Cong. Fert. Steril.*, Madrid (A 032), 1980.
122. J. A. Andrada, F. von der Walde, J. C. Hoschoian, J. C. Comini, and H. E. Mancini, *Andrologia* *9*:207 (1977).
123. R. Haensch, *Andrologia* *5*:147 (1973).
124. G. Daugaard, H. D. Petersen, U. Abildgaard, H. Marcussen, M. Wallach, P. Jess, T. Hjort, and S. G. Johnsen, *Arch. Androl.* *10*:245 (1983).
125. S. S. Witkin and J. Sonnabend, *Fertil. Steril.* *39*:337 (1983).
126. G. M. Mavligit, M. Talpaz, F. T. Hsia, W. Wong, B. Lichtiger, P. W. A. Mansell, and D. M. Mumford, *JAMA* *251*:237 (1984).
127. P. Rümke, in *Oligozoospermia: Recent Progress in Andrology* (G. Frajese, E. S. E. Hafez, C. Conti, and A. Fabbrini, eds.), Raven Press, New York, 1981, p. 185.

128. S. Shulman, in *Oligozoospermia:Recent Progress in Andrology* (G. Frajese, E. S. E. Hafez, C. Conti, and A. Fabbrini, eds.), Academic Press New York, 1981, p. 199.
129. P. Rümke, in *Immunology of Reproduction* (R. G. Edwards, ed.), International Planned Parenthood Federation, London, 1968, p. 251.
130. F. Dondero, F. Mazzilli, P. Giovenco, A. Lenzi, and A. Isidori, in *Recent Progress in Andrology* (A. Fabbrini and E. Steinberger, eds.), Academic Press, New York, 1978, p. 427.
131. B. Fjällbrant, *Acta Obstet. Gynecol. Scand. 47*(Suppl. 4) (1968).
132. W. F. Hendry, H. Morgan, and J. Stedronska, *Br. J. Urol. 49*:757 (1977).
133. J. Friberg, *Am. J. Obstet. Gynecol. 139*:587 (1981).
134. Y. Ainmelk, M. Nemirowsky, S. Belisle, N. Kandalaft, D. McClure, and M. El Hilali, *Int. J. Fertil. 27*:52 (1982).
135. J. Kremer and S. Jager, *Fertil. Steril. 27*:335 (1976).
136. J. Kremer, S. Jager, and J. Kuiken, in *Immunological Influence on Human Fertility* (B. Boettcher, ed.), Academic Press, New York, 1977, p. 47.
137. S. Jager, J. Kremer, J. Kuiken, T. van Slochteren-Draaisma, I. Mulder, and I. W. de Wilde-Janssen, *Fertil. Steril. 36*:784 (1981).
138. T. Hjort, K. B. Hansen, and F. Poulsen, in *Spermatozoa, Antibodies and Infertility* (J. Cohen and W. F. Hendry, eds.), Blackwell Scientific, Oxford, 1978, p. 101.
139. N. J. Alexander, *Fertil. Steril. 41*:433 (1984).
140. S. Mathur, H. O. Williamson, M. E. Baker, P. F. Rust, G. L. Holtz, and H. H. Fudenberg, *Fertil. Steril. 41*:81 (1984).
141. R. A. Bronson, G. W. Cooper, and D. L. Rosenfeld, *Fertil. Steril. 41*:609 (1984).
142. R. A. Bronson, G. W. Cooper, and D. L. Rosenfeld, *Fertil. Steril. 38*:724 (1982).
143. A. C. Menge and C. S. Black, *Fertil. Steril. 32*:214 (1979).
144. G. G. Haas, J. E. Sokoloski, and D. P. Wolf, *Am. J. Reprod. Immunol. 1*:40 (1980).

145. R. A. Bronson, G. W. Cooper, and D. L. Rosenfeld, *Fertil. Steril. 40*:91 (1983).
146. W. R. Jones, in *Immunology of Human Reproduction* (J. S. Scott and W. R. Jones, eds.), Academic Press, New York, 1976, p. 375.
147. O. S. El-Alfi and F. Bassili, *J. Reprod. Fertil. 21*:23 (1970).
148. D. M. Mumford, P. B. Barsales, K. D. Ball, and H. L. Gordon, *J. Urol. 105*:858 (1971).
149. J. R. Wall, J. Stedronska, R. D. David, R. F. Harrison, D. Goriup, and M. Lessof, *Fertil. Steril. 26*:1035 (1975).
150. K. Thestrup-Pedersen, K. Husted, and T. Hjort, *Int. J. Fertil. 21*:218 (1976).
151. S. K. Husted, K. Thestrup-Pedersen, and T. Hjort, *Int. J. Fertil. 21*:226 (1976).
152. R. Polidori, F. Ambrogi, P. L. Izzo, M. Mariani, B. Grassi, and G. F. Menchini Fabirs, *Andrologia 12*:141 (1980).
153. P. S. Nagarkatti and S. S. Rao, *Clin. Exp. Immunol. 26*:239 (1976).
154. G. Valesini, A. Lenzi, R. Pastore, M. Picardo, and F. Dondero, in *Autoimmune Aspects of Endrocrine Disorders* (A. Pinchera, D. Doniach, G. F. Fenzi, and L. Baschieri, eds.), Academic Press, New York, 1980, p. 409.
155. Z. H. Marcus, J. H. Frishaim, J. L. Houlk, J. H. Herman, and E. V. Hess, *Clin. Immunol. Immunopathol. 9*:318 (1978).
156. E. M. Lord, G. F. Sensabaugh, and D. P. Stites, *J. Immunol. 118*:1704 (1977).
157. F. Dondero, A. Lenzi, M. Picardo, R. Pastore, and G. Valesini, *Andrologia 12*:25 (1980).

5
Immunologic Effects of Vasectomy in Men

PIERLUIGI E. BIGAZZI

University of Connecticut Health Center
Farmington, Connecticut

Vasectomy is an effective, simple, rapid, relatively inexpensive male sterilization procedure, usually devoid of serious medical complications. As a result, it has become an increasingly popular and demographically important method of fertility control in several countries. In particular, its prevalence rate is 5–10% of fertile couples in countries with large populations, such as China, India, and the United States (reviewed in Ref. 1). In the People's Republic of China, 2,616,000 vasectomies were performed in 1977 and a total of 13.8 million between 1971 and 1978 (2). In India, 6 million men were vasectomized in the years from 1968 to 1972 in large-scale government-sponsored programs and more recently 590,000 vasectomies were performed in the years 1982–1983. In the United States, approximately 15 million men were vasectomized in the period between 1970 and 1981 and 455,000 in 1983 (1). Overall, it has been estimated that about 35 million men have had a vasectomy in the last 10 years (3) and that the world total for vasectomies is well above 50 million (4).

The wide acceptance of vasectomy has raised some concerns, since this surgical procedure has the rather special characteristic of eliciting an immune response to self-antigens of spermatozoa.

However, numerous epidemiologic studies of vasectomy have consistently found *no increase* in the risk of cardiovascular disease, autoimmune disease, neoplasia, or other diseases in vasectomized men. As stated in a recent review, "at this time, epidemiologic studies of vasectomy in man are strongly reassuring" (5). Considering the large populations involved, it is indeed reassuring that vasectomy is not causing in humans some of the problems (autoimmune orchitis and glomerulonephritis observed in experimental animals. The reasons for this fortunate difference are at present obscure but should be carefully investigated as they can reveal important aspects of autoimmune responses and disease.

Vasectomized men and animals experience a variety of autoimmune responses to antigens of spermatozoa (reviewed in Ref. 6). To date, humoral responses have been documented more extensively than delayed hypersensitivity responses. Thus, sperm-agglutinating and sperm-immobilizing antibodies, as well as numerous other antibodies to various components of the spermatozoon, have been demonstrated in the sera of approximately 50% or more of vasectomized subjects. Antibodies directed to surface antigens of the spermatozoal membrane may interfere with the function of the spermatozoon and therefore have special interest in the vasovasostomized subjects. Antibodies directed to internal components of the spermatozoon have less importance from this point of view, since they cannot bind to unexposed epitopes. However, they may react with autoantigens released from spermatozoa and form in situ immune complexes. Ongoing studies should clarify the clinical relevance of both types of autoantibodies. Recently, human monoclonal antibodies to spermatozoa have been obtained by the fusion of peripheral blood lymphocytes from vasectomized subjects and murine myeloma cells (7). These monoclonal antibodies should greatly facilitate the analysis of sperm autoantigens as well as the identification of relevant idiotopes of antisperm antibodies.

I. HUMORAL IMMUNE RESPONSES TO SPERMATOZOA AND OTHER ANTIGENS

A. Sperm-Agglutinating Antibodies (SAA)

As previously mentioned in Chapter 2, the tests most commonly used to detect SAA are based on the Kibrick method (macroagglutination) and the Franklin-Dukes method (microagglutination). Results obtained by these procedures often vary among different laboratories, which may explain variations in incidence of SAA reported in different groups of vasectomized men.

The first study on the immunologic effects of vasectomy in men was published in 1959 by Rümke (8), who, in collaboration with Hellinga, tested sera from four vasectomized men and found that one contained SAA. A few years later, Phadke and Padukone (9) investigated a larger group of vasectomized men and showed that circulating SAA were present in 32% of 25 individuals. In both studies, no tests were performed on sera obtained prior to surgery; thus, although the association of sperm antibodies and vasectomy was suggestive, a causal relationship was by no means demonstrated. Studies from Shulman's laboratory (10) provided the necessary evidence, obtained in a group of 22 men, whose sera were examined by a modification of the Kibrick test. Significant increases in sperm-agglutinating activity were shown in 12 subjects (55%), and 2 subjects had a very slight increase and therefore were considered marginal (the incidence would reach 64% if they were included within the positive group). A time course study in 7 subjects with SAA showed that 4 had a peak between the second and the sixth month after vasectomy, and the other 3 had a later response at about postoperative months 5–6. In 1 of the 12 positive subjects SAA were present even before vasectomy, but titers increased after surgery.

In the following years, these observations have been confirmed by numerous other investigators. Ansbacher showed that between 50 and 70% of vasectomized subjects have SAA. In a first study, performed on men 6 months after vasectomy, 26 of 48 men (54.2%) had SAA in their sera, with titers ranging from 2 to 128

(11). In a later study, it was found that the incidence of SAA was 51.3% after 6 weeks (with titers ranging between 2 and 128), 51.9% after 6 months (with titers between 2 and 64), and 55.5% after 1 year (titers 2-1024) (12). Similar results were obtained when a group of vasectomized subjects was followed for a longer period of time (13); i.e., 38.9% had SAA at 6 months (titers 4-16), 44.4% at 12 months (titers 2-64), 50% at 18 months (titers 8-128), 44.4% at 24 months (titers 4-256), and 38.9% at 36 months (titers 4-128). Finally, a study of vasectomized men through their first 5 postoperative years showed that SAA had a peak incidence of 69.7% after 12 months, with a subsequent decrease in both incidence and titers after 24 months (14). Percentages of SAA between 30 and 70% have also been reported by other laboratories (15-20).

Finally, the results of a series of long-term studies on the immunologic effects of vasectomy in men were presented in 1978 at a meeting organized by the National Institute of Child Health and Development of the NIH. Percentages of SAA were reported to vary between 52 and 68% at 6 months and 52 and 60% after 1 year (21-24).

Thus, the association between vasectomy and circulating SAA has been firmly established by reproducible investigations. These antibodies persist in the circulation for long periods of time; however, there is no proof that they have a pathogenetic role.

B. Sperm-Immobilizing Antibodies (SIA)

As described in Chapter 2, antibodies capable of immobilizing spermatozoa are detected by the Isojima procedure, based on calculation of the percentage of immobile spermatozoa after incubation with patients' sera and complement. There are some problems with the reproducibility of the sperm-immobilization test, which may account for differences reported in the incidence of SIA in vasectomized subjects.

Ansbacher (11) first utilized the Isojima test with sera from vasectomized subjects and found that 15 of 48 (31.3%) had circulating SIA 6 months after vasectomy, with titers ranging between

2 and 128. Further studies showed that, 6 months after vasectomy, 37% of the sera contained SIA (titers 2–128) and, 1 year post-vasectomy, 40.7% (titers 2–1024) (12). However, when vasectomized subjects were followed for longer periods, a sudden decrease in the incidence of these antibodies was noted at 18 months (13): in a group of 18 vasectomized men the incidence of SIA was 22.2% at 6 months (titers 2–64), 33.3% at 12 months (titers 4–256), 5.6% after 18 months (titer 128), and 5.6% after 24 and 36 months (titer 4). This decrease was later confirmed in a group tested for up to 5 years (14). Other groups have confirmed these data and reported an incidence of circulating SIA varying between 24 and 62% (17–25).

C. Antibodies to Spermatozoa Detectable by Indirect Immunofluorescence (IIF-ASA)

As described in Chapter 2, circulating antibodies to various components of spermatozoa are detectable by indirect immunofluorescence on methanol-fixed or swollen spermatozoa. Methanol-fixed spermatozoa are used to demonstrate antibodies to antigenic determinants of the acrosome, equatorial region, midpiece, and tail of the spermatozoon. On the other hand, spermatozoa with swollen heads are the substrate for the detection of antibodies to nuclear antigens (protamines) specific to spermatozoa. The value of indirect immunofluorescence for the detection of ASA is still uncertain.

Tung (26) first reported that 61% of 114 subjects had circulating IIF-ASA before vasectomy. The incidence rose significantly after surgery, reaching 77% 2 months after vasectomy and 90% after 6–9 months. The IIF-ASA observed before vasectomy were directed to the acrosome, with a diffuse pattern of staining (detected in 30% of subjects), equatorial region (24%), postacrosomal region (11%), midpiece (19%), and main piece (3%) of the tail. Usually the titers of IIF-ASA observed in normal subjects were low: titers of 10 or less were detected in 59%, titers of 20–40 in 36%, and titers over 80 in 5%. After vasectomy, the incidence of all IIF-ASA increased. Circulating antibodies to the acrosome with diffuse staining) were observed in 61% of subjects, to the equatorial region in 49%, to the postacrosomal region in 24%, to the main piece of the tail in 31%, and to the midpiece in 22%. Other antibodies, usually not detected in normal subjects before vasectomy, were found in the circulation 6-9 months after vasectomy. These included IIF-ASA to the sperm nucleus (33%) and to a second antigen of the acrosome (speckled staining, 7%). Antibody titers also increased, so that 40% of vasectomized subjects had titers of 10 or less, 49% between 20-40, and 11% over 80. The immunoglobulin classes of IIF-ASA were mostly IgM for antiacrosomal, IgG for antiequatorial and antinucleus, and otherwise equally distributed between IgG and IgM. Interestingly, Tung noted that only a few of a small group of positive sera bound complement.

Other investigators have performed similar studies, reporting percentages from 11% for all types of circulating IIF-ASA (27) to 23-25% for antiprotamine IIF-ASA (25,28).

D. Antibodies to Spermatozoa Detectable by ELISA (ELISA-ASA)

Circulating antibodies to spermatozoa are detectable by the enzyme-linked immunosorbent assay (ELISA-ASA) using human spermatozoa or purified spermatozoal antigens fixed to wells of microtiter plates. This type of assay in general has several advantages, such as sensitivity, simplicity, suitability for large-scale testing, and no need for radioactive isotopes. Unfortunately, as discussed in Chapter 2, there are still some problems with the various ELISA used to detect antibodies to spermatozoa.

Witkin et al. (29) demonstrated that only 6.6% of vasectomized subjects had developed ELISA-ASA 4 months postvasectomy. A prospective study (30) has shown that the percentage of vasectomized subjects positive for ELISA-ASA increases to 25% at 15-20 months and 27% at 21-26 months postvasectomy. However, a collaborative effort between various laboratories using ELISA has revealed variability in the results obtained (31). Much work is still needed to improve reproducibility and reduce nonspecific reactions with normal control sera, but a satisfactory ELISA may be successfully developed in the long term.

E. Antibodies to Stem Cells

Antibodies to hematopoietic progenitor cell antigens were found in the sera from two vasectomized subjects with high titers of SAA (32). Both sera reduced the number of granulocyte colony-forming units of cultures from human marrow and also affected the growth of colony-forming units, erythroprotein-dependent progenitors of erythrocyte colonies, and precursors of colony-forming units in culture progenitors of granulocyte colonies. No reactions were observed with normal peripheral leukocytes and tonsil (predominantly B) lymphocytes. Further studies by positive enrichment using a fluorescence-activated cell sorter confirmed these findings and showed that hematopoietic stem cells possess "unique" surface antigens cross-reactive with sperm, brain, and embryonic antigens (33). Similar antihematopoietic progenitor cell antibodies have been noted in the sera of five additional vasectomized men (25).

F. Antibodies to HLA Antigens

Some investigators have reported that vasectomy is followed by the development of lymphocytotoxic antibodies with HLA specificity. Henry (34) noted that 1 of 12 vasectomized men had lymphocytotoxic antibodies, considered to be specific for or cross-reactive with HLA antigens. Studies on a second group of 10 vasectomized subjects (35) also showed that the sera of 6 men had a significant increase in lymphocytotoxic antibody activity against a 40-donor panel of normal lymphocytes. This increase was detected 2–6 months after vasectomy and then disappeared in the following months. Similarly, 9 men had lymphocytotoxic antibodies against a panel of leukemic B cells and 3 had weak reactions against their own lymphocytes. Jennings et al. (36) observed that sera from 2 of 32 vasectomized men had a definite increase in lymphocytotoxic antibodies 6–12 months after surgery. The sera of 4 men had slight increases. The serum of 1 man once had a positive reaction against his own lymphocytes. When some of the same subjects were examined again 21–44 months after vasectomy, their sera did not have significant lymphocytotoxic activity (37). Of the 2 subjects whose sera were positive in the previous study, 1 was negative at 27 and 35 months after surgery and the other had weak reactivity against 1 of a 29-member lymphocyte donor panel. Lymphocytotoxic antibodies have also been detected by an antiglobulin cytotoxic assay in approximately 20% of vasectomized subjects compared with 15% of controls (38).

On the other hand, these findings have not been confirmed by White et al. (39), who did not observe any significant difference in lymphocytotoxic antibodies present in prevasectomy and postvasectomy sera. In addition, Law et al. (40) found that in a group of vasectomized subjects investigated within 1 year of surgery, there was a significantly elevated frequency of reactions with the subjects' own lymphocytes and various lymphoid lines. However, they did not notice any significant difference between the prevalence before and after vasectomy and concluded that there was no evidence of increased production of anti-HLA-A, B, or C or anti-Ia antibodies after vasectomy.

G. Antibodies to Other Autoantigens

Most investigators have not observed any significant difference between vasectomized subjects and controls for a variety of serum autoantibodies, such as ANA, rheumatoid factor, autoantibodies to mitochondria, smooth muscle, parietal cells, glomerular basement membrane, or thyroglobulin (22,24,26,27). In our laboratory, we tested a total of 150 sera from vasectomized subjects and did not detect antibodies to steroid-producing cells of adrenals and testis (Bigazzi and Rose, unpublished data).

On the other hand, significant increases in the incidence of autoantibodies to thyroglobulin and an unidentified connective tissue antigen have been reported by other investigators (25,41). Similarly, "weak" autoantibody reactions to several antigens have been noted in another group of vasectomized subjects (42).

H. Circulating Immune Complexes

Tung et al. (43) searched for circulating immune complexes (CIC), using both the Raji cell method (RCM) and the C1q solid-phase assay (C1qSPA), in sera from 160 men, vasectomized 2–4 years earlier, and 59 age-matched controls. No CIC were detected in any sera by the RCM, but 12% of vasectomized and 3.5% of control subjects were positive by C1qSPA (a difference that was not statistically significant). However, the levels of CIC were considerably higher in vasectomized men than in controls. A similar study performed in three different laboratories using three different procedures (indirect phagocytosis, C1q inhibition, and C1q deviation test) gave rather inconclusive results that seemed to suggest the absence of CIC in vasectomized men (44); another study by the C1q-binding assay gave a percentage of positivity of 3.8%, similar to that found in the general male population (4.3%) or in the family members used as controls (6.9%) (25).

More recently, a Task Force in the Indian Council for Medical Research has found CIC in 12% of vasectomized men and 4% of controls (45), and Witkin et al. (30) have reported that 11% of vasectomized Austrian men had CIC before surgery, 24% at 2–3 months, 10% at 4–6 months, and 0% at 15–26 months. Finally, Linnet et al (46) detected no significant difference in CIC between vasectomized subjects (5 years after surgery) and age-matched controls.

II. DELAYED HYPERSENSITIVITY REACTIONS

Very few studies of cell-mediated immunity have been performed in vasectomized men, and the results available are contrasting and inconclusive. A decrease in lymphocyte responses after stimulation with phytohemagglutinin (PHA) has been observed in some men after vasectomy (23), but normal skin test reactions as well as normal responses to mitogen stimulation were detected in other vasectomized subjects (24,47).

Similarly inconclusive are the studies of delayed hypersensitivity to sperm antigens. In India, Nagarkatti and Rao (48) found that 32.2% of 62 vasectomized men had leukocyte migration inhibition reactions to a crude spermatozoal extract, but no reactions were observed in the other vasectomized men and 22 controls. Approximately 22% of the men produced leukocyte migration inhibition factor in the first 5 years after surgery, and this percentage increased to 46% after 6–10 years. A similar incidence of delayed hypersensitivity reactions was noted by Mumford et al (23), who, using the lymphocyte transformation test, detected cell-mediated immunity to spermatozoa in 24% of subjects after vasectomy.

These results are in contrast to those reported by other investigators, who used leukocyte migration inhibition and/or lymphocyte transformation tests and found no significant differences in cell-mediated immunity to spermatozoa between vasectomized men and controls (22,24,47). In view of these findings, the statement that "results of the lymphocyte transformation test with sperm antigens were erratic and difficult to interpret" (22) is not surprising. It is obvious that studies of delayed hypersensitivity to spermatozoa in vasectomized subjects should be pursued further, utilizing more sophisticated techniques and purified antigens. Well-controlled investigations of general immune competence should also be continued. A few years ago, it was hypothesized that "sperm" could have immunosuppressive effects in male homosexuals and vasectomized men (49). The discovery of the viral cause of acquired immune deficiency syndrome (AIDS) later attenuated the impact of that suggestion. In addition, recent evidence showing that the in vitro immunosuppressive activity of seminal plasma is observed only in the presence of bovine serum (50) has reduced the rather mystical importance sometimes attributed to products of the male genital tract. Luckily for the many millions of vasectomized men, there are no significant data indicating that tumor development or infections increase after vasectomy (4). However, we agree with Linnet (4) that this line of research should be continued, and even "negative" results be given a high publication priority.

III. IMMUNOGENETIC STUDIES

The relation between the HLA system and immune responses observed after vasectomy has been investigated by Law et al (40). A group of 188 vasectomized men and a control group of 100 men (about to undergo the operation) were tested for circulating SAA, SIA, IF-ASA, and a variety of other autoantibodies. At the same time, their lymphocytes were typed for HLA-A and B locus antigens. This study showed that HLA antigen A28 was associated with SAA (head agglutination pattern), with a significance at less than the 0.1% level. In addition, associations between A28 and strong SIA and IF-ASA (equatorial) were found at the 5% and the 1% level, respectively. An association at the 1% level was found between B17 and strong IF-ASA (acrosomal) as well as between Bw22 and SAA (head agglutination pattern). No other associations were found between other autoantibodies to spermatozoa and HLA. The association between head agglutinating antibodies and antigen A28 of the HLA system may be of particular importance, as "one of the first clear-cut examples of antibody production associated with the HLA system (40). Further studies are obviously needed to determine possible associations between HLA-D and/or DR antigens and the autoimmune responses to spermatozoa observed after vasectomy.

IV. TESTICULAR HISTOPATHOLOGY AND IMMUNOHISTOPATHOLOGY

It is clearly impossible to investigate the kinetics of histopathological changes in the testes of vasectomized men, since it would be unethical to perform testicular biopsies of normal subjects at regular intervals. Therefore, the only studies available to date are limited to biopsies performed on volunteers at a single time after vasectomy, usually at the moment of surgical recanalization. In this case the procedure is morally justifiable, since the histopathology of the testis may provide indications predicting fertility after surgically successful reversal.

A summary of the various reports, from a grand total of 185 vasectomized subjects, is provided in Table 1. The results indicate that significant morphological changes occur in the human testis after vasectomy. It is also evident that a definitive investigation, correlating immunology, immunopathology, and histopathology in an adequate sample of vasectomized men, is still lacking.

Kubota (51) examined testicular biopsies from 8 vasectomized subjects and 34 healthy male controls and found that most of them were normal. However, the biopsies obtained from two vasectomized men (3 and 7 years after surgery) showed degenerative changes of spermatocytes. Hagedoorn and Davis (52) also studied testicular biopsies obtained 3-7 years after vasectomy and noted that the germinal epithelium was present, with normal stages of spermatogenesis. Spermatids were observed in the usual culsters of four to five, while spermatozoa were not in their typical location close to the lumen, but rather abutting the basal part of the Sertoli cells, often close to the basement membrane of the tubules. The Sertoli cells appeared intact but contained a large number of lysosomes in the area between nucleus and basement membrane. They interpreted these findings as suggestive of normal spermatogenesis as well as phagocytic absorption and/or elimination of spermatozoa by Sertoli cells. Another group of investigators (53) also reported normal or reduced spermatogenesis after vasectomy in men.

More complex are the findings observed by Gupta et al. (54), who studied the histopathology of the testis in 20 young men 1 month after vasectomy and noted significant changes in all subjects. There was marked degeneration of germinal epithelium, with spermatogenesis arrested at the level of spermatocytes and thickening of basement membranes (several layers of connective tissue) but no evidence of inflammatory reactions. These changes were more marked and widespread in the testes of 10 men over 50 years of age who showed spermatogenesis arrested at the spermatocyte stage in most of the tubules. Thickening of the tubular basement membranes and intertubular fibrosis, which are observed in normal males over 50 years of age, were further accentuated in vasectomized men at this age. Finally, the testes of 10 young subjects undergoing vasovasostomy were also investigated. Full differentiation of germ cells and active spermatogenesis were observed, as well as moderate Leydig cell hyperplasia. In 4 cases, vacuolating degeneration in a few tubules, thickening of basement membranes, and intertubular fibrosis were noted. Testis biopsies obtained at the time of vasovasostomy in another group of 11 subjects (2–10 years after vasectomy) showed intertubular edema and reduced spermatogenesis, in a patchy pattern (47). There was occasional vacuolization and, in some biopsies, hypertrophy of spermatogonia, less mature spermatozoa, and a few intraluminal giant cells. Histological abnormalities did not seem related to the subsequent fertility of these subjects.

In our laboratory we have performed a study correlating testis histopathology, immunohistopathology, and autoimmune responses to spermatozoa. To this aim, we examined both sera and testicular biopsies obtained from 21 vasectomized subjects undergoing vasovasostomy (55). Of the sera collected, 3 contained SAA and 1 SIA, and IIF-ASA were detected in 10 (antiprotamine in 4, antiequatorial in 5, antiacrosomal in 5, and antitail in 5). Direct IF studies showed that none of the testicular biopsies contained immune deposits, which might be because none of our subjects had strong autoimmune responses to spermatozoa. Histopathological observations showed that the majority of the biopsies contained relatively normal tissue. However, alterations of the seminiferous tubules and/or the interstitial tissue were noted in 4 cases. Of these, 2 showed severe disruption of the germ cell layers, with thickening of the tubular basement membrane, and the other 2 showed fibrosis in the interstitial tissue.

Similar results were obtained by another group of investigators, who were unable to demonstrate immune deposits in 36 testicular biopsies examined by direct immunofluorescence (56). Light microscopy of 62 biopsies also showed that normal spermatogenesis was well preserved in most subjects and was impaired in only 4 biopsies. In contrast with our findings, no interstitial fibrosis or thickening of basement membranes was reported. However,

Table 1 Summary of Studies on Testicular Biopsies from Vasectomized Men[a]

Number of subjects	Histopathology	%	ASA	CMI	Testis immuno-pathology	Reference
8	Degenerative changes of spermatocytes	25	ND	ND	ND	51
?	Phagocytosis of spermatozoa?	?	ND	ND	ND	52
13	Normal or reduced spermatogenesis	?	ND	ND	ND	53
40	Spermatogenetic arrest thickening of TBM, interstitial fibrosis	85	ND	ND	ND	54

11	Intertubular edema and reduced spermatogenesis	100	ND	-	ND	47
21	Thickening of TBM, interstitial fibrosis	19	+	ND	-	55
56	Mostly normal, but impaired spermatogenesis in 4 biopsies	7	+	ND	-	56
5	Interstitial fibrosis, thickened TBM	60	ND	ND	ND	57
31	Interstitial fibrosis thickening of TBM, spermatogenic arrest	23	ND	ND	ND	58

[a] Abbreviations: %, percentage of vasectomized men with histopathological changes; ASA, antisperm antibodies; CMI, cell-mediated immunity to spermatozoa; ND, not done; TBM, basement membrane of seminiferous tubules.

more recently, Mehrotra et al. (57) have reported diffuse interstitial fibrosis and thickening of the lamina propria in testicular biopsies from three of five vasectomized subjects undergoing vasovasostomy. There was no evidence of inflammatory reactions in the interstitial tissue. Similarly, Jarow et al. (58) have observed focal interstitial fibrosis in 23% of 31 vasectomized subjects, compared with a control group of 21 healthy volunteers. In addition, they noted increased tubular wall thickness: collagen deposition was increased within the basement membrane of the tubular wall, and the basal lamina was thicker. Spermatogenetic arrest was noted in 6% of the subjects who had significantly reduced numbers of mature spermatids and Sertoli cells. There was no evidence of inflammatory reactions. Even though not mentioned in the report, one must also assume that electron-opaque deposits were not present at the level of the tubular basement membranes. Interestingly, the interstitial fibrosis was the only finding that correlated with infertility after reversal of the vasectomy.

Thus, studies of testicular biopsies from vasectomized men seem to indicate that thickening of basement membranes and interstitial fibrosis are the major histopathological consequences of vasectomy, at least in some subjects. It should be noted here that a similar thickening of the collagenous basal lamina, with increased amounts of collagen fibrils, has also been observed in the testes of vasectomized rabbits (59) (see also Chap. 8) and patients with sterility (60,61) (see also Chap. 6). At present, the pathogenesis of the testicular changes observed after vasectomy is unknown and remains an interesting subject for future research (62).

V. EPIDEMIOLOGICAL STUDIES OF VASECTOMY

Studies in rabbits and monkeys suggested that in these animals vasectomy may be related to the development and severity of atherosclerosis, possibly through the mediation of immune mechanisms (63). Similarly, studies in vasectomized mice detected an increased incidence of neoplasias (64). Even though the evidence was rather limited (see Chap. 8), these observations raised considerable concern because of the large populations at risk. However, several epidemiological studies have found no increase in the risk of cardiovascular or other disease in vasectomized men (reviewed in Ref. 5).

Walker et al. (65) have found that the incidence of nonfatal myocardial infarction in 4830 vasectomized men was slightly lower than in matched controls. They also examined the incidence of first-time hospitalizations for a variety of diagnoses in a group of 6092 vasectomized men and found no statistically significant elevations in diseases of the cardiovascular system (66). The only interesting finding in this group was a higher incidence of various diseases of the genitourinary system during the early postvasectomy period. Similar results were obtained by Wallace et al. (67), who, in a small group of vasectomized men, found no association of coronary disease with vasectomy, and by Goldacre et al. (68), who found no epidemiological evidence of any overall excess of cardiovascular, endocrine, autoimmune, or other disorders. In contrast with these rather reassuring observations, Fahrenbach et al. (69) discovered a significant increase of retinal arteriolar constrictions in nonhypertensive vasectomized men, but a similar study by Linnet et al. (46) revealed no difference whatsoever in the distribution of arteriolosclerotic retinopathy in 46 men 5 years after vasectomy, compared with 46 age-matched controls.

More recent reports have provided the results obtained from investigations of large populations of vasectomized subjects and the appropriate controls. Cross-sectional studies of more than 4000 vasectomized men and cohort studies of more than 10,000 subjects have detected no increase in the risk of cardiovascular disease (5).

VI. IMMUNOLOGICAL EFFECTS OF VASECTOMY REVERSAL

In recent years, the large number of vasectomies has created a demand for surgical recanalization procedures. In the United States, this phenomenon has occurred because of a rising divorce and remarriage rate. In other countries, such as India, where adoption is not well accepted, vasectomy reversal may be required in case of death of children or remarriage (70). Initial statistics varied in success rates, but the introduction of a sophisticated microsurgery procedure by Silber (71) has provided more comforting results. In a series of about 1000 vasovasostomies (including patients who had previously undergone unsuccessful operations), 88% of patients developed normal semen parameters and 71% of their partners achieved pregnancies. To date, these are the best reported results. Other groups have obtained recanalization rates between 80 and 88% and pregnancy rates between 41 and 62% (72,73). Several variables, besides surgical expertise, affect the outcome: for example, vas patency was 100% in subjects who had been vasectomized for less than 6 years (pregnancy rate, 60%), 74% in subjects vasectomized for 6–10 years (pregnancy rate, 33%), and 33% in those vasectomized for more than 10 years (pregnancy rate, 0%) (73). Other variables may relate to the presence or absence of sperm granulomas and the possibility of epididymal "blowouts" (71). Finally, changes in the vasectomized testis (interstitial fibrosis) (58) and/or persisting autoimmune responses to spermatozoa may be responsible for the lack of fertility in those subjects who fail to recover normal sperm counts or remain infertile in spite of normal semen parameters.

In initial studies, Gupta et al. (70) found low fertility rates in 25 vasovasostomized males: 52% became normospermic after successful recanalization, 16% were oligospermic, and 32% remained azoospermic. Except 3 oligospermic subjects, all had circulating antisperm antibodies. Among 13 normospermic vasovasostomized subjects, a significant correlation was found between the titers of circulating spermagglutinins and autoagglutination of spermatozoa in their ejaculates as well as between circulating sperm-immobilizing antibodies and degree of sperm motility. Of these men 3 had low levels of spermagglutinins, no sperm-immobilizing antibodies, and normal semen: their partners achieved pregnancies. Sullivan and Howe (74) also found that serum autoantibodies to spermatozoa were significantly more frequent in those men who remained infertile after recanalization but detected no autoagglutination in the ejaculate. Other investigators have reported an immediate rise in titers of circulating sperm antibodies after vasovasostomy, with a return to preoperative levels by 1 year after vasectomy reversal (75,76). Hellema also demonstrated sperm agglutinins in the seminal plasma of 4 of 18 vasovasostomized subjects (76). The study of sperm agglutinins in the seminal plasma was pursued by Linnet and his co-workers (77–79). In a prospective investigation of 29 men before and after reconstructive vasovasostomy (77), it was found that 90% of the subjects had spermatozoa in their ejaculate after vasovasostomy and 69% had sperm agglutinins in their serum, with no significant changes in titers after recanalization of the vas deferens. However, 28% of subjects had sperm agglutinins in the seminal plasma after vasovasostomy. A strong association between the presence of sperm agglutinins in the seminal fluid and failure to impregnate over a period of 14–33 months was described in a later report (78). The presence of sperm agglutinins in the seminal fluid was always associated with their presence in the serum, usually in a higher titer, suggesting leakage from the circulation, but the investigation of the immunoglobulin classes of sperm-agglutinating antibodies present in the seminal fluid of four vasovasostomized men has shown that in two subjects the major part of the seminal agglutinins was IgA and, in one, IgG (79). Thus, both local production and diffusion of sperm agglutinins from serum to the testis-epididymis compartment may take place.

Rather contrasting results have been obtained in studies of larger groups of vasovasostomized subjects. Antisperm antibodies have been measured in serum and seminal plasma in 130 males before and after vasectomy reversal, followed for at least 1 year (80). Circulating sperm-agglutinating antibodies were found in 70% of subjects before and 89% after vasovasostomy. Seminal plasma antibodies were present in only 9.5% before and 29.5% after reversal. Patency of the vas deferens was achieved in almost all cases, as shown by sperm counts. Overall, pregnancies occurred in the partners of 45% of those subjects who were trying to produce children. Pregnancies were less likely to occur when the preoperative serum levels of sperm antibodies were high, but similar numbers of pregnancies were obtained by patients with or without low titers of seminal plasma antibodies. On the other hand, Sutherland et al. (81) have demonstrated a statistically significant association between infertility following reversal of vasectomy and the presence of sperm-agglutinating activity in semen samples. They found that the reversal of vasectomy results in a significant increase in the percentage of patients whose semen contains agglutinating activity, but serum levels do not show such marked changes. About 65% of men whose semen lacked sperm-agglutinating activity were fertile following reversal of vasectomy, but only 7% of those with sperm antibodies in their semen samples were fertile. Interestingly, the examination of segments of surgically removed vas deferens in 37 subjects undergoing vasovasostomy has shown that vasitis nodosa (a ductular proliferation originating from the lumen of the proximal obstructed end of the vas) is present in 66% of patients (82).

In summary, vasectomy does not seem to be a reversible procedure in all subjects, even when the more sophisticated reconstruction approaches are employed. The persistence of infertility in the presence of apparently normal semen may be caused by autoantibodies to spermatozoa acting within the seminal fluid or by changes within the testis. This area obviously deserves additional investigations aimed at the determination of the parameters capable of predicting a successful outcome of vasectomy reversal. Another topic that deserves further studies relates to the persistence of autoimmune responses to spermatozoa even when the flow of the semen has resumed its normal course after vasovasostomy. If spermatozoa were once more separated from the immune system, autosensitization to sperm antigens should eventually disappear. Since this does not actually occur, one possible explanation is that permeability changes have taken place at some level, either in the testis or in the excurrent tract, and are not reversible even when the vas deferens is recanalized.

VII. CONCLUSIONS

In the present chapter we have attempted to review the most significant of the numerous studies on the immunologic effects of vasectomy in men and will now summarize what we consider the "lessons of vasectomy" (83). The first conclusion we can reach, based on extensive epidemiological studies, is that, in humans, vasectomy seems to be a safe procedure. Should we be surprised by the finding that there is no increased incidence and severity of atherosclerosis in vasectomized subjects? Perhaps we should not, considering the numerous other opportunities available to human beings for immune complex formation, caused by vaccination, infectious diseases, and even autoimmune responses. Indeed, if the idiotype-anti-idiotype network is really operative under physiologic circumstances (84), immune complexes should be formed continuously in humans and animals. It is obvious that additional factors (genetics, functional status of the reticuloendothelial system, electrostatic charge of the antigens, antigen to antibody ratios, and others) are necessary for the development of immune complex-mediated disease.

The second conclusion that can be reached is that, without doubt, vasectomy can induce autoimmune responses to spermatozoa in a large percentage of otherwise normal human subjects. This is an extremely interesting occurrence, since in general (and with the exception of "spontaneous" autoimmune disease) it is rather difficult to experimentally obtain strong and persistent immune responses to autoantigens. The administration of certain chemicals may be followed by autoimmune responses in both humans and experimental animals (85). Similarly, some surgical procedures or irradiation of certain organs may be followed by autoimmune responses, usually of short duration (86–88). However, immune responses to autoantigens are usually better obtained after stimulation of the immune system with such adjuvants as complete Freund's adjuvant and/or *Bordetella pertussis*, routinely used in animal experiments. In men, there is only one published study (89) in which volunteer patients with prostatic carcinoma were injected with testicular antigens in adjuvant or testicular antigens alone and only the group treated with adjuvant became immunized. Therefore, that surgical interruption of the vas deferens causes strong and persistent autoimmune responses to spermatozoa is extremely interesting. The simplest explanation may be that previously "sequestered" autoantigens become available to the immune system through leakage at some level of the excurrent tract or from the seminiferous tubules themselves. If this explanation is correct, successful reversal of vasectomy should eventually result in the termination of autoimmune responses to spermatozoa, since the antigens should no longer be available to the immune system. Unfortunately, this does not seem to occur, casting some doubt on the validity of the original assumption. In fact, we still ignore many of the events leading to the initial sensitization against spermatozoa. Observations from patients with disorders of the genital tract may provide some help: subjects with congenital absence of the vas deferens produce antisperm antibodies (90), but patients with Young's syndrome, i.e., obstructive azoospermia due to inspissated secretions in the epididymis, do not produce high levels of such antibodies (91). It appears that autoimmune responses to spermatozoal antigens are more likely to occur if sperm goes through the epididymis before coming into contact with the immune system. Thus, studies on the immunologic effects of vasectomy might benefit from a focus on initial events at the level of the excurrent tract.

A third conclusion is that vasectomy may not be a reversible procedure in every subject. Indeed, thickening of basement membranes of seminiferous tubules and interstitial fibrosis are observed more frequently in testicular biopsies from vasectomized subjects than in controls. The pathogenesis of these alterations is unknown and deserves to be investigated. In view of the findings of immune deposits in the testes of infertile men, it would perhaps be worthwhile to search for similar deposits in testicular biopsies from vasectomized men with strong and persistent autoimmune responses to spermatozoa.

Finally, the major lesson of vasectomy may be provided by the wealth of information generated on this topic within the span of a few years. Through the use of NIH and other funds allocated to the study of the effects of vasectomy because of the concern about the safety of this procedure, we currently know much more not only about vasectomy, but also about the pathophysiology and immunology of the male reproductive system, an area that for years had not received adequate attention. It would be a pity if both research funding and scientists' efforts were to decrease at this point in time, when sophistication in the study of male reproductive immunology has finally reached a satisfactory level.

ACKNOWLEDGMENTS

Our research on the immunologic effects of vasectomy is supported by U.S. Public Health Service Grant HD17546 from the National Institute of Child Health and Human Development of the NIH. We thank Drs. Kosuda, Takami, and Zanetti for their expert collaboration and Ms. Ruth Conrod and Laura Henricks for excellent secretarial assistance.

REFERENCES

1. D. G. Huber, S. Hong and J. A. Ross, The international experience with vasectomy. In *Male Contraception* (G. I. Zatuchni, A. Goldsmith, J. M. Spieler, and J. J. Sciarra, eds.), Harper and Row, Philadelphia, 1986, pp. 7-18.
2. Population and birth planning in the People's Republic of China. *Popul. Rep.* [*J*] 590, 1982.
3. B. Stokes, Men and family planning. *Worldwatch Paper 41*:11, 1980.
4. L. Linnet, Clinical immunology of vasectomy and vasovasotomy. *Urology 22*:101-114, 1983.
5. D. B. Petitti, Epidemiologic studies of vasectomy. In *Male Contraception* (G. I. Zatuchni, A. Goldsmith, J. M. Spieler, and J. J. Sciarra, eds.), Harper and Row, Philadelphia, 1986, pp. 24-33.
6. P. E. Bigazzi, Immunologic effects of vasectomy in men and experimental animals. *Prog. Clin. Biol. Res. 70*:461-476, 1981.

7. J. C. Herr, J. E. Fowler, Jr., S. S. Howards, M. Sigman, W. M. Sutherland, and D. J. Koons, Human antisperm monoclonal antibodies constructed postvasectomy. *Biol. Reprod. 32*: 695-711, 1985.
8. P. Rümke and G. Hellinga, Autoantibodies against spermatozoa in sterile men. *Am. J. Clin. Pathol. 32*:357-363, 1959.
9. A. M. Phadke and K. Padukone, Presence and significance of autoantibodies against spermatozoa in the blood of men with obstructed vas deferens. *J. Reprod. Fertil. 7*:163-170, 1964.
10. S. Shulman, E. Zappi, U. Ahmed, and J. E. Davis, Immunologic consequences of vasectomy. *Contraception 5*:269-278, 1972.
11. R. Ansbacher, Sperm-agglutinating and sperm-immobilizing antibodies in vasectomized men, *Fertil. Steril. 22*:629-632, 1971.
12. R. Ansbacher, K. Keung-Yeung, and J. C. Wurster, Sperm antibodies in vasectomized men. *Fertil. Steril. 23*:640-643, 1972.
13. R. Ansbacher, Bilateral vas ligation: Sperm antibodies. *Contraception 9*:227-237, 1974.
14. R. Ansbacher, P. Hodge, A. Williams, and D. M. Mumford, Vasligation: Humoral sperm antibodies. *Int. J. Fertil. 21*:258-260, 1976.
15. P. H. Howard and L. P. James, Immunologic implications of vasectomy. *J. Urol. 109*:76-78, 1973.
16. A. Halim and D. Antoniou, Autoantibodies to spermatozoa in relation to male infertility and vasectomy. *Br. J. Urol. 45*:559-562, 1973.
17. N. J. Alexander, B. J. Wilson, and G. D. Patterson, Vasectomy: Immunologic effects in rhesus monkeys and men. *Fertil. Steril. 25*:149-156, 1974.
18. N. J. Alexander, S. S. Schmidt, M. J. Free, M. V. Danilchik, and W. T. Hill, Sperm antibodies after vasectomy with fulguration. *J. Urol. 115*:77-78, 1976.
19. N. J. Alexander and D. J. Anderson, Vasectomy: Consequences of autoimmunity to sperm antigens. *Fertil. Steril. 32*:253-260, 2979.

20. W.-B. Schill, A. Hofstetter and M. Stock, Zur Frage der Autoantikoerperbildung nach freiwilliger Vasektomie. *Urologe [Ausg. A] 14*:194–198, 1975.
21. H. W. J. Hellema and P. Rümke, Sperm autoantibodies as a consequence of vasectomy. I. Within 1 year post-operation. *Clin. Exp. Immunol. 31*:18–29, 1978.
22. G. S. Bernstein, R. Chopp, M. Cosgrove, A. Coulgon, W. Kiely, G. Friou, J. Korelitz, F. J. Massey, Jr., R. Mendez, J. Mestman, R. Nakamura, F. Quismorio, and R. Takano, A controlled prospective study of the effects of vasectomy. In *Vasectomy. Immunologic and Pathophysiologic Effects in Animals and Man* (I. H. Lepow and R. Crozier, eds.), Academic Press, New York, 1979, pp. 473–489.
23. D. M. Mumford, R. Ansbacher, and J. S. Sung, Longitudinal immune studies in vasectomized men. In *Vasectomy. Immunologic and Pathophysiologic Effects in Animals and Man* (I. H. Lepow and R. Crozier, eds.), Academic Press, New York, 1979, pp. 491–508.
24. E. V. Hess, J. H. Herman, J. L. Houk, and Z. H. Marcus, Studies on the immune system in human vasectomy. In *Vasectomy. Immunologic and Pathophysiologic Effects in Animals and Man* (I. H. Lepow and R. Crozier, eds.), Academic Press, New York, 1979, pp. 509–519.
25. N. R. Rose and P. L. Lucas, Immunological consequences of vasectomy. II. Two-year summary of a prospective study. In *Vasectomy. Immunologic and Pathophysiologic Effects in Animals and Man* (I. H. Lepow and R. Crozier, eds.), Academic Press, New York, 1979, pp. 533–560.
26. K. S. K. Tung, Human sperm antigens and antisperm antibodies. I. Studies on vasectomy patients. *Clin. Exp. Immunol. 20*:93–104, 1975.
27. P. Crewe, L. Dawson, R. D. Barnes, E. Tidmarsh, I. Chanarin, T. Hjort, and J. Ingerslev, Lack of association of the development of anti-sperm antibodies and other autoantibodies as a consequence of vasectomy. *Int. J. Fertil. 22*:104–109, 1977.
28. H. W. H. Hellema, T. Samuel, and P. Rümke: Sperm autoantibodies as a consequence of vasectomy. II. Long-term follow-up studies. *Clin. Exp. Immunol. 38*:31–36, 1979.

29. S. S. Witkin, G. Zelikovsky, A. M. Bongiovanni, N. Geller, R. A. Good, and N. K. Day, Sperm-related antigens, antibodies and circulating immune complexes in sera of recently vasectomized men. *J. Clin. Invest. 70*:233–40, 1982.
30. S. S. Witkin, N. J. Alexander, and J. Frick, Circulating inmune complexes and sperm antibodies following vasectomy in Austrian men. *J. Clin. Lab. Immunol. 14*:69–72, 1984.
31. L. Mettler, A. B. Czuppon, N. Alexander, M. De Almeida, G. G. Haas, Jr., T. Hjort, J. Møller Jensen, R. Ing, W. R. Jones, S. X. Wang, S. S. Witkin, and A. M. Bongiovanni, Antibodies to spermatozoa and seminal plasma antigens detected by various enzyme-linked immunosorbent (ELISA) assays. *J. Reprod. Immunol. 8*:301–312, 1985.
32. R. L. Krogsrud, J. Bain, and G. B. Price, Serologic identification of hemopoietic progenitor cell antigens common to mouse and man. *J. Immunol. 119*:1486–1492, 1977.
33. R. L. Krogsrud and G. B. Price, Hemopoietic stem cells bear sperm-associated antigens. *Exp. Hematol. 7*:377–382, 1979.
34. J. B. Henry, Immunological effects of vasectomy. *JAMA 225*:642, 1973.
35. Y. J. Choi, L. Reiner, and C. Ney, Immunological observations following vasectomy. *Experientia 35*:1243–1244, 1979.
36. P. B. Jennings, M. K. McCarthy, S. R. Plymate, and J. N. Wettlaufer, Prevalence of circulating HL-A lymphocytotoxic antibodies in men after vasectomy. *Fertil. Steril. 26*:53–56, 1975.
37. P. B. Jennings, J. N. Wettlaufer, and C. A. Paulsen, Absence of circulating HL-A lymphocytotoxic antibodies in men 21 to 44 months after vasectomy. *Fertil. Steril. 228*:446–447, 1977.
38. D. M. Mumford, H. L. Gordon, R. Ansbacher, J. S. Sung, R. D. Rossen, and S. Farrow, Incidence of lymphocytotoxins in vasectomy patients. In *Control of Male Fertility* (J. J. Sciarra, C. Markland, and J. J. Speidel, eds.), Harper and Row, Hagerstown, Maryland, 1975, pp. 196–202.
39. A. G. White, G. S. Watson, C. Darz, and P. Edmond, Lymphocytotoxins in vasectomized men. *J. Urol. 114*:240–241, 1975.

40. H. Y. Law, W. F. Bodmer, J. D. Mathews, and D. C. G. Skegg, The immune response to vasectomy and its relation to the HLA system *Tissue Antigens 14*:115–139, 1979.
41. H. W. J. Hellema, I. R. J. M Sondag-Tschroots, P. Rümke, and T. E. W. Feltkamp, Somatic autoantibodies as a consequence of vasectomy. In *Immunological consequences of vasectomy in men*, Thesis, University of Leiden, The Netherlands, 1978, pp. 99–109.
42. J. D. Mathews, D. C. G. Skegg, M. P. Vessey, M. Konice, E. J. Holbrow, and J. Guillevaud, Weak autoantibody reactions to antigens other than sperm after vasectomy. *Br. Med. J. 2*:1359–1360, 1976.
43. K. S. K. Tung, R. K. Bryson, L. P. B. Han, and L. C. Walker, Circulating immune complexes in vasectomy. In *Vasectomy. Immunologic and Pathophysiologic Effects in Animals and Man* (I. H. Lepow and R. Crozier, eds.), Academic Press, New York, 1979, pp. 301–335.
44. P. Rümke and H. W. Hellema, Immunologic studies in long-term follow-up of vasectomized men. In *Vasectomy. Immunologic and Pathophysiologic Effects in Animals and Man* (I. H. Lepow and R. Crozier, eds.), Academic Press, New York, 1979, pp. 521--532.
45. Long-term effects of vasectomy. Part II. Immunological parameters. *Contraception 28*:527–541, 1983.
46. L. Linnet, N. P. Hundahl Moller, P. Bernth-Petersen, N. Ehlers, I. Brandslund, and S. E. Svehag, No increase in arteriolosclerotic retinopathy or activity in tests for circulating immuno complexes 5 years after vasectomy. *Fertil. Steril. 37*:798–806, 1982.
47. I. L. Jenkins, V. Y. Muir, N. J. Blacklock, J. L. Turk, and H. G. Hanley, Consequences of vasectomy: An immunological and histological study related to subsequent fertility. *Br. J. Urol. 51*:406–410, 1979.
48. S. Nagarkatti and S. S. Rao, Cell-mediated immunity to homologous spermatozoa following vasectomy in the human male. *Clin. Exp. Immunol. 26*:239–242, 1976.
49. G. M. Shearer and V. Hurtenbach, Is sperm immunosuppressive in male homosexuals and vasectomized men? *Immunol. Today 3*:153–154, 1982.

50. R. C. Rees and P. J. Vallely, Immunosuppression mediated by seminal plasma–fact or artefact? *Immunol. Today 7*:190, 1986.
51. R. Kubota, Electron microscopic studies of the testis after vasectomy in rats and men. *Jpn. J. Urol. 60*:373-397, 1969.
52. J. P. Hagedoorn and J. E. Davis, Fine structure of the seminiferous tubules after vasectomy. *Physiologist 17*:236, 1974.
53. F. C. Derrick, W. L. Glover, Z. Kanjuparamban, C. B. Jacobson, M. McDougall, K. McCowin, H. D. Mercer, and L. D. Rollins, Histologic changes in the seminiferous tubules after vasectomy. *Fertil. Steril. 25*:649-658, 1974.
54. A. S. Gupta, L. K. Kothari, A. Khruno, and R. Bapna, Surgical sterilization by vasectomy and its effect on the structure and function of the testis in man. *Br. J. Surg. 62*:59-63, 1975.
55. P. E. Bigazzi, N. J. Alexander, and S. J. Silber, Studies on testicular biopsies from vasectomized men. In *Vasectomy. Immunologic and Pathophysiologic Effects in Animals and Man* (I. H. Lepow and R. Crozier, eds.), Academic Press, New York, 1979, pp. 459-469.
56. H. A. Bagshaw, J. R. W. Masters, and J. P. Pryor, Factors influencing the outcome of vasectomy reversal. *Br. J. Urol. 52*:57-60, 1980
57. R. Mehrotra, T. Path, P. Tandon, K. M. Singh, and H. Kumar, Ultrastructural appearances of interstitial tissue of testis in vasectomized individuals. *Indian J. Med. Res. 77*:347-352, 1983.
58. J. P. Jarow, R. E. Budin, M. Dym, B. R. Zirkin, S. Noren, and F. F. Marshall, Quantitative pathologic changes in the human testis after vasectomy. *N. Engl. J. Med. 313*:1252-1256, 1985.
59. P. E. Bigazzi, L. L. Kosuda, K. C. Hsu, and G. A. Andres, Immune complex orchitis in vasectomized rabbits. *J. Exp. Med. 143*:382-404, 1976.
60. F. Salomon and C. E. Hedinger, Abnormal basement membrane structures of seminiferous tubules in infertile men. *Lab. Invest. 47*:543-554, 1982.

61. F. Salomon, P. Saremaslani, M. Jakob, and C. E. Hedinger, Immune complex orchitis in infertile men. Immunoelectron microscopy of abnormal basement membrane structures. *Lab. Invest. 47*:555-567, 1982.
62. C. J. Flickinger, The effects of vasectomy on the testis. *N. Engl. J. Med. 313*:1283-1284, 1985.
63. T. B. Clarkson and N. J. Alexander, Effect of vasectomy on diet-induced atherosclerosis. In *Vasectomy. Immunologic and Pathophysiologic Effects in Animals and Man* (I. H. Lepow and R. Crozier, eds.), Academic Press, New York, 1979, pp. 121-162.
64. D. J. Anderson, N. J. Alexander, D. L. Fulghan, and J. L. Palotay, Spontaneous tumors in long-term vasectomized mice: Increased incidence and association with antisperm immunity. *Am. J. Pathol. 111*:129-139, 1983.
65. A. M. Walker, J. R. Hunter, R. N. Watkins, H. Jick, A. Danford, L. Alhadeff, and K. J. Rothman, Vasectomy and nonfatal myocardial infarction. *Lancet 1*:13-15, 1981.
66. A. M. Walker, H. Jick, J. R. Hunter, A. Danford, and K. J. Rothman, Hospitalization rates in vasectomized men. *JAMA 245*:2315-2317, 1981.
67. R. B. Wallace, J. Lee, W. L. Gerber, W. R. Clarke, and R. M. Lauer, Vasectomy and coronary disease in men less than 50 years old: Absence of association. *J. Urol. 126*:182-184, 1981.
68. M. Goldacre, M. Vessey, J. Clarke, and M. Heasman, Record linkage study of morbidity following vasectomy. In *Vasectomy. Immunologic and Pathophysiologic Effects in Animals and Man* (I. H. Lepow and R. Crozier, eds.), Academic Press, New York, 1979, pp. 567-579.
69. H. B. Fahrenbach, N. J. Alexander, J. W. Senner, D. L. Fulgham, and L. J. Coon, Effect of vasectomy on the retinal vasculature of men. *J. Androl. 1*:299-303, 1980.
70. I. Gupta, S. Dhawan, G. D. Goel, and K. Saha, Low fertility rate in vasovasostomized males and its possible immunologic mechanism. *Int. J. Fertil. 20*:183-191, 1975.
71. S. J. Silber, Reversal of vasectomy and the treatment of male infertility: Role of microsurgery, vasoepididymostomy and pressure induced changes of vasectomy. *Urol. Clin. North Am. 8*:53-62, 1981.

72. A. M. Belker, Techniques and results of microsurgical vasectomy reversal. *J. Kentucky Med. Assoc. 82*:507–510, 1984.
73. K. W. Aldridge, A. J. Bueschen, L. K. Lloyd, and J. R. Burns, Microsurgical vasovasostomy for reversal of elective bilateral segmental vasectomy. *South. Med. J. 78*:967–969, 1985.
74. M. J. Sullivan and G. E. Howe, Correlation of circulating antisperm antibodies to functional success in vasovasostomy. *J. Urol. 117*:189–191, 1977.
75. R. Ansbacher, Sperm antibodies after vas reanastomosis. *Landet 1*:204, 1977.
76. H. W. J. Hellema, Post-vasectomy sperm autoantibodies and fertility after vasovasostomy. A preliminary report. In *Immunological consequences of vasectomy in men*, Thesis, University of Leiden, The Netherlands, 1978, pp. 113–126.
77. L. Linnet, T. Hjort, and P. Fogh-Andersen, Vasovasostomy: Sperm agglutinins in operatively obtained epididymal fluid and in seminal plasma before and after operation. *J. Clin. Lab. Immunol. 2*:245–248, 1979.
78. L. Linnet, T. Hjort, and P. Fogh-Andersen, Association between failure to impregnate after vasovasostomy and sperm agglutinins in semen. *Lancet 1*:117–119, 1981.
79. L. Linnet, P. Fogh-Andersen, T. Hjort, and N. P. Hundahl Moller, Immunoglobulin classes, secretory component, and sperm agglutinins in semen after vasovasostomy. *Am. J. Reprod. Immunol. 2*:13–17, 1982.
80. J. M. Parslow, M. G. Royle, M. M. B. Kingscott, D. M. A. Wallace, and W. F. Hendry, The effects of sperm antibodies on fertility after vasectomy reversal. *Am. J. Reprod. Immunol. 3*:28–31, 1983.
81. P. D. Sutherland, P. L. Matson, J. R. W. Masters, and J. P. pryor, Association between infertility following reversal of vasectomy and the presence of sperm agglutinating activity in semen. *Int. J. Androl. 7*:503–508, 1984.
82. J. B. Taxy, F. F. Marshall, and R. J. Ehrlichman, Vasectomy. Subclinical pathologic changes. *Am. J. Surg. Pathol. 5*:767–772, 1981.
83. T. Samuel and N. R. Rose, The lessons of vasectomy. A review. *J. Clin. Lab. Immunol. 3*:77–83, 1980.

84. P. E. Bigazzi, Anti-idiotypic immunity in autoimmunity. *Ann. N.Y. Acad Sci. 476*:66–80, 1986.
85. P. E. Bigazzi, Mechanisms of chemical-induced autoimmunity. In *Immunotoxicology and Immunopharmacology* (J. H. Dean, M. I. Luster, A. E. Munson, and H. Amos, eds.), Raven Press, New York, 1985, pp. 277–290.
86. M. A. Engle, Humoral immunity and heart disease: Postpericardiotomy syndrome. *Adv. Exp. Med. Biol. 161*:471–478, 1983.
87. W. J. Irvine, Thyroid auto-immunity as a disorder of immunological tolerance. *Q. J. Exp. Physiol. 49*:324–337, 1964.
88. J. Jonsson, N. Einhorn, A. Fagraeus, and J. Einhorn, Organ antibodies after local irradiation. *Radion 90*:536–540, 1968.
89. R. E. Mancini, J. A. Andrada, D. Saraceni, A. E. Bachmann, J. C. Lavieri, and M. Nemirowsky, Immunological and testicular response in man sensitized with human testicular homogenate. *J. Clin. Endocrinol. Metabol. 25*:859-875, 1965.
90. R. D. Amelar, L. Dubin, and C. Schoenfeld, Circulating sperm-agglutinating antibodies in azoospermic men with congenital bilateral absence of the vasa deferentia. *Fertil. Steril. 26*:228-231, 1975.
91. D. J. Handelsman, A. J. Conway, L. M. Boyland, and J. R. Turtle, Young's syndrome. Obstructive azoospermia and chronic sinopulmonary infections. *N. Engl. J. Med. 310*:3-9, 1984.

6
Histopathology of Immunologic Lesions of the Human Testis

FRANCO SALOMON * and CHRISTOPH E. HEDINGER

University of Zurich
Zurich, Switzerland

**Present affiliation*: St. Thomas's Hospital Medical School, London, England

The study of immunologically mediated diseases in the testis is characterized by long-standing and vast experimental knowledge but a paucity of morphological investigations in infertile men. This gap is due partly to the impossibility of transferring to clinical situations the results of experimental autoimmune orchitis (EAO) induced by the injection of different purified testicular homogenates. On the other hand, the monotony of the histological picture, with only subtle signs of an inflammatory process in biopsies from infertile men, provoked widespread skepticism among examining pathologists whether immunologically mediated processes really do occur in the human testis.

In the histopathologic study of immunologic lesions in testicular biopsies, several important limitations must be considered. In experimentally induced autoimmune orchitis (see Chap. 8) histopathological changes display a wide spectrum of changes depending on the species studied and the different purifications and applications of the antigens. No pathognomonic light microscopic features are found except mononuclear interstitial infiltrates that invade the tubules (1). This inflammatory reaction is transient and can easily be missed unless sequential studies are performed. With the exception of rare cases, the duration of the process in infertile men is unknown, and as repeated biopsies are lacking for obvious reasons its course has to be reconstructed by analogy to experimental studies and by analyzing large numbers of cases. Testicular biopsies, usually taken far away from the rete testis, yield information on small pieces of peripheral tissue, not on the rete testis itself, which in some animal models has emerged as one of the primarily involved sites (1). In addition, owing to the often focal distribution of the lesions, sampling errors must also be taken into consideration.

Immunofluorescent methods are the main instrument in the morphological study of immunologically mediated diseases. Several studies on testicular biopsies of infertile men have been undertaken in the attempt to elucidate immunopathogenetic mechanisms leading to testicular failure (2–12). Rabin et al. (8) studied 20 patients with idiopathic oligospermia and found positive staining for IgG and/or C3 in 75%. In 11 cases the tubular wall and in 9 cases undefined cells within the seminiferous tubules were positive. In a control group of 14 patients who had undergone orchidectomy for prostatic cancer, IgG and C3 each were found in 2 cases and in another they were present together. Jadot-van de Casseye et al. (11) investigated 50 patients with different degrees of abnormal seminal parameters. Positive staining for IgG was found in the tubular wall in 6 cases, in vessels in 3, and in 1 case each in germ cells and Leydig cells. In the cases with positively stained germ cells, ischemic necrosis was present at light microscopy. Complement was detected in two vessels, in one of them with IgG corresponding to PAS-positive staining. Morenz and Donat (12) performed immunofluorescence on biopsies of 190 patients: 18 revealed normal spermatogenesis, 91 hypospermatogenesis without and 62 with maturation arrest, 14 had the picture of Sertoli cell only syndrome, and 5 had Klinefelter's syndrome. Diffuse tubular wall staining was observed in 19 cases, mostly to IgG, and in 3 of them together with a complement factor. Germ cells were positive for C3, C4, IgA, and IgD in one case each.

As pointed out by all authors, the interpretation of immunofluorescent findings is difficult and inconclusive. This is due partly to the absence of an appropriate animal model as a source of basic understanding; surprisingly, the fundamental work of Bigazzi et al. (13) is not cited in the publications after 1976. Moreover, the presence of antibodies without complement suggests trapping rather than an active immunopathogenetic mechanism. Judging from the published photographic documentation and from our experience (unpublished results), however, the main problems are of a technical nature. Testicular tissue is easily distorted and needs to be processed immediately by strong fixatives (e.g., Bouin's solution) for light microscopic investigation. For the problems discussed above, Bouin's fixation was not suitable (personal observations). Frozen sections exhibit many artifacts, which interfere with a conclusive interpretation. The most intriguing difficulties arise from the interpretation of tunica propria luminescence. The considerable autofluorescence of the usually enlarged collagen fraction, the positive stainging of myoid and germ cells, mostly spermatogonia, cannot be distinguished from immune deposits in the basement membrane (BM) of seminiferous tubules. These difficulties could not be overcome by pretreatment with trypsin. The reasons that immunofluorescence does not give as satisfactory results in human tissue as it does in animals are not clear. Comparison of immunofluorescent findings with the results of electron and immunoelectron microscopy in our material showed no adequate correlation and compelled us to abandon this simple and quick method (unpublished results).

I. IMMUNE COMPLEX ORCHITIS

A major advance in the complex field of testicular immunology was the demonstration of immune complex orchitis in vasectomized rabbits by Bigazzi et al. (13): first, because the experimental approach corresponded to a common clinical problem, and second, because a specific and well-known ultrastructural marker became available. Briefly, some of the vasectomized animals developed a

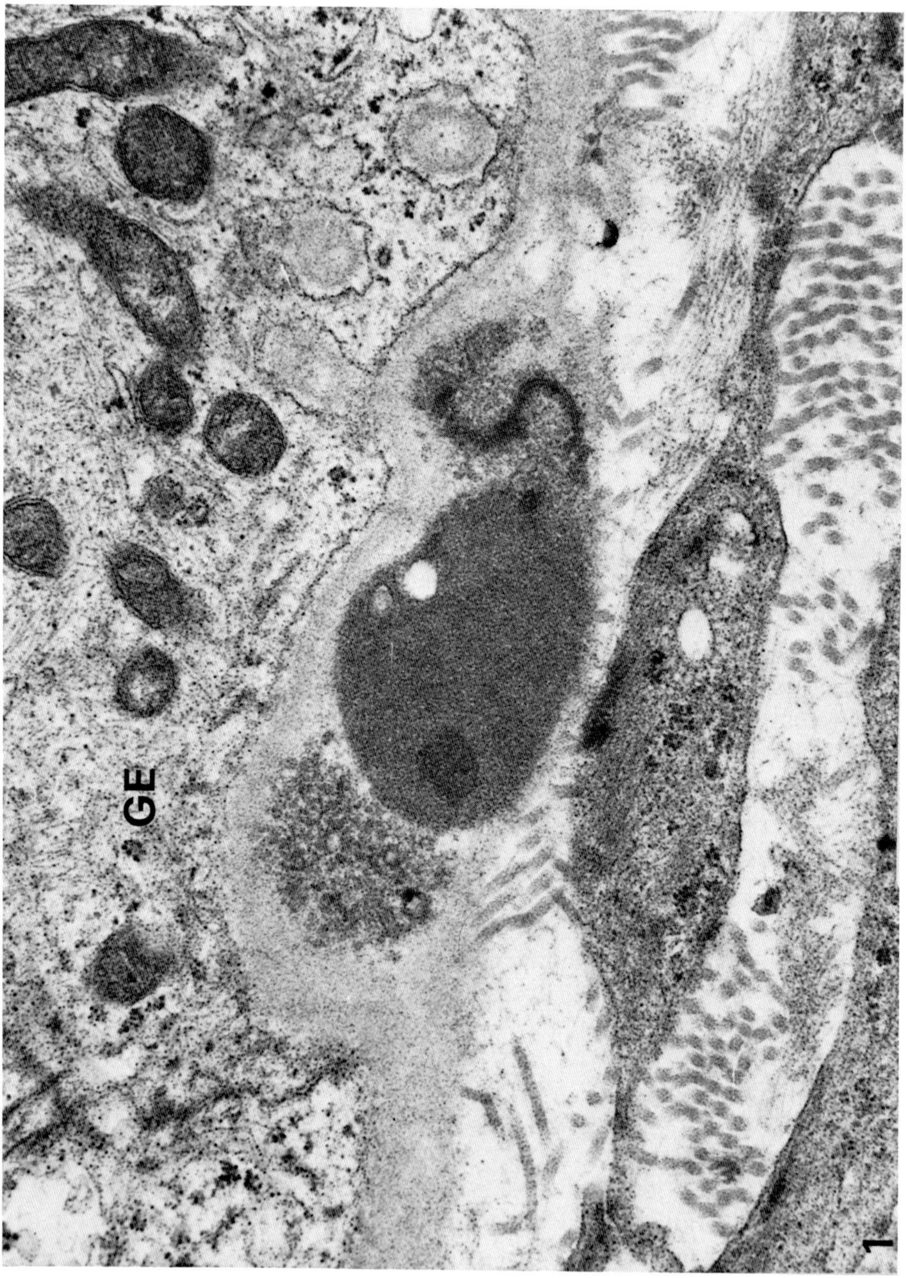
GE
1

humoral response to sperm antigens after a year. Histologically, an orchitis with variable degrees of tubular atrophy was present, rarely accompanied by mononuclear cell infiltrates. By immunofluorescence, IgG, C3, and sperm antigens could be localized in the tunica propria near the BM, probably representing immune complexes formed in situ. These antigen-antibody complexes corresponded at ultrastructural levels to electron-dense deposits in the BM of seminiferous tubules. Similar changes have been observed in dark mink with secondary infertility, representing an animal model with a spontaneous autoimmune testicular disease (14). Furthermore, immune deposits were reported in the testes of vasectomized guinea pigs (1). In rhesus macaques vasectomized 1-12 years earlier, no immune deposits could be demonstrated at the level of the testis but they were present in the efferent ducts (15). In these ducts, positive staining for IgG and C3 was found in the BM together with electron-dense deposits.

The electron microscopic investigation of seminiferous tubules BM in testicular biopsies of infertile men revealed findings almost identical to those of rabbit immune complex orchitis (16). In addition, other BM changes were observed, which are similar to those known from glomerular BM pathology. Indeed, the correspondence was to such a degree that the classification of Olsen et al. (17) for glomerular BM changes could be applied with ease (16). The extended version of this classification comprises six instead of five types of abnormal BM structures (ABMS). Type 1 are electron-lucent areas in the BM, which is broken up in multiple layers and partly filled with flocculent material. Type 2 are classic immune-type deposits (Figs. 1 and 2). Type 3 are small viruslike and type 4 large vesicular particles (Figs. 1 and 3). Type 5 represent membranous profiles (Figs. 1, 2, and 3) and type 6, microfilamentous material.

Figure 1 BM of seminiferous tubules with ABMS type 2 in the middle showing a membranous profile (ABMS type 5) on the right side. Left, ABMS type 4. GE, germinal epithelium. (Magnification x26,300.) (From Ref. 16.)

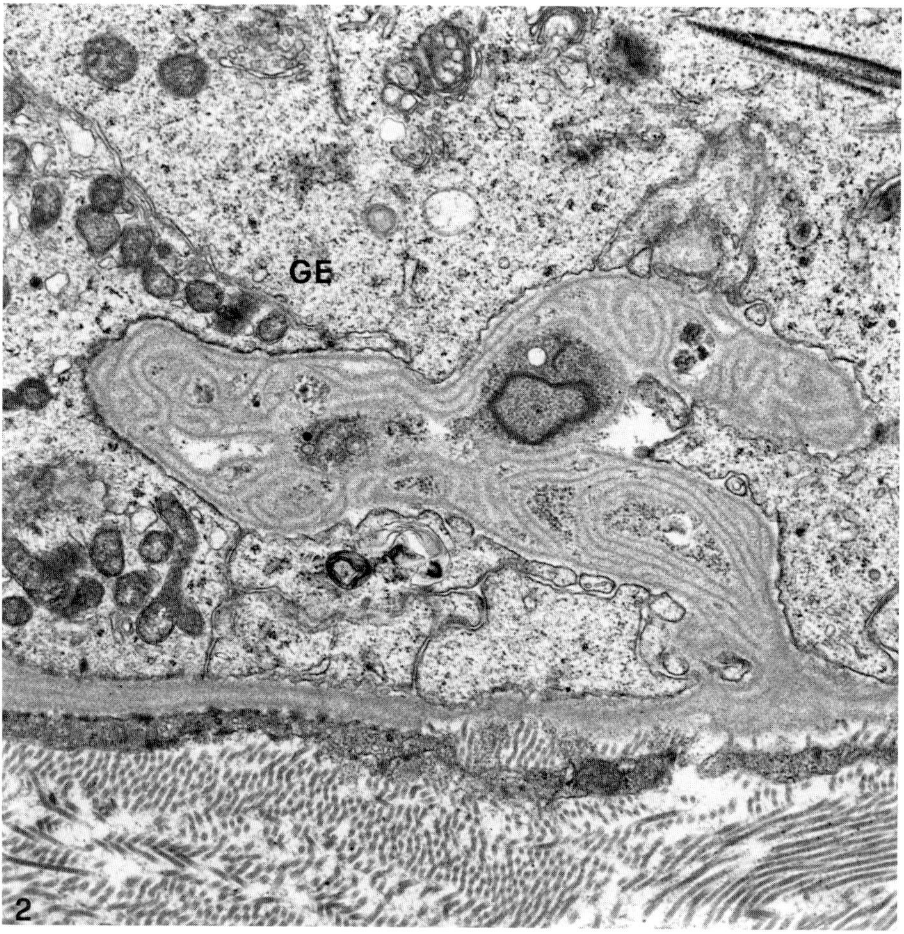

Figure 2 BM protrusion into germinal epithelium (GE) with ABMS type 2 containing membranous profiles. Additionally, small ABMS type 4 with large vesicular particles can be seen. (Magnification x12,600.) (From Ref. 16.)

By immunoelectron microscopy, three of them, types 2, 4, and 5, turned out to be positive for IgG and C3 (Figs. 4, 5, and 6) and are therefore of immunopathogenetic relevance (18). They occurred in 30 of 67 cases studied by electron microscopy and were not present in normal biopsies. In severe diffuse tubular atrophy, 11 of 13 cases and in focal tubular atrophy, 9 of 11 cases showed immune complex orchitis. In light and moderate diffuse atrophy, 5 of 15 had ABMS types 2, 4, and 5, as did 6 of 28 cases with azoospermia.

The ABMS varied considerably in number and size. A correlation between the light microscopic changes and the predominance and frequency of the AMBS could be established. BM lesions in membranous glomerulonephritis show many similarities to those in immune complex orchitis. On this basis, a classification of immune complex orchitis into four stages is proposed with reference to those for membranous glomerulonephritis by Ehrenreich and Churg (19).

A. Staging of Immune Complex Orchitis

For staging, light and electron microscopic features are considered. Stage I represents the early lesion; in stage II it is fully developed and in stage III advanced, and stage IV represents the late state.

1. Stage I

a. Electron microscopy (EM) All three types of ABMS can occur in this stage, but they are very rare and typically found only after long and careful scrutiny.

The pathological significance of stage I is not clear. In experimental studies the presence of immune deposits around the seminiferous tubules is always the result of a pathological process (1). Deposits in the rete testis and in the efferent ducts, however, are not in all cases of pathological significance and are probably to a certain degree the result of a physiological process. In the rete testis the blood-testis barrier is less developed than in the seminiferous tubules (20) and permeable to antibodies (21). At the level of seminiferous tubules the barrier is formed by extensive tight

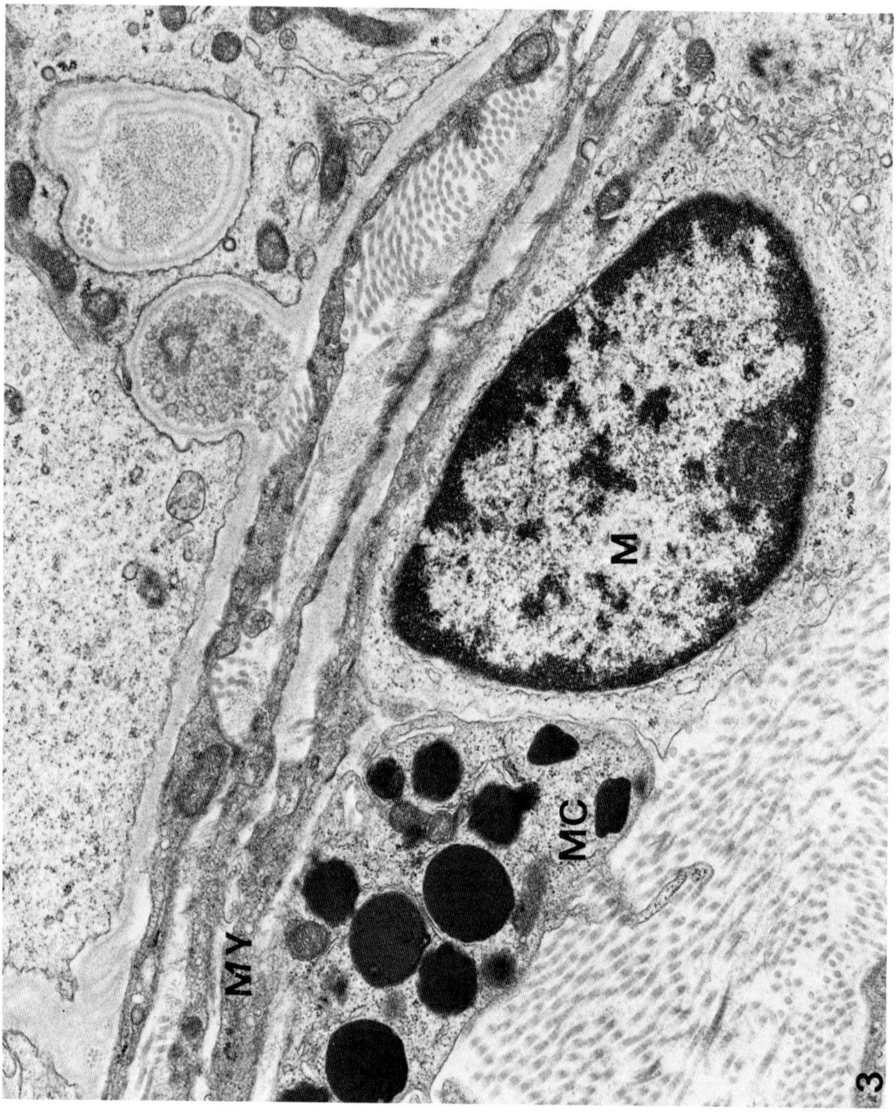
M
MC
MY
3

junctions between Sertoli cells (22) representing perhaps one of the tightest of the body. Circulating antibodies are excluded from the antigen-bearing adluminal compartment, and given an intact barrier, antigen leakage is probably insignificant (23). The immune complexes found in postvasectomy orchitis have been demonstrated to be testis specific and most probably formed in situ (13). Conceivably, for the formation of the immune deposits, an at least temporary disruption of the blood-testis barrier by whatever mechanism must be assumed. Therefore, it can be postulated that the lesions in stage I represent a pathological process, which can be interpreted as an early stage or a light form of an evolving autoimmune destruction. That all three types of ABMS may be found argues for the latter possibility. It cannot be excluded on the basis of our studies that stage I is only an accompanying phenomenon of another unidentified process. Further studies are needed to clarify this important problem.

b. Light Microscopy (LM) The tubules show only slight signs of atrophy. The number of spermatozoa is diminished. All stages of spermatogenesis, however, are well preserved. There are no hyalinized tubules. The interstitial tissue is not increased, and Leydig cells show no alterations (Fig. 7).

2. Stage II

a. EM ABMS type 2 is present almost exclusively and readily noted. ABMS types 4 and 5 are seldom found. Type 2 lies more on the outer side of the BM, often covered by only one newly formed BM layer. At immunoelectron microscopy, there is distinct staining for IgG and C3. Small deposits stain uniformly; larger ones show a clearing in the center.

Figure 3 BM of seminiferous tubule with combined ABMS type 2 and type 4. Additionally, ABMS type 6. Beneath BM, processes of myoid cells (MY), mast cell (MC), and mononuclear cell (M). (Magnification x15,200.) (From Ref. 16.)

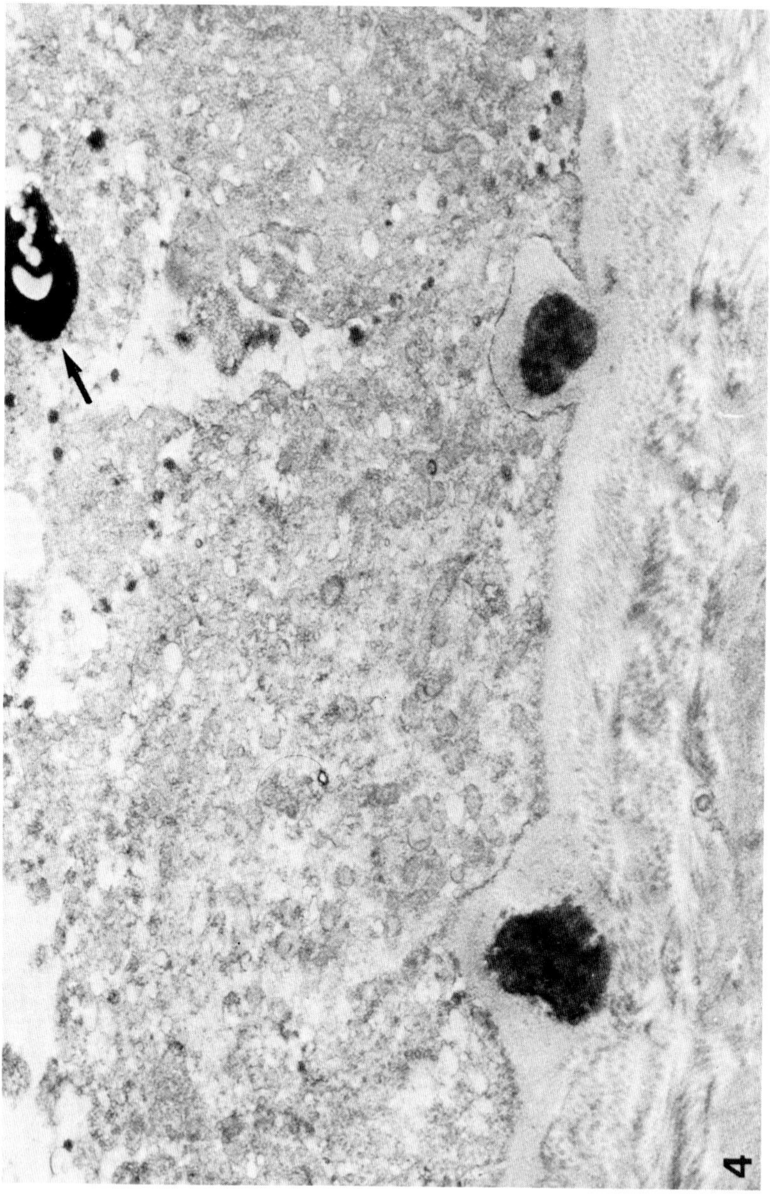

Figure 4 ABMS type 2 positive for C3. Positive lysosomal vesicles of Sertoli cell (arrow). (Original magnification × 10,500.) (From Ref. 18.)

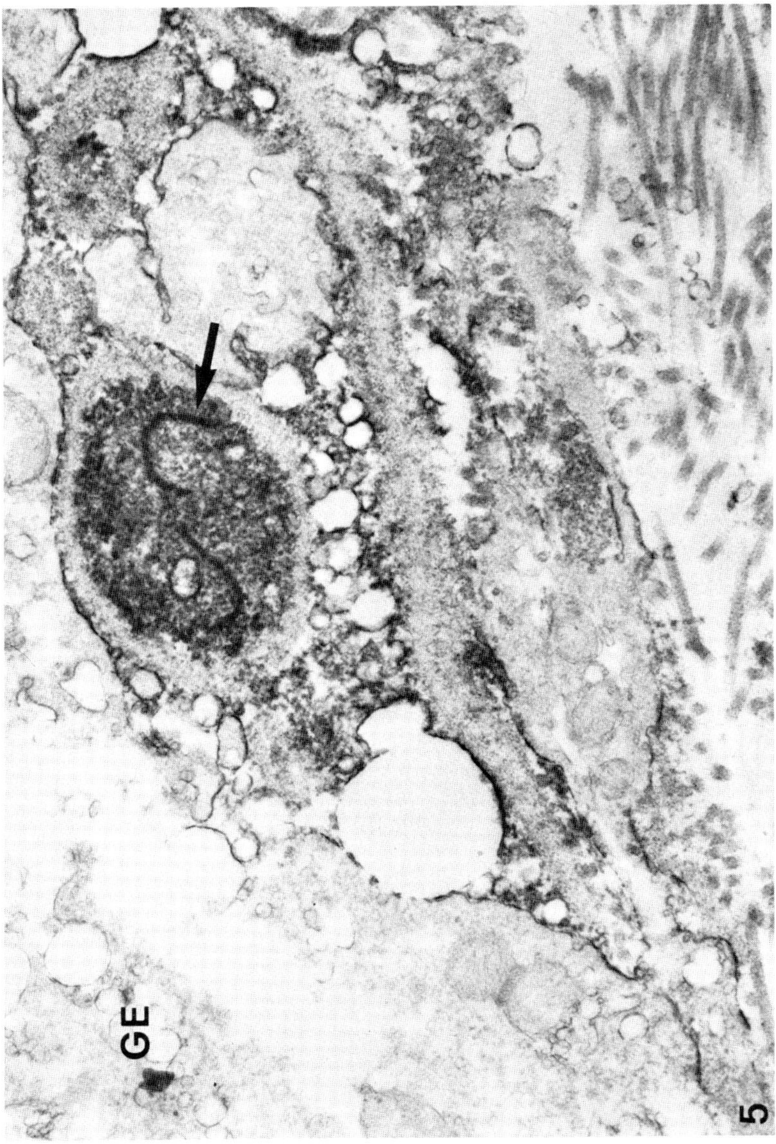

Figure 5 Combined ABMS types 2, 4, and 5 (arrow) positive for IgG. GE, germinal epithelium. (Magnification ×23,900.) (From Ref. 18.)

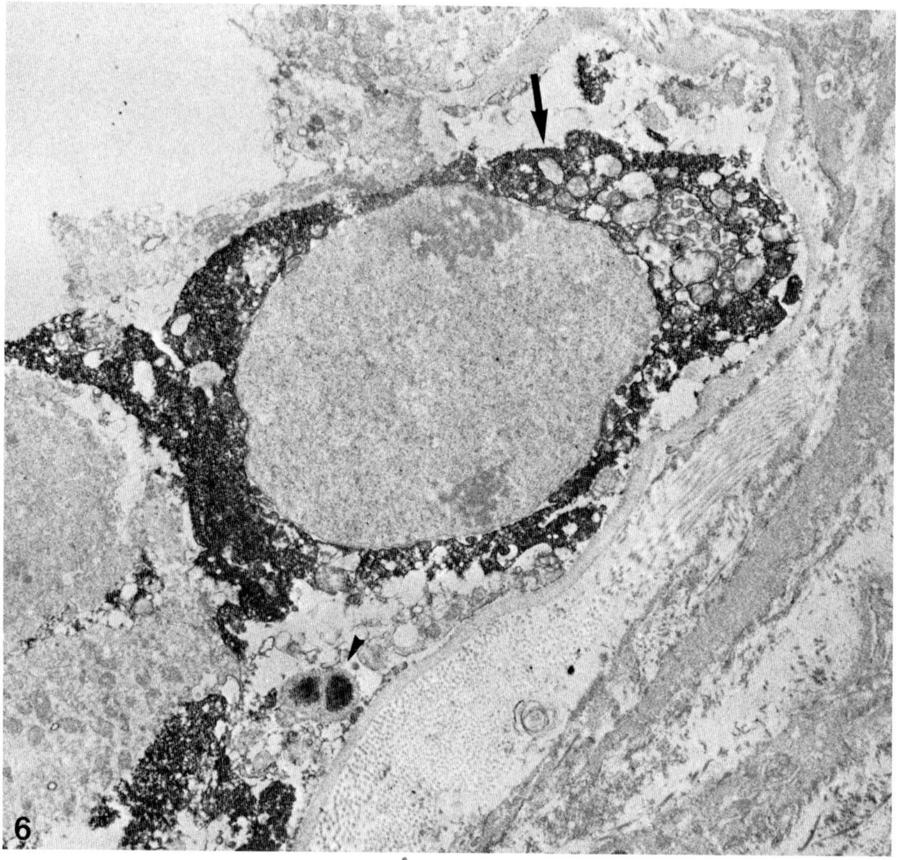

Figure 6 Spermatogonia with cytoplasm positive for IgG except mitochondria (arrow). ABMS type 2 in basement membrane (arrowhead). (Magnification x5000.) (From Ref. 18.)

Except in rare cases, the latency between the occurrence of the causative factors and the appearence of the testicular lesions is not known to be due to the indolent clinical course. We studied a patient with left-sided epididymectomy for tuberculous involvement 5 years before biopsy (18, case 51/81) when immune com-

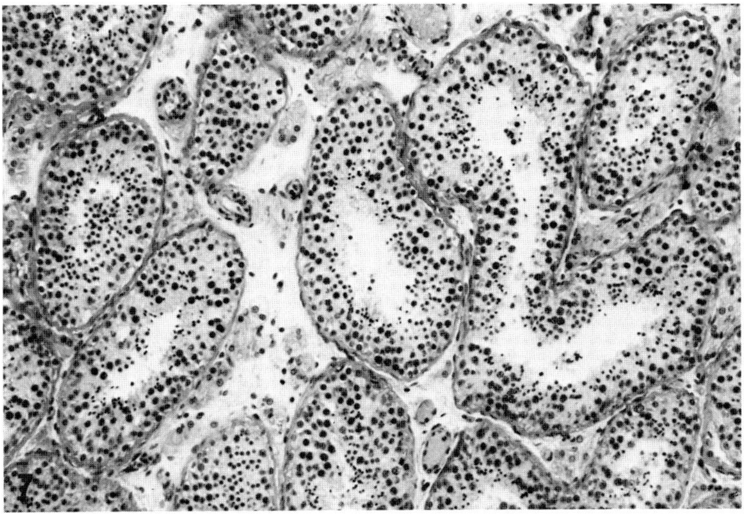

Figure 7 Testicular biopsy, stage I. Slight tubular atrophy with reduced number of spermatozoa (33-year-old man, HE, original magnification × 140).

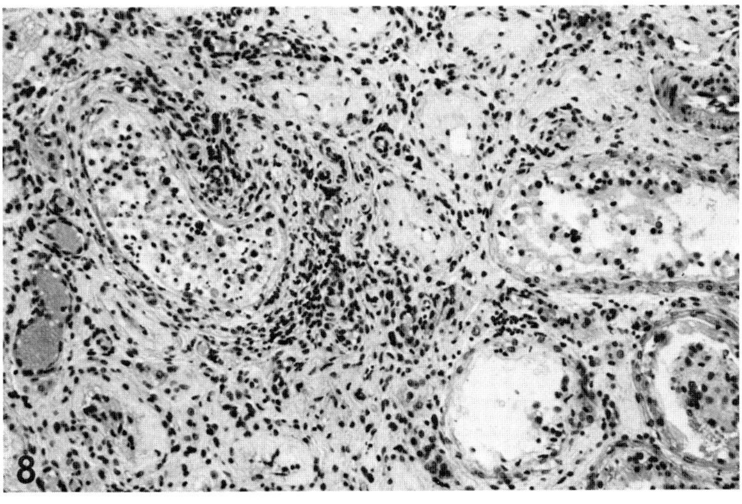

Figure 8 Testicular biopsy, left side. Left-sided epididymectomy for tuberculous involvement 5 years before testicular biopsy. Severe tubular atrophy with focal inflammation (26-year-old man, HE, original magnification × 140).

plex orchitis stage II was found bilaterally. Light microscopy showed severe focal atrophy with sparse infiltrates on the side of the obstruction (Fig. 8) and slight diffuse atrophy on the right side (Fig. 9). Therefore, the development of stage II took at least 5 years, probably longer, since unilateral obstruction from the inflammatory process can be assumed to have had its effect before the operation. The temporal relation in this paradigmatic case indicates that protracted and continuous contact of the antigens with the immune apparatus is necessary for the development of autoimmune testicular lesions. Moreover, this case demonstrates the occurrence of sympathetic immune complex orchitis in the contralateral, primarily unaffected testis–a phenomenon that is well known from experimental studies (24,25) and has been suspected to occur in humans (11).

b. LM The tubular atrophy is somewhat more pronounced than in the testes of stage I. As Figure 20 demonstrates, spermatogenesis is slightly disturbed. Spermatozoa are largely missing. In some tubules giant spermatogonia indicate impaired proliferation. In some cases, however, tubular atrophy is already pronounced. Foci of inflammation may be observed (Figs. 11 and 12).

3. Stage III

a. EM This stage is characterized by the simultaneous presence of all three types of ABMS in large numbers. Type 2 often displays a more granular form. Types 4 and 5 are found in many cases within deep protrusions of the BM into the seminiferous tubules. Unspecific changes of germinal epithelial cells become more evident but are better quantified by light microscopy.

b. LM The tubular atrophy is much more pronounced. Figure 13 demonstrates rare tubules with preserved spermatogonia and inflammatory infiltrates. In the case shown in Figure 14, there is complete loss of the germinal epithelium corresponding to a Sertoli cell only syndrome. Eccentric intimal deposits in small arteries are frequently observed (Fig. 15). These lesions, however, are not specific (26). Immunoperoxidase reactions for IgG and C3 give negative results (unpublished data).

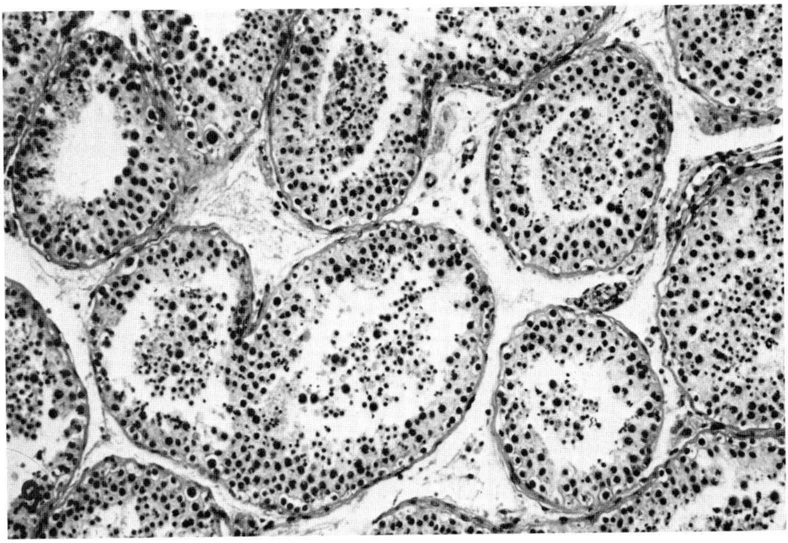

Figure 9 Same patient as Fig. 8. Testicular biopsy, right side. Only slight diffuse tubular atrophy (HE, original magnification × 140).

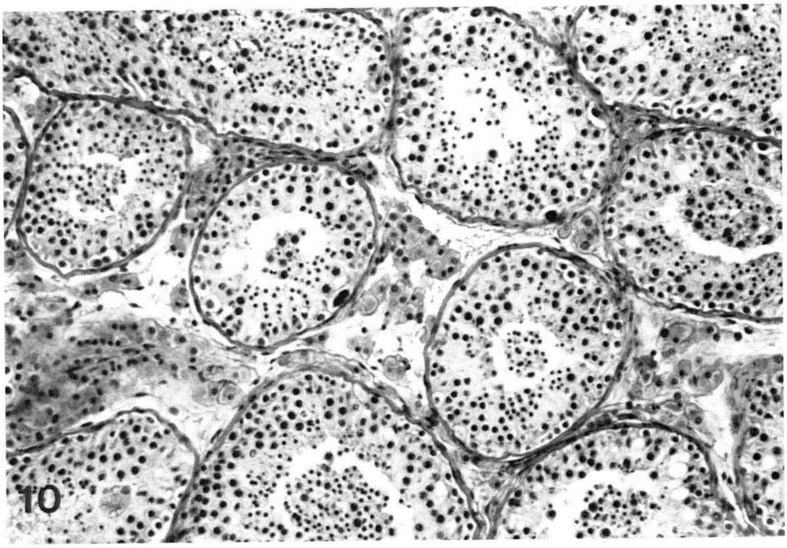

Figure 10 Testicular biopsy, stage II. Slight tubular atrophy. Giant spermatogonia as sign of impaired spermatogenesis (31-year-old man, van Gieson stain, original magnification × 140).

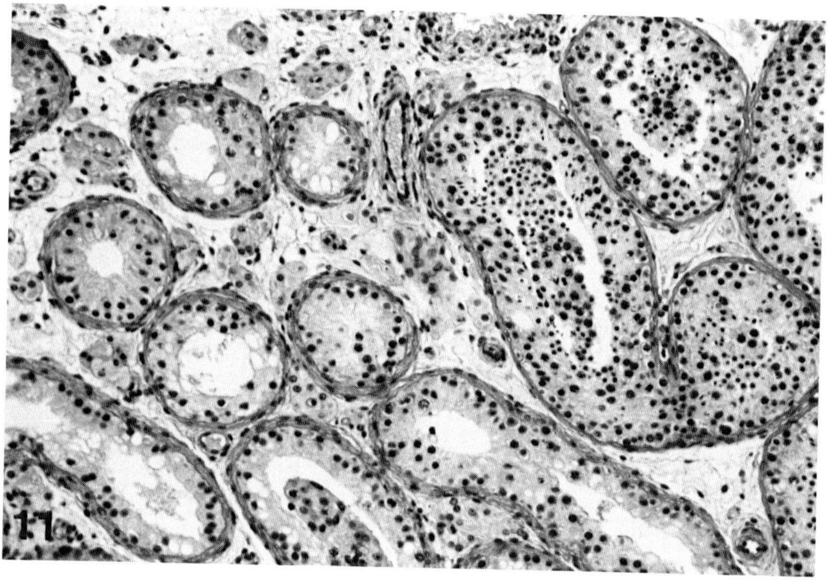

Figure 11 Testicular biopsy, stage II. Pronounced focal tubular atrophy (29-year-old man, PAS stain, original magnification × 140).

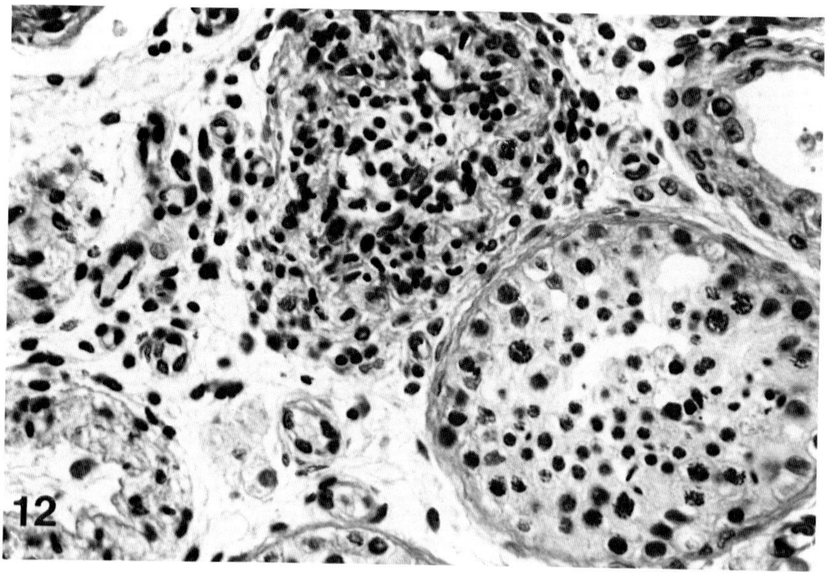

Figure 12 Same patient as Fig. 11. Focal inflammation (PAS stain, original magnification × 360).

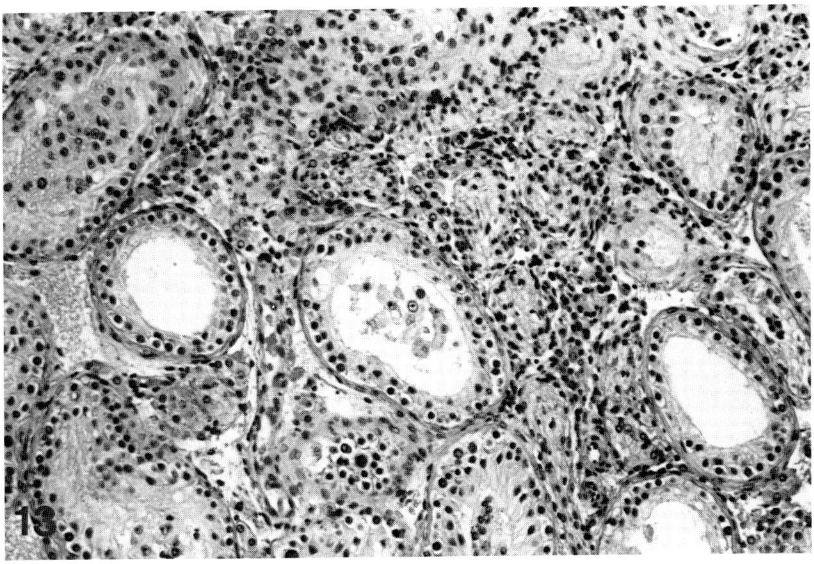

Figure 13 Testicular biopsy, stage III. Pronounced tubular atrophy, focal inflammation (44-year-old man, original magnification × 140).

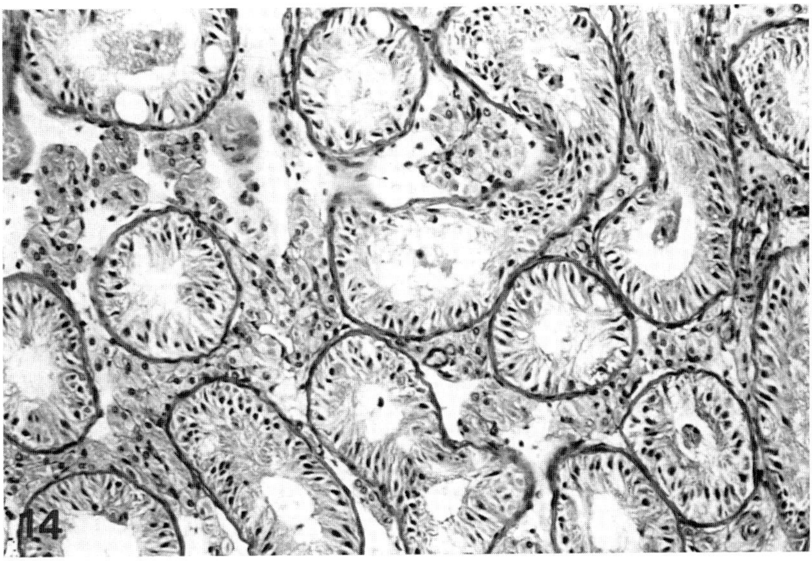

Figure 14 Testicular biopsy, stage III. Severe tubular atrophy, Sertoli cell only syndrome (28-year-old man, PAS stain, original magnification × 140).

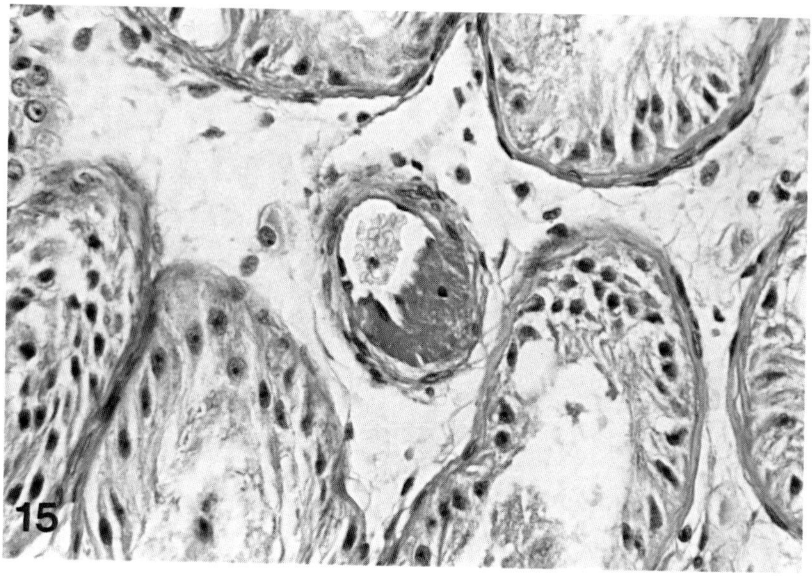

Figure 15 Same patient as Fig. 14. Eccentric intimal deposit, PAS positive, in small testicular artery (PAS stain, original magnification × 360).

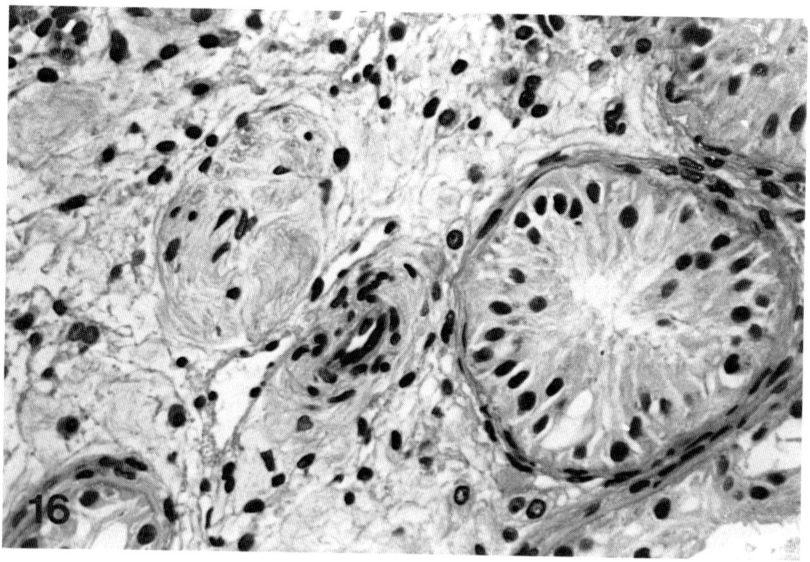

Figure 16 Testicular biopsy, stage IV. Severe tubular atrophy with completely hyalinized tubules (27-year-old man, original magnification × 360).

4. Stage IV

a. EM Types 4 and 5 largely predominate in stage IV. BM alterations indicating severe tissue damage as microcalcifications or BM gaps with protrusions of Sertoli cells are frequent.

The changing pattern of the demonstrable ABMS, together with the increasing severity of tubular atrophy, indicates the natural course of immune complex orchitis in infertile men. Unfortunately, we do not know whether a progression to stage IV is an inevitable result once the process is started.

b. LM The lesion resembles those of stage III. As Figure 16 demonstrates, completely hyalinized tubules occur.

B. Further Immunopathological Findings

Myoid cells, normally separated by a collagen layer, are often found in direct contact with the BM (Fig. 17). Morphologically, they cannot be distinguished from migrated macrophages. The presence of IgG and C3 in their cytoplasm was observed mainly in cases with immune complex orchitis but also in the absence of immune deposits (Fig. 18). Direct phagocytic activity could not be demonstrated, but the numerous pinocytic vesicles and their position near BM makes phagocytosis of immune deposits most likely. Mere trapping seems improbable.

An unexplained finding is the staining of spermatogonia for IgG in cases with and without immune complex orchitis (Fig. 6). Whether antibodies were present in more mature germ cells could not be determined. This phenomenon is well known from immunofluorescent studies (8,11,12). After perfusion with peroxidase Willson et al. (27) found peroxidase within spermatogonia and proposed a carrier mechanism for antibodies by the spermatogonia through the blood-testis barrier. Teleologically, this Trojan horse hypothesis seems very improbable. On the other hand, the absence of degeneration of the IgG-positive cells makes the assumption of an artifact unlikely.

Immunoelectron microscopy revealed two cases with linear staining for IgG and C3 in a few tubules, in one case associated

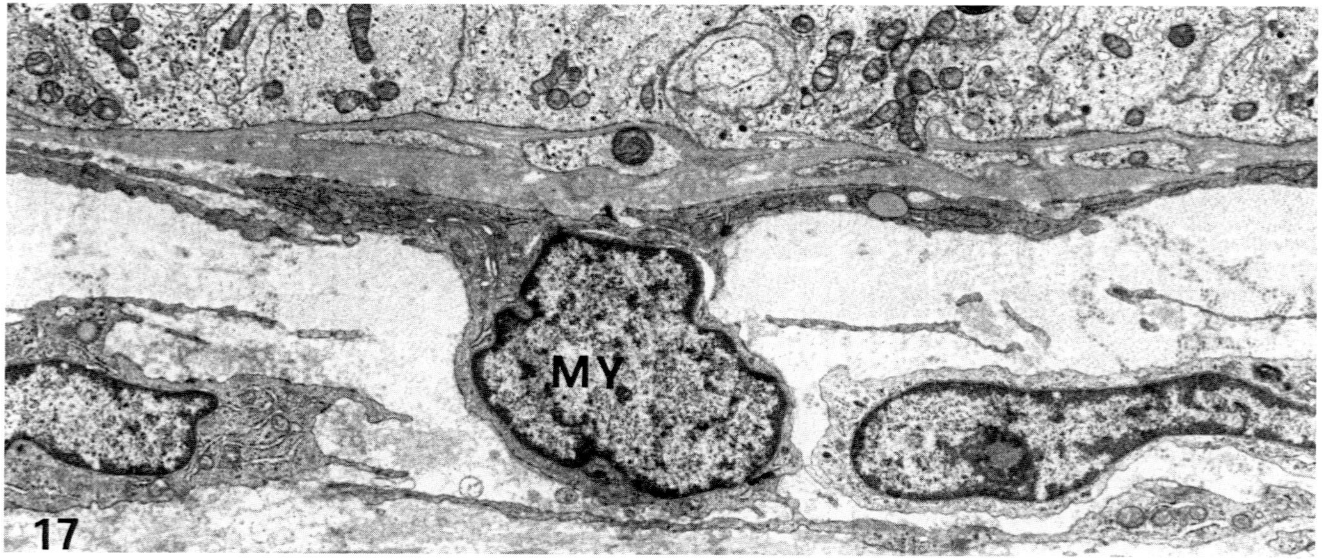

Figure 17 Myoid cell (MY) in close contact with BM (original magnification × 5300). (From Ref. 16.)

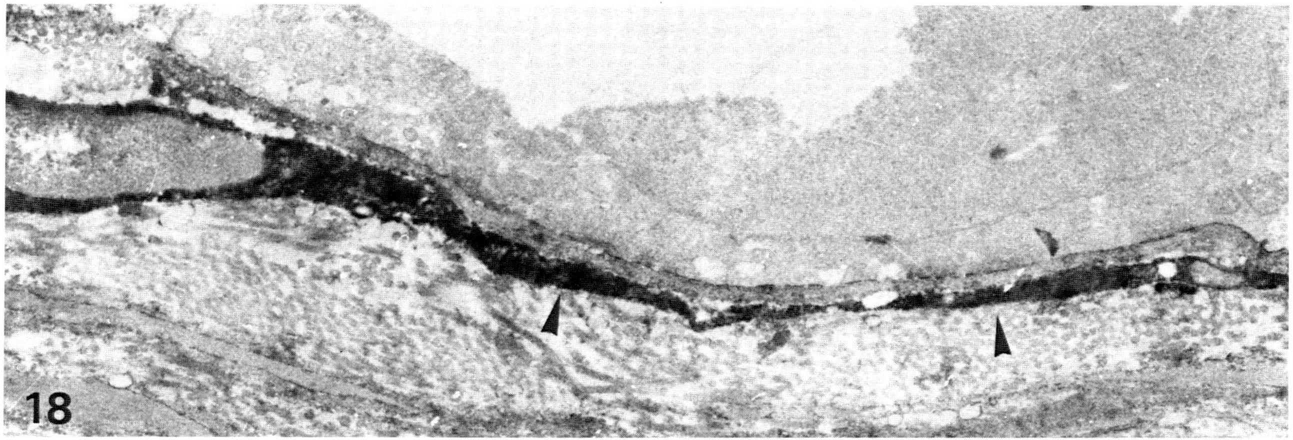

Figure 18 Peritubular cell with positive cytoplasm for IgG (arrowheads) ($\times$10,500). (From Ref. 18.)

with negatively stained ABMS types 2 and 5 (18). The BM showed lamellation, a very frequent and unspecific finding (16,28). Similar changes have been observed in rats after the injection of an antiserum to seminiferous tubules BM (29). The presence of IgG and C3 in our cases argue for an immunologically active process. Whether it truly represents a diverse immunopathogenetic mechanism, i.e., a primary reaction against BM constituent(s), cannot be determined. The simultaneous occurrence of negatively stained ABMS in one of the cases indicates a situation similar to that in cases of membranous glomerulonephritis, in which the transition to antiglomerular BM glomerulonephritis was observed (30).

On light microscopy, three of our cases with severe diffuse tubular atrophy and an insignificant amount of ABMS were found to have a large number of mast cells in their interstitium. Mast cells are the target cells of IgE antibodies, which have been found in high levels in the serum and sperm of infertile men (31). Hypothetically, destruction of germ cells, directly or indirectly, by mediators released from sensitized testicular mast cells may occur. Such an anaphylactic reaction would explain the virtual absence of ABMS.

II. COMMENT

The demonstration of immune deposits in the BM of seminiferous tubules in infertile but otherwise healthy young men, together with the pertinent experimental models, leaves little doubt about the presence of immunologically mediated processes in the human testis. To assess the significance of immune deposits in the testis, it is helpful to distinguish causative factors, primary immunopathogenetic mechanisms, and secondary pathogenetic mechanisms, such as those that McCluskey (32) has proposed for glomerular diseases. In our context, causative factors can trigger an autoimmune response to testicular antigens in susceptible patients. Primary immunopathogenetic mechanisms are those that initiate the lesions in the testis, e.g., the reaction of antibodies with germ cell antigens. They type of primary immunopathogenetic mechanisms appears to depend on the predominant antigen (33). Secondary pathogenetic mechanisms actually mediate the injury, e.g., through complement activation or the release of proteolytic enzymes from damaged germ cells. Thereby, secondary immunopathogenetic mechanisms can be triggered owing to the multitude of antigens present or altered antigenicity of structures, such as the BM discussed above. In the following we will briefly comment on possible causative factors and immunopathogenetic mechanisms from a morphological point of view.

A well-established causative factor is the spontaneous or artificial obstruction of the efferent sperm ducts (see Chaps. 4, 5). In our series only two cases were known to have an obstruction, but considering the crude methods used in assessing it, their number is probably much higher. The typical clinical situation is that of normally sized testes, intact endocrine parameters, and azoospermia. In testicular biopsies, occlusive azoospermia is suspected when histologically only slight changes or none at all are present. It is evident that, in cases of azoospermia with advanced testicular lesions, obstruction can only be diagnosed by additional vasography. Unilateral occlusion evades recognition in many cases without bilateral vasography. It is important to diagnose this situation because of the possible subsequent development of bilateral immune complex orchitis.

Apart from obstruction, traumatic and vascular injury of the testes are known to induce EAO in animals (24,25). In our series, only one case with a past history of torsion showed immune complex orchitis stage III in a unilateral biopsy on the side of torsion. Whether sympathetic lesions occur after torsion cannot be answered definitely but seems most likely.

Signs of any type of infection were not present in our cases, except in one in whom viruslike particles (ABMS type 3) were found. Other virus-associated phenomena, however, were lacking. Testicular infections (for review, see Ref. 34) may break the blood-testis barrier and thus promote an autoimmune response and immunologically mediated damage to the remaining tissue. Mumps orchitis, on the other hand, one of the most frequent types of testicular inflammation, seems to be the result of a cross-reactive mechanisms, since EAO could be induced by injection of parotid gland extract (35,36).

The role of cryptorchidism in autoimmune testicular diseases is not clear. The two investigated cases in our series with bilateral congenital cryptorchidism showed no ABMS. Tung et al. (14) found no immune complexes in primary infertile black mink, which have a high rate of cryptorchidism.

The primary immunopathogenetic mechanism involved in immune complex orchitis appears to be an antibody-mediated reaction able to activate complement. The occurrence of an anaphylactoid reaction needs further investigation.

About the pathogenesis of human immune complex orchitis little or nothing is known, and the possible pathways are proposed by analogy to the results of animal studies. The pathogenesis is closely related to anatomic and functional conditions in the testis. For the understanding of immunologic processes, the means by which the sequestered antigens are protected from the immune apparatus are very important. The isolation is not only guaranteed by mechanical means, i.e., the blood-testis barrier, but also by local immunosuppressive factors (37). Once the autoimmune response is triggered, the protective mechanisms can be overwhelmed, probably at the weakest point of the mechanical barrier. From experimental studies it seems to be the rete testis that in most cases is the primarily affected site (1). In guinea pigs, Johnson (38) demonstrated by serial sections the spreading of inflammation from the rete testis to the periphery, relating focal lesions away from the rete testis to changes in the rete. The local manifestation of the lesions is characterized by the destruction of the adluminal germ cells, breakdown of the blood-testis barrier, and focal lymphocytic infiltrates (38,39). The focal lesions often encountered in early stages of immune complex orchitis in men suggest an analogous pathogenesis. Hatakeyama et al. (40) found a similar distribution of focal tubular atrophy in sections of the entire testes of men who died in accidents. The progression of the focal lesions from the rete testis to the testicular periphery correlated with increasing age. Together with the higher incidence of antisperm antibodies in aged men (41), it leads to speculation whether immune complex orchitis in infertile men represents the premature counterpart of an aging process.

Immune deposits in the BM therefore represent the footprint of immunologically mediated damage to testicular cells, most probably germ cells. On the basis of testicular findings alone, it is difficult to establish if these immune deposits are the expression of a primary or secondary immunopathogenetic process. Taking in consideration the well-known humoral response to sperm antigens in the human, especially in cases with obstruction of the sperm ducts and the well-documented experimental models, immune complex orchitis seems to represent the result of a primary immunopathogenetic mechanism triggered by different causes. Judging from our findings of frequent immune deposits in testicular biopsies, immunologically mediated damage is probably the leading cause of tubular atrophy in patients with disturbed fertility.

Although the antigenicity of testis products has been one of the first to be demonstrated in men, immune complex orchitis is the youngest member in the large family of autoimmune phenomena that affect endocrine organs.

This work was supported by a grant from the Wilhelm Sander-Stiftung, Neustadt, Donau.

REFERENCES

1. K. S. K. Tung, *Dev. Immunol. 9*:34 (1980).
2. A. Isidori, F. Dondero, and D. Lombardo, *Experientia 26*:1375 (1970).
3. W. Michalkiewicz, K. Mietkiewski, T. Rucki, and J. B. Warchol, *Folia Histochem. Cytochem.* (*Krakow*) *9*:277 (1971).
4. F. Dondero and A. Isidori, *Ann. Endocrinol. 33*:417 (1972).
5. G. Pousset, D. Andre, J. C. Monier, M. Cognat, and Z. Papathanassiou, *Lion Med. 228*:255 (1972).
6. G. Lüders, *Med. Welt 27*:1086 (1976).
7. S. M. Girgis, E. M. Ekladios, and M. M. Melek, *J. Egypt. Med. Assoc. 60*:351 (1977).
8. B. S. Rabin, H. R. Nankin, and P. Troen, in *The Testis in*

Normal and Infertile Men (P. Troen and H. R. Nankin, eds.), Raven Press, New York, 1977, p. 435.
9. T. A. Taylor, D. G. Scott, C. K. Anderson, N. Jones, and P. A. H. Stewart, *Br. J. Urol. 50*:419 (1978).
10. H. Vu Van, J. A. Grimaud, and M. Cognat, *Arch. Androl. 1*:351 (1978).
11. M. Jadot-van de Casseye, G. de Bled, W. Gepts, and R. Schoysman, *Andrologia 12*:122 (1980).
12. J. Morenz and H. Donat, *Int. J. Fertil. 26*:94, (1981).
13. P. E. Bigazzi, L. L. Kosuda, K. C. Hsu, and G. A. Andres, *J. Exp. Med. 143*:382 (1976).
14. K. S. K. Tung, L. Ellis, C. Teuscher, A. Meng, J. C. Blaustein, S. Kohno, and R. Howell, *J. Exp. Med. 154*:1016 (1981).
15. L. D. Marsh and N. J. Alexander, *Am. J. Pathol. 107*:310 (1982).
16. F. Salomon and C. E. Hedinger, *Lab. Invest. 47*:543 (1982).
17. S. Olsen, S.-O. Bohman, and V. P. Petersen, *Lab. Invest. 30*:176 (1974).
18. F. Salomon, P. Saremaslani, M. Jakob, and C. E. Hedinger, *Lab. Invest. 47*:555 (1982).
19. T. Ehrenreich and J. Churg, *Pathol. Annu. 3*:145 (1968).
20. F. Suzuki and T. Nagano, *Anat. Rec. 191*:503 (1978).
21. K. S. K. Tung, E. R. Unanue, and F. J. Dixon, *J. Immunol. 106*:1463 (1971).
22. T. Nagano and F. Suzuki, *Cell Tissue Res. 166*:37 (1976).
23. D. W. Fawcett, in *Vasectomy: Immunologic and Pathophysiologic Effects in Animals and Men* (I. H. Lepow and R. Crozier, eds.), Academic Press, New York, 1979, p. 3.
24. L. Fainboim, C. N. Barrera, and R. E. Mancini, *Andrologia 8*:243 (1976).
25. R. G. Harrison, D. I. Lewis-Jones, M. J. Moreno de Marval, and R. C. Connolly, *Lancet 2*:723, (1981).
26. D. Frei and C. Hedinger, *Virchows Arch.* [*Pathol. Anat.*] *381*:269 (1979).
27. J. T. Willson, N. A. Jones, S. Katsh, and S. W. Smith, *Anat. Rec. 176*:85 (1973).
28. G. B. Pierce and P. K. Nakane, *Lab. Invest. 21*:27 (1969).
29. L. Lustig, B. Denduchis, N. N. Gonzales, and R. P. Puig, *Arch. Androl. 1*:333 (1978).

30. J. Klassen, C. Elwood, A. L. Grossberg, F. Milgrom, M. Montes, M. Sepulveda, and G. A. Andres, *N. Engl. J. Med. 290*: 1340 (1974).
31. S. Mathur, H. O. Williamson, E. R. Baker, and H. H. Fudenberg, *Am. J. Obstet. Gynecol. 140*:923 (1981).
32. R. T. McCluskey, in *Pathology of the Kidney* (R. H. Heptinstall, ed.), Little, Brown, Boston, 1983, p. 301.
33. G. A. Voisin and F. Toullet, *Folia Allergol. 18*:310 (1971).
34. G. Mikuz and I. Damjanov, *Pathol. Annu. 17*:101 (1982).
35. T. Nagano and K. Okumura, *Virchows Arch.* [*Cell. Pathol.*] *14*:223 (1973).
36. J. A. Andrada, F. von der Walde, J. C. Hoschoian, E. Comini, and E. Mancini, *Andrologia 9*:207 (1977).
37. U. Hurtenbach, F. Morgenstern, and D. Bennett, *J. Exp. Med. 151*:827 (1980).
38. M. H. Johnson, *J. Reprod. Fertil. 22*:119 (1970).
39. S. Kohno, J. A. Munoz, T. M. Williams, C. Teuscher, C. C. A. Bernard, and K. S. K. Tung, *J. Immunol. 130*:2675 (1983).
40. S. Hatakeyama, T. Takizawa, and Y. Kawahara, *Acta Pathol. Jpn. 29*:901 (1979).
41. B. Fjällbrant, *J. Reprod. Fertil. 43*:145 (1975).

7
Treatment of Immunologic Infertility in Men

JAN FRIBERG

Mount Sinai Hospital Medical Center
and Rush Medical College
Chicago, Illinois

The clinical concept of autoimmunity to spermatozoa in men was introduced in 1954 by Wilson (1) in the United States and Rümke (2) in Holland. Prior to 1954, the presence of isoimmunity in the human (production of sperm antibodies in females) as well as the immunogenicity of sperm after injection into experimental animals had been well documented and studied for over 50 years. However, the induction of immunity in females as well as after injection of sperm into experimental animals is fundamentally different from the concept of an autoimmune phenomenon in the male. It is quite likely that different types of antibodies would be produced under such circumstances, and also the approach to treatment of isoimmunized women is different. Therefore, it is important to emphasize that this presentation only refers to autoimmunity in men.

I. FREQUENCY OF SPERM ANTIBODIES IN MEN

The first more comprehensive study of the presence of sperm antibodies in men was represented by Rümke and Hellinga (3), who studied 2015 unselected infertile men. They found that approximately 3% of these men had sperm-agglutinating antibodies in their serum in a titer of more than 1:32, whereas such high titers were never seen among 416 fertile men. Approximately one-third of these patients were azoospermic, one-third oligozoospermic, and one-third normozoospermic.

A few years later, Fjällbrant (4–6) published a comprehensive evaulation of sperm-agglutinating and sperm-immobilizing antibodies in unselected infertile men as well as fertile men and blood donors. He came to approximately the same conclusion as previously found by Rümke and Hellinga and noted that 7% of the infertile men and 2½% of the fertile men had sperm antibodies in their serum. Low titers were noted among both fertile and infertile men, whereas high titers were significantly more often found among the infertile men. However, it must be pointed out that, occasionally, fertile men were found to have a titer above 1:32. In principle most of the subsequent studies have supported the findings in these early studies (7–13).

II. PROGNOSIS FOR FERTILITY IN MEN WITH SPERM ANTIBODIES

Very few follow-up studies have been reported in the literature on men with sperm-agglutinating antibodies in serum. The only comprehensive study was performed by Rümke et al. (14), who followed 133 men previously found to have sperm-agglutinating antibodies in serum and recorded the fertility status of these men. It was noted that the partners of men with a serum titer above 1:512 never achieved pregnancy whereas men with serum titers 1:64 to 1:256 occassionally were able to induce a conception. With the use of lifetime tables, these authors were able to document that with titers less than 1:32 pregnancy rates were reasonably good, whereas with moderate titers it decreased significantly, and with titers above to 1:512 no conception was recorded and sterility was considered present (Table 1). This study referred to serum titers, and only isolated reports have been related to a simultaneous

Table 1 Clinical Evaluation of Sperm-Agglutinating Antibodies in Serum[a]

	Titer range			
	⩽ 1:16	⩽ 1:32	1:64–1:512	⩾ 1:1024
Serum				
clinical interpretation		Minor interference with fertility	Markedly decreases fertility	Probability sterility
clinical approach		May not need any treatment	Suggest treatment	Recommend treatment
Seminal fluid				
clinical interpretation	Markedly decreased fertility	Probability sterility		
clinical approach	Suggest treatment	Recommend treatment		

[a]Clinical evaluation of a reported sperm-agglutinating antibody titer in serum and seminal fluid. If both a serum and seminal fluid titer are present, the seminal fluid titer appears to be more important than the serum titer.

evaluation of both serum and seminal fluid titers of sperm-agglutinating antibodies. However, Husted and Hjort (15) followed 26 men with high serum titers and moderate to low seminal fluid titers and reported that a conception occurred in the partners of three men in whom the highest seminal fluid titers were 1:16.

III. CLINICAL EVALUATION

In the clinical evaluation of men with sperm-agglutinating antibodies in serum, it is important to consider the serum titer as well as the seminal fluid titer. Since the degree of autoagglutination in the ejaculate seems to be closely related to the invasion of spermatozoa into the cervical mucus both in vivo and vitro, the degree of autoagglutination is important to record. It is quite likely that the amount of antibodies attached to spermatozoa in the ejaculate as determined by the MAR test would be clinically significant, and such evaluations are recommended. Since sometimes a determination of autoagglutination in the ejaculate or the performance of MAR test is difficult to obtain, a postcoital test with evaluation of invasion of spermatozoa into the cervical mucus would be important. Some clinical guidelines for the patient with sperm-agglutinating antibodies would therefore be possible to give, and this information should serve as a baseline for the selection of patients for treatment (Table 2). From a clinical point of view it has been noted that men with antibody titers of less than 1:32 may only have a slightly reduced chance of conception and the importance of the treatment of these men needs further study. However, sterility is considered the case if the titer is above 1:512, and here treatment is essential.

It is also important to consider the findings in the ejaculate in the clinical evaluation of men with sperm-agglutinating the antibodies. In men with an oligozoospermia and a moderate to low serum and seminal fluid titer of antibodies, even a low titer may be quite important in inducing poor function of the spermatozoa. In men with a high sperm count and moderate to high serum titers but a low antibody titer in seminal fluid, enough free and unaf-

Table 2 Chances to Achieve a Pregnancy[a]

	After attempting pregnancy for	
Titer of sperm-agglutinating antibody in serum	5 years (% pregnancy)	10 years (% pregnancy)
⩽1:32	26	46
1:64–1:512	5	15
⩾1:1024	0	0

[a]Prognosis for fertility in men with circulating sperm-agglutinating antibodies.
Source: From Rümke et al., 1974 (14).

fected spermatozoa may be present so that the function of the spermatozoa is almost normal.

IV. TREATMENTS

For many years after the discovery of sperm autoimmunity in men, no effective treatment was available. However, over the past 10 years this situation has changed quite considerably and the physician treating the couple in which the male partner has sperm autoimmunity as a likely cause for the infertility now has several different reasonably effective treatments from which to choose.

V. TREATMENT OF MEN WITH PROSTATITIS OR EPIDIDYMITIS

In the clinical histories of men with sperm antibodies, it is frequently noticed that the presence of a genital infection is not uncommon (16). The etiologic association between sperm antibodies and genital infection has not been well established, but it is easy to assume that an obstruction with extravasation of spermatozoa may occur if a severe prostatitis or epididymitis causes edema and obstruction in the wall of the efferent sperm transportation pathways. In association with these infections, sperm antibody production has been seen to develop and, after healing of the infection, spontaneous disappearance of the antibodies has been noted (17). It appears, however, to be more usual that the antibodies persist, a phenomenon related to the possible persistence of a low-grade infection. The infection may also serve as an adjuvant and promote the development of sperm antibodies.

Several authors have reported that if intensive antibiotic treatment of chronic prostatitis is given the antibody titer sometimes may decrease. However, the decreased antibody titer does not always seem to be equal to a return of fertility, but in a series of patients studied by Fjällbrant and Nilsson (18) a decrease in the antibody titers occurred after long and extensive treatment with different antibiotics as well as low doses of methyltestosterone. Here, treatment periods of up to 6 months were used; in eight men a marked drop in the serum titer of sperm-agglutinating antibodies was noted, and in five couples with improved sperm penetration of the cervical mucus a conception was reported.

In view of the fact that sperm antibodies seem to be fairly frequently associated with a genital infection, aggressive treatment of these infections at an early stage seems to be important. Prolonged treatment if symptoms do not immediately disappear is of outmost importance, and treatment for 6–12 months may be necessary as the titers may not start to decrease until after such long treatment periods. The coexistence of an infection in the female partner should also be considered by the treating physician so that a simultaneous treatment of both partners, when applicable, should be performed.

VI. SURGICAL CORRECTION

When the clinical examination of men with sperm antibodies indicates the presence of damaged or degenerated testicular tissue or abnormalities of the epidydimis, it may be appropriate to perform a surgical correction of this abnormality in the hope that the antibody titers would decrease following surgery. Rümke and Hellinga

(3) removed one atrophied testis from an infertile man but noticed no change in the antibody titer. However, Bandhauer (17) reported the removal of an epididymal cyst from one man and an epididymectomy in another man with tuberculosis epididymitis that resulted in a subsequent decrease in the sperm antibody tiers, but whether this resulted in an effect on the fertility of the men was not reported. A similar patient who had developed cytotoxic sperm antibodies after epididymoorchitis had a disappearance of these antibodies that took place after orchiectomy and a normalization of the sperm sample during a 9-month follow-up after the surgery (19).

In an evaluation of men with high titers of circulating sperm-agglutinating antibodies but normal sperm samples, Friberg and Fritiofsson (20) noted that several of these men had a previous inguinal herniorrhaphy. From this selected group, 10 men underwent surgical exploration of the area where the herniorrhaphy had been performed. In 5 men normal anatomy was recorded, but in the other 5 a unilateral obstruction of the vas deferens was noted. In 4 of these men reconstructive surgery with re-establishment of patency in the vas deferns was possible to perform, and these men were followed for over a year after the surgical procedure. None of the men showed any change in the serum or seminal fluid antibody titers after the surgery and no conceptions were reported in the female partners during the observation period.

Surgical treatment of infertile men with sperm antibodies cannot at present be considered realistic to induce fertility. However, certain subgroups may be identified who may be suitable for surgical correction, perhaps in combination with some of the treatments suggested below.

VII. SPERM WASHING AND INTRAUTERINE INSEMINATION

The area in the male genital tract where antibodies against spermatozoa are produced is at present unknown. It has been suggested that the antibodies are both produced locally and secreted from the circulation in the prostatic gland (21) but it has also been reported that sperm antibodies may be synthetized all along the male reproductive genital tract (22,23). If the antibodies are produced in the epididymis, fairly long exposure of the spermatozoa to the antibodies may take place and therefore a firm attachment between the spermatozoa and the antibodies could be expected. However, if the spermatozoa and the antibodies are just combined at the time of the ejaculation, then a quick washing of the spermatozoa and suspension of the washed spermatozoa in another sperm-supportive medium would be of benefit. With the last possibility in mind, washing the spermatozoa immediately after the ejaculation and subsequent intrauterine insemination of these washed spermatozoa have been performed. This fairly simple procedure has been used by several authors with a moderate amount of success. Halim et al. (24) reported 3 pregnancies in 12 such treated couples. This method was also used by Shulman et al. (25,26), and his group achieved one pregnancy in seven treated couples. Some success was also reported by Kremer et al. (27,28), who performed intrauterine inseminations in couples in which the male partner had high titers of sperm-agglutinating antibodies in the serum (titers 1:32–1:4096) and, in addition, high seminal fluid titers combined with poor sperm penetration of the cervical mucus. In their attempts three couples conceived, indicating that even with high sperm antibody titers some success is achieved with intrauterine insemination.

Intrauterine insemination of washed spermatozoa may be beneficial since most of the spermatozoa from men with sperm antibodies are inhibited from further penetration of the female genital tract in the cervix (28,29), but if spermatozoa are deposited in the uterus they may not be affected and may migrate up into the Fallopian tube and fertilize an ovum. If the inseminations are performed with unwashed spermatozoa, uterine cramps may frequently ensue and therefore a safer procedure is to use washed spermatozoa from which the seminal fluid (including prostaglandins) is removed.

Recently, the use of spermatozoa washed in Ham's F10 have proved to be of some additional advantage and is probably currently the technique of choice (30). The insemination should be performed at the appropriate time in the ovulatory cycle, and frequently in the use of human chorionic gonadotropin (HCG) may be helpful in order to perform the intrauterine insemination at the time when the ovulation takes place. The procedure is relatively easy to perform and probably deserves an initial approach in the treatment of the couples in which the male partner has sperm antibodies. It may be reasonable to perform intrauterine insemination at the time of the ovulation for three to six menstrual cycles before a more aggressive treatment protocol would be used, such as high- or low-dose corticosteroids.

VIII. LOW-DOSE CORTICOSTEROID TREATMENT

Soon after it was realized that agglutination in male ejaculates were caused by sperm antibodies, corticosteroid treatment of these infertile males was attempted. This was based upon the well-known immunosuppressive effects of corticosteroids. No success was achieved either in reducing the antibody titer or in inducing a pregnancy. This was probably related to the fairly low doses and short treatment periods that were used. Not until long treatment periods were employed did a reduction in the sperm antibody titer with subsequent pregnancies turn out to be achievable. De Almeida and Soufir (31) gave 2 mg dexamethasone daily for 6 months to a man with a high serum titer and, in addition, a high seminal fluid titer of sperm antibodies as well as a pronounced autoagglutination in the ejaculate. A reduction in the titer was noted, and after 5 months of therapy a conception occurred. Later, Hendry et al. (32) used 15 mg prednisone daily for the treatment of 15 oligozoospermic and 14 normozoospermic men. In a substantial number of the oligozoospermic men (sperm count less than 20 million per milliliter), the sperm counts normalized, and they recorded two conceptions in this group. In the normozoospermic group two conceptions occurred. Another three conceptions occurred when sperm washing and intrauterine inseminations were added to the regimen. It is of particular interest to note that many oligozoospermic men became normozoospermic during the corticosteroid treatment, and it is possible, as pointed out by the authors, that the use of low-dose corticosteroids would be preferable in men with sperm counts less than 20 million per milliliter (as recorded on repeated examinations). However, Hendry et al. (32) also used high-dose corticosteroid treatment (see below) and considered this the preferred treatment in normozoospermic patients.

IX. HIGH-DOSE CORTICOSTEROID TREATMENT

The immunosuppressive effect of corticosteroids has been unknown for over 30 years, but the fact that high doses of corticosteroids actually could depress immunoglobulin levels substantially was not realized until Butler and Rossen (33) treated human volunteers with high doses of corticosteroids (methylprednisolone) for 3–5 days and noticed a marked drop in the IgG levels and a more subtle decrease in the IgA levels, whereas no change in the IgM levels were recorded over an ensuing 2- to 3-week period.

The idea of using this high-dose corticosteroid treatment to suppress sperm antibody production was first introduced by Shulman (34), who, when treating a man with a high serum and seminal fluid titer, noticed a decrease in the titer of antibodies; when the seminal fluid antibody titer had disappeared and the serum titer substantially dropped, a conception was reported. Shulman et al. (26,35) later extended these studies to two smaller groups of men with circulating sperm antibodies and they also observed conceptions in these groups. They recorded four pregnancies in the partners of 18 treated men and in the later series five conceptions in the partners of 15 men with circulating sperm antibodies. Kremer et al. (27) also used the high-dose methylprednisolone treatment. In single treatment cycles they were not impressed with the results, and only with repeated courses of methylprednisolone did they note success with one conception in the partners of five treated men. An even more promising pregnancy rate was recorded by Katz and Newill (36), who recorded four pregnancies in seven treated couples. These authors used repeated treatments if conception did not occur after an initial treatment cycle. A 33%

pregnancy rate was also reported by Haas et al. (12) when they used intermittent high-dose methylprenisolone treatment.

Over the past few years three major studies comprising 123 adequately followed men have been published in which the high-dose corticosteroid regimen has been given. Hendry et al. (32) followed 18 men and achieved a 39% pregnancy rate, and Shulman and Shulman (37) in a followup of 71 patients reprted a 44% pregnancy rate. Hargreave and Elton (38) used intermittent high-dose methylprednisolone as well as intermittent high-dose betamethasone treatment regimens and noticed that the titers of antibodies fell after treatment with both regimens. They reported a significantly increased pregnancy rate (38%) when these treated patients were compared with other infertile patients followed for a similarly long period of time.

The high-dose steroid treatments are not without side effects, and this has been documented in almost all the cited publications. Mild side effects are reported by about two-thirds of the patients, with such complaints as weight gain, dyspepsia, irritability, acne, mood changes, rash, edema, limb pain, urinary frequency, and gastrointestinal distress. Only a few percentage of the patients have had side effects that were so severe that they had to stop the treatment. This includes exacerbation of a peptic ulcer with hematemesis and melena, as well as reported hip problems that have been described as aseptic hip necrosis. For this reason careful selection of patients for the high-dose corticosteroid treatment is essential. It is important to inform the patient about the potential side effects and also have the patient immediately report if any of the severe side effects are noticed. Prophylatic antacids may be considered in selected individuals, and it is important to emphasize that careful medical control of the patients must be given during the treatment.

In view of the minimal effects the corticosteroid regimens have on IgM antibodies it, is probably of value to document that circulating antibodies in men undergoing treatment are of the IgG or the IgA class. After a 5- to 7-day corticosteroid treatment, the maximum inhibition of the immunoglobulin synthesis takes place approximately 21 days later. Treatments started in the luteal phase of the menstrual cycle would therefore give a maximal inhibition of antibody production just at the periovulatory phase of the next cycle. From currently available data, repeated treatments seem to be recommended and up to six courses are suggested. Which of the steroid regimens, methylprednisolone or betamethasone, that should be recommended is at present unknown, but Hargreave and Elton (38) had the impression that betamethasone had fewer side effects than methylprednisolone.

X. TESTOSTERONE REBOUND PHENOMENON WITH INHIBITION OF SPERM PRODUCTION AND SUBSEQUENT SUPPRESSION OF SPERM ANTIBODY PRODUCTION

The stimulus for sperm antibody production seems to be the presence of mature spermatozoa. If the production of spermatozoa could be suppressed, the production of antibodies would be inhibited and the titers fall. This approach was first used by Schoysman (39,40), who treated 29 men with serum titers of more than 1:32 with testosterone and noticed that in 17 of these men a suppression of the antibody titers was seen to titers below 1:32 after at least 6 months of treatment. The testosterone treatment was then stopped and sperm returned in the ejaculate, but in the majority of the men the antibodies returned at the same time as the spermatozoa and no conceptions were reported in these couples. However, in 7 men, the antibodies did not return until sperm had been present in the ejaculate for some time, and in five of these couples conceptions were reported.

Rümke et al. (41) tried to repeat this success, and they treated 12 men with high titers of sperm-agglutinating antibodies for 6 months to over a year; with their treatment they were unable to document any decrease in antibody titers. They therefore stopped the treatment, and in fact noted three pregnancies, but the authors did not believe that these three pregnancies were directly related to the testosterone treatment.

Dondero et al. (42) performed a large-scale evaluation of 48 men with sperm-agglutinating antibodies who were treated with 250 mg Depo-Testosterone once a week until azoospermia had been maintained for approximately 1-2 months. When the Depo-Testosterone treatment was stopped, the men were treated with a moderate dose of methylprednisolone for 8 weeks. In 26 men, either the antibody titers did not change or they returned to the original values as soon as the azoospermia was relieved after stopping the Depo-Testosterone, but in 22 men the titers disappeared and remained absent for approximately 1 year. In this group, 12 conceptions had occurred when a follow-up was performed 1 year later.

Suppression of sperm production with the use of Depo-Testosterone seems to be beneficial in certain patients in reducing the amount of sperm antibodies in the circulation. However, in view of the potential possibility of persistent azoospermia after testosterone treatment is discontinue, caution with this treatment is recommended. Certainly, in the situation in which a couple is considering donor insemination, testosterone suppression of sperm production may be considered as a last resort.

XI. IN VITRO FERTILIZATION

During the last few years an enormous development of in vitro fertilization programs have taken place, and in these programs the evaluation of men with poor sperm samples has taken a prominent place. The man with sperm antibodies may be considerd in the same category as an oligozoospermic man in whom only a few sperm may be free and unaffected by the sperm antibodies. In the in vitro fertilization system in which only a few hundred thousand motile sperm are employed, this would be enough to induce conception. Very little work has so far been presented in this area, but in a few programs men with high titers of sperm antibodies in serum and seminal fluid have produced conceptions (43,44). The next few years will demonstrate the place for in vitro fertilization in the treatment of men with sperm antibodies.

XII. CONCLUSION

It has to be pointed out clearly that no treatment of choice is available although sperm washing followed by intrauterine insemination, as well as steroid treatments, seems to be the most recommended therapy. All treatments have some disadvantages, and it is important for the treating physician to inform the couple so that an intelligent approach may be used in order to optimize the treatment with the fewest possible side effects.

REFERENCES

1. L. Wilson, Sperm-agglutinins in human semen and blood. *Proc. Soc. Exp. Biol. Med. 85*:652-655 (1954).
2. P. Rümke, The presence of sperm antibodies in the serum of two patients with oligo-zoospermia. *Vox Sang. 4*:135-140 (1954).
3. P. Rümke and G. Hellinga, Autoantibodies against spermatozoa in sterile men. *Am. J. Clin. Pathol. 32*:357–363 (1959).
4. B. Fjällbrant, Immunoagglutination of sperm in cases of sterility. *Acta Obstet. Gynecol. Scand. 44*:474–490 (1965).
5. B. Fjällbrant, Sperm agglutinins in sterile and fertile men. *Acta Obstet. Gynecol. Scand. 47*:89–101, (1968).
6. B. Fjällbrant, Sperm agglutinins in male blood donors. *Acta Obstet. Gynecol. Scand. 48*:64–70 (1969).
7. R. Ansbacher, S. Manarange-Pangan, and S. Srivannaboon, Sperm antibodies in infertile couples. *Fertil. Steril 22*:298–302 (1971).
8. A. Halim and D. Antoniou, Autoantibodies to spermatozoa in relation to male infertility and vasectomy. *Br. J. Urol. 45*:559–562 (1973).
9. S. Shulman, H. Jackson, and M. L. Stone, Antibodies to spermatozoa. VI. Comparative studies of sperm agglutination activity in groups of infertile and fertile women. *Am. J. Obstet. Gynecol. 123*:139–144 (1975).
10. W. F. Hendry, H. Morgan, and J. Stedronska, The clinical significance of anti-sperm antibodies in male subfertility. *Br. J. Urol. 49*:757–762 (1977).
11. T. Hjort and S. Husted, Autoimmunity to sperm. *Proc. R. Soc. Med. 68*:253–255 (1975).

12. G. G. Haas, D. B. Cines, and A. D. Schreiber, Immunologic infertility. Identification of patients with antisperm antibody. *N. Engl. J. Med. 303*:722-727 (1980).
13. T. B. Hargreave, The incidence of sperm agglutinating and immobilizing activity in couples complaining of an infertile marriage. *Int. J. Fertil. 27*:90-94 (1982).
14. P. Rümke, N. van Amstel, E. N. Messer, and P. D. Bezemer, Prognosis of fertility of men with sperm-agglutinins in the serum. *Fertil. Steril. 25*:393-398 (1974).
15. S. Husted and T. Hjort, Sperm antibodies in serum and seminal plasma. *Int. J. Fertil. 20*:97-105 (1975).
16. J. Friberg, Immunological infertility in men: Clinical and therapeutic considerations. In *Treatment of Male Infertility* (J. Bain, W. B. Schill, and L. Schwarzstein, eds.), Springer-Verlag Berlin, 1982, pp. 153-168.
17. K. Bandhauer, Immunreaktionen bei Fertilitätsstörungen des Mannes. *Urol. Int. 21*:247-282 (1966).
18. B. Fjällbrant and S. Nilsson, Decrease of sperm antibody titer in males, and conception after treatment of chronic prostatis. *Int. J. Fertil. 22*:255-256 (1977).
19. C. Laurenti, A. Fagioli, A. Lenzi, and F. Dondero, Antisperm antibodies in a case of secondary unilateral testicular atrophy. *Br. J. Urol. 50*:352 (1978).
20. J. Friberg and Å. Fritiofsson, Inguinal herniorrhaphy and sperm-agglutinating antibodies in infertile men. *Arch. Androl. 2*:317-322 (1979).
21. P. Rümke, The origin of immunoglobulins in semen. *Clin. Exp. Immunol. 17*:287-297 (1974).
22. L. Linnet, P. Fogh-Andersen, T. Hjort, and N. P. Hundahl Møller, Immunoglobulin classes, secretory component and sperm agglutinins in semen after vasovasostomy. *Am. J. Reprod. Immunol. 2*:13-17 (1982).
23. J. Friberg, Seminal immunoglobulins, autoagglutination in ejaculates, and infertility in men. In *Reproductive Immunology* (N. Gleicher, ed.), Alan R. Liss, New York, 1981, pp. 423-435.
24. A. Halim, D. Antoniou, P. W. Leedham, J. P. Blandy, and G. C. Tresidder, Investigation and treatment of the infertile male. *Proc. R. Soc. Med. 66*:373-378 (1973).

25. S. Shulman, P. Davis, P. Lade, and J. V. Reyniak Immune infertility and new approaches to treatment. In Immunological Influence of Human Fertility (B. Boettcher, ed.), Academic Press, Sydney, 1977, pp. 281-288.
26. S. Shulman, B. Harlin, P. Davis, and J. V. Reyniak, Immune infertility and new approaches to treatment. *Fertil. Steril.* *29*:309–313 (1978).
27. J. Kremer, S. Jager, and J. Kuiken, Treatment of infertility caused by anti-sperm antibodies. *Int. J. Fertil. 23*:270–276 (1978).
28. J. Kremer, S. Jager, J. Kuiken, and T. van Slochteren-Draaisma, Recent advances in diagnosis and treatment of infertility due to anti-sperm antibodies. In *Spermatozoa Antibodies and Infertility* (J. Cohen and W. F. Hendry, eds.), Blackwell Scientific, Oxford, 1978, pp. 117–127.
29. J. Friberg, Post-coital tests and sperm-agglutinating antibodies in men. *Am. J. Obstet. Gynecol. 141*:76–80 (1980).
30. J. F. P. Kerin, J. Peek, G. M. Warnes, C. Kirby, C. Jeffrey, and R. Jeffrey Improved conception rate after intrauterine insemination of washed spermatozoa from men with poor quality semen. *Lancet 1*:533–535 (1984).
31. M. De. Almeida and J. C. Soufir, Corticosteroid therapy for male autoimmune infertility. *Lancet 2*:815–816 (1977).
32. W. F. Hendry, J. Stedronska, L. Hughes, K. M. Cameron, and R. C. B. Pugh, Steroid treatment of male subfertility caused by anti-sperm antibodies. *Lancet 2*:498–501 (1979).
33. W. T. Butler and R. D. Rossen, Effects of corticosteroids on immunity in man. I. Decreased serum IgG concentration caused by 3 or 5 days of high-dose of methylprednisolone. *J. Clin. Invest. 52*:2629–2640 (1973).
34. S. Shulman, Treatment of immune male infertility with methylprednisolone. *Lancet 2*:1243 (1976).
35. S. Shulman, D. T. Mininberg, and J. E. Davis, Significant immunologic factos in male infertility. *J. Urol. 119*:231–234 (1978).
36. M. Katz and R. Newill, Steroid treatment for infertility associated with antisperm antibodies. *Lancet 1*:1306 (1980).

37. J. F. Shulman and S. Shulman, Methylprednisolone treatment of immunologic infertility in the male. *Fertil. Steril. 38*:591-599 (1982).
38. T. B. Hargreave and R. A. Elton, Treatment with intermittent high dose methylprednisolone or intermittent betamethasone for antisperm antibodies. Preliminary communication. *Fertil. Steril. 38*:586-590 (1982).
39. R. Schoysman, Treatment of male infertility due to autoagglutination of spermatozoa. In *VIth World Congress Fertility and Sterility*. Tel Aviv (Abstr) 1968, pp. 112-113.
40. R. Schoysman, Immunologie du testicle et des spermatozoides. In *Endocrinopathies et immunologie.* Masson, Paris, 1971, pp. 345-365.
41. P. Rümke, N. van Amstel, E. N. Messer, and P. D. Bezemer, Prognosis of men with auto-sperm-agglutinins in the serum and the unsuccessful treatment with testosterone. In *Immunology of Reproduction*, proceedings of the Second International Symposium, Varna, Bulgaria, 1971 (K. Bratanov, R. G. Edwards, V. H. Vulchanov, V. Dikov, B. Somlev, eds.), Bulgarian Academy of Sciences, Sofia, 1973. pp. 319-324.
42. F. Dondero, A. Isidori, A. Lenzi, M. Cerasaro, F. Mazzilli, P. Giovenco, and C. Conti, Treatment and follow-up of patients with infertility due to spermagglutinins. *Fertil. Steril. 31*:48-51 (1979).
43. R. G. Edwards, personal communication (1984).
44. N. Naaktgeboren, P. Devroey, and A. C. Van Steirteghem, Successful in vitro fertilization with sperm cells from a man with immune infertility. *J. In Vitro Fertil. 1*:128 (1984).

8
Animal Models of Testis Autoimmunity

LINDA L. KOSUDA and PIERLUIGI E. BIGAZZI

University of Connecticut Health Center
Farmington, Connecticut

Immunology has made great progress through the study of human "experiments of nature," especially certain primary immunologic deficiency diseases and, more recently, the acquired immune deficiency syndrome (AIDS) (1,2). Vasectomy, a procedure used for population control, may also be considered a rather unique example of human experimentation, since it causes autoimmune responses to spermatozoa that can be investigated to gain information about basic principles of autoimmunity (3). Otherwise, experimentation on humans is rarely feasible or ethically justifiable, and even in the case of vasectomized men there are obvious limits to the kind of studies that can be performed (see Chap. 5).

Animal models of autoimmune disease are therefore not only useful, but in some cases an absolute necessity. Such investigations have been extensive and in general have provided valuable and often illuminating information (4-9). Autoimmune responses and autoimmune disease can be obtained in experimental animals by the administration of drugs and other chemicals or following x-irradiation and surgical manipulations (e.g., thymectomy). More commonly, experimental models of autoimmunity result from the immunization of laboratory animals with antigens obtained from another species (heterologous or xenogeneic) or from other animals of the same species (homologous or allogeneic). Such antigens are usually administered in combination with adjuvants. Immunizations have also been performed with antigens obtained from animals of the same inbred strain (syngeneic) or, occasionally, from the same animal (autologous). Historically, the first animal model of autoimmunity was developed in guinea pigs immunized with spermatozoa in the early experiments of Metalnikoff (10). This was later followed by models of autoimmunity to antigens of the nervous system, thyroid, other endocrine tissues, and practically any other known autoantigen (11-13). The information and the suggestions provided by studies in experimental models are quite valuable, particularly the immunogenetic investigations and the more recent and very elegant work with T-cell clones in autoimmune diseases of rats and mice (14-17). One must recognize, however, that those models are biased by the immunization procedures, requiring strong adjuvants and/or the use of heterologous antigens. This criticism was once well presented by Burnet, who noted that "an elderly woman with Hashimoto's disease of the thyroid has not been injected with rabbit thyroid in Freund's complete adjuvant" (18). Therefore, there is a need for animal models of autoimmune disease that are not obtained through the artificial administration of antigens and adjuvant, but occur spontaneously, resembling more closely the situation occurring in humans. For these reasons, we include in the present review both experimentally induced models and those arising naturally, i.e., without any manipulation.

Experimentally induced testis autoimmunity may be produced by immunization (active or passive), infection with microorganisms, administration of chemicals, physical trauma to the testis, and surgical procedures, such as vasectomy or neonatal thymectomy. "Spontaneous" or "natural" testis autoimmunity occurs in various animal species, such as minks, mice, beagles, and monkeys. We briefly review these models, underlying the insights that can be gained from each. First, let us consider the human relevance of animal models of testis autoimmunity. Autoimmune responses to spermatozoa have been detected in men with infertility from unknown causes as well as in vasectomized men. On the other hand, inflammatory testis damage of an autoimmune nature does not seem to occur very frequently in humans, even though an autoimmune pathogenesis may be postulated for both granulomatous orchitis and the atrophy that follows mumps orchitis in some individuals. However, the recent findings of immune deposits in the testes of infertile men suggest that many cases of male infertility may be the consequence of earlier episodes of testis autoimmunity. Therefore, animal models of testis autoimmunity are useful in the study of male infertility. In addition, they can be used for investigations of immunologic procedures of population control, as can be obtained by immunization with spermatozoal antigens. Second, in our review we compare results obtained in different species and use them in an attempt to unravel the existing obscurities in the field of autoimmunity to the testis, if not autoimmune disease in general. Too often, in our perusal of the immunologic literature we note that observations in one animal species are not correlated with those obtained in other species but are used to draw general conclusions that may not be warranted.

I. EXPERIMENTALLY INDUCED MODELS OF AUTOIMMUNITY TO TESTIS

We include in this section all the models of testis autoimmunity that are experimentally induced, irrespective of the manipulations involved (Table 1). It should be noted at the outset that in some models only autoimmune responses have been obtained, but in others both immune responses and histopathological changes in the testis and other reproductive tract organs have been reported. In addition, the histopathological lesions observed in some of these models may be of an inflammatory nature (classic orchitis and epidydimitis), but in others one may find aspermatogenesis alone or various modifications of testis structure (e.g., thickening of basement membranes of seminiferous tubules and interstitial fibrosis) that are not usually considered characteristic features of

Table 1 Experimental Induction of Testis Autoimmunity

Method	Species	References
Active immunization	Guinea pig	10, 19, 37, 42-46, 55-60, 63–72, 76-82, 87-94
	Rabbit	100, 102, 107, 115
	Rat	123, 132-134, 147, 149, 150,153-155
	Mouse	163, 185-188, 197, 198, 202-203, 205-211, 215
	Monkey	220
Passive transfer with antibodies	Guinea pig	90
	Rat	166, 153-155
	Mouse	204, 212
Adoptive transfer		
Cells sensitized in vivo	Guinea pig	86, 89-94
	Rat	164
	Mouse	209, 213, 214
Cells sensitized in vitro	Rat	152, 168, 172
Trauma or surgery		
Thermal injury	Guinea pig	21, 22
Cryoinjury	Rabbit	102, 103
Injection	Rabbit	104
Torsion	Rat	145
Vasectomy	Guinea pig	61, 70-72, 84, 85, 87
	Rabbit	100, 106, 112-115, 121
	Rat	132, 135-144, 148, 156-160
	Mouse	181, 189-195, 196, 199
	Monkey	221-228
Thymectomy, neonatal	Rat	146, 151
	Mouse	195, 196
Infection with		
Listeria	Guinea pig	73, 74
BCG	Rat	161

Table 1 (Continued)

Method	Species	References
Administration of chemicals		
Cadmium	Guinea pig	83
α-Chlorohydrin	Rat	83

inflammation. In a sense, this is a situation similar to that observed in kidney pathology, where the term "glomerulonephritis" covers a number of immunologically mediated pathologic conditions, some frankly inflammatory and others that do not show the classic signs of inflammation. We particularly refer to the entity termed "membranous glomerulonephritis," which some pathologists prefer to name "membranous nephropathy" because of the absence of an inflammatory component.

A. Induction of Testis Autoimmunity

A summary of the various methods utilized for the experimental induction of testis autoimmunity is presented in Table 1. The most investigated experimental model, and historically the first to be developed, is the so-called experimental allergic orchitis (EAO) or autoimmune aspermatogenic orchitis (AIOA). Most immunologists prefer to use the term "experimental autoimmune orchitis," in analogy to other models of autoimmune disease, such as experimental autoimmune thyroiditis (EAT). This is the "classic" model, developed over the years through the efforts of famous immunologists, such as Voisin and Freund, and obtained by active immunization with testicular or spermatozoal antigens emulsified in adjuvants. The experimental production of autoimmunity to the testis has been associated with the use of adjuvants since the initial description by Voisin et al. (19). However, other investigators have succeeded in inducing histopathologic changes in the testis by repeated immunization without the use of adjuvants or utilizing thermal injury (20-22). In addition, EAO can be produced by passive immunization, transferring into untreated recipients specific antibodies or (more often) sensitized cells. In the latter case, lymphocytes can be obtained from actively immunized animals or can be sensitized in vitro.

Other models, less investigated but quite interesting, are those obtained after unilateral bacterial infection, administration of chemicals, trauma, or vasectomy. Postinfectious orchitis has been produced experimentally in guinea pigs infected with Listeria and is intriguing because of its similarity to the situation occurring in humans during and after mumps infection. Chemicals, such as cadmium and α-chlorohydrin, cause lesions in the rete testis and efferent duct system that may result in immune aspermatogenesis. Posttraumatic and postvasectomy testis autoimmunity also provide interesting models, especially since the latter has an obvious counterpart in vasectomized men. Finally, the orchitis induced by neonatal thymectomy has fascinating features, because it suggests that the elimination of certain populations (or subpopulations) of lymphocytes may generate testis autoimmunity. On the other hand, one should not forget that the thymus microenvironment or thymic hormones may have influences on endocrine organs and other tissues. Therefore, the removal of the thymus may have effects on the testis independent of the effects on thymic lymphocytes.

B. Guinea Pig Models

Over the years, studies of guinea pigs have provided a wealth of information on testis autoimmunity. The literature on EAO in this species is practically impossible to cover in detail, and we refer to previous reviews for a more extensive commentary (23-31). It should be noted that lately guinea pigs have become less attractive to investigators, in part because of their relatively high maintenance costs, but most importantly because only a limited number of inbred strains are available. At this point in time, a critical analysis of the results obtained in this species may be necessary to decide which avenues if any, warrant further investigation.

1. Testis-Specific Antigens

Attempts at purification and characterization of guinea pig testis and/or spermatozoal antigens go back in time and have generated a copious literature (32-34) (see Chap. 1). Although the early studies on sperm autoimmunity in guinea pigs were performed in animals injected with spermatozoa, experimental autoimmune orchitis was induced in this species for the first time after immunization with testis homogenate in complete Freund's adjuvant (CFA) (19). Eventually four autoantigens of guinea pig spermatozoa were identified (23). The first, soluble in trichloroacetic acid (TCA) and termed S, may be a large glycoprotein molecule. S reacts with anaphylactic and hemagglutinating antibodies, but not with precipitating, complement-fixing, or spermotoxic antibodies. The second, P, is insoluble in TCA and reacts with precipitating antibodies that fix complement but are not spermotoxic. It is smaller than serum albumin and is resistant to heat, peptidases, and TCA. The third, Z, is soluble in TCA and induces precipitating antibodies. The fourth, T, insoluble in water, reacts with complement-fixing and spermotoxic antibodies. Later studies showed that S and P are water-soluble acrosomal autoantigens, but T is an insoluble membrane autoantigen, localized on the plasma membrane of spermatozoa and testicular cells (35,36). The plasma membrane T antigen is the only guinea pig spermatozoal antigen known to be involved in spermotoxicity and spermagglutination. Voisin's group has managed to solubilize it without altering its biologic properties. Starting from a crude insoluble T-containing cell membrane preparation, it was possible to obtain a soluble T-purified fraction, free of S and P, that remained capable of inducing EAO. Solubilization of T antigen was only partially obtained with 8 M urea, and a more purified soluble preparation could be obtained by affinity chromatography on an anti-T immunoabsorbent column. Their results suggest that the T antigen is an integral part of the plasma membrane and contains proteins, carbohydrates, and lipids.

Many other investigators soon joined in the search for testis-specific antigens, utilizing a variety of methods usually based on combinations of acid or phenol extraction, ammonium sulfate or ethanol precipitation, and treatment with trichloroacetic acid (37,38). The antigens purified in this fashion were usually glycoproteins, but a testicular sorbitol dehydrogenase and a lactate dehydrogenase-X isozyme have also been obtained (39-41). More recently, purification and characterization of guinea pig antigens has been accomplished through the utilization of modern immunochemical procedures. A highly soluble protein has been isolated from the testes of guinea pigs and found to be a potent inducer of EAO, since as little as 0.2 μg induced orchitis in 60% of guinea pigs (42). This protein, called AP1, is relatively small and neutral, stable under acid conditions, and homogeneous by gel electrophoresis, immunoelectrophoresis, and immunodiffusion. Antisera to this protein, used in indirect immunofluorescence on guinea pig spermatozoa, have produced acrosomal fluorescence. Thus, the AP1 protein probably occupies a position within the acrosomal membrane. Compared with other guinea pig spermatozoal antigens previously isolated by other investigators, AP1 is not a glycoprotein and is a much more powerful inducer of EAO. The same investigators isolated four glycoproteins (GP1, 2, 3, and 4) from guinea pig testes (43). Of these glycoproteins, three (GP1, 2, and 4) are localized in the acrosome and two (GP1 and GP4) can induce allergic aspermatogenic orchitis with a time course and pathology identical to that induced by AP1.

Equally interesting are the results obtained by Tung's group. Antibodies induced in guinea pigs by immunization with testis homogenates were observed to react with antigens in two different locations of the guinea pig sperm (44–46). One group of antibodies reacts with intracellular acrosomal components of spermatozoa and testicular cells, and the other reacts with the surface of testicular cells and spermatozoa. These surface antigens are clearly present only in the late stages of testicular cell differentiation, are male specific, and are found exclusively on spermatozoa and testicular cells. They have been defined as testicular cell-sperm differentiation antigens. Other spermatozoal antigens, termed AP2 and AP3, have also been purified (45). The first was obtained by heat inactivation of enzymatic activity of soluble acrosomal content, followed by chaotropic solubilization and ultracentrifugation, gel filtration on Sephadex G-50, preparative isoelectric focusing, and SDS-polyacrylamide gel electrophoresis (PAGE). Approximately 80 μg of AP2 were obtained from 1-2 $\times 10^{10}$ spermatozoa. AP2 has a weight of 9500 as determined by unreduced SDS-PAGE and an isoelectric point of 5.52. Amino acid analysis indicated that it is a protein, and not likely to be a glycoprotein since there is no detectable hexose or hexosamine as determined by liquid chromatography. A total of 5 μg AP2 is capable of inducing EAO in 100% of guinea pigs. Another protein, AP3, has been isolated from guinea pig testes by sequential delipidation, acid extraction, pH precipitation, ammonium sulfate fractionation, TCA precipitation, and gel filtration on Sephadex G-75. These procedures are followed by preparative isoelectric focusing from pH 3 to 10, followed by isoelectric focusing from pH 7 to 10, gel filtration on Sephadex G-75 Superfine under reducing conditions, and reduced acid urea gel electrophoresis. Approximately 250 μg of AP3 was obtained from 500 g of guinea pig testes. Amino acid analysis of AP3 indicates that it is a protein, and gas liquid chromatography suggests that it is not a glycoprotein. A total of 2–5 μg is capable of inducing EAO in 100% of guinea pigs. A comparison of the physicochemical characteristics, amino acid composition, and carbohydrate analysis of AP3 with other aspermatogenic antigens (AP1, AP2, GP1, and GP4) purified from guinea pig spermatozoa and/or testes supports the uniqueness of AP3. Ultrastructural studies have localized autoantigens of guinea pig spermatozoa on the plasma membrane over the spermatozoal head, in the acrosomal contents, within structural components of the tail filament, and on the inner acrosomal membrane (47). Galactose oxidase and periodate oxidation followed by tritiation revealed two major plasma membrane glycoprotein autoantigens with molecular weights of 35,000 and 32,000 daltons (D) and one sialoglycoprotein of 34,000 D. Immune precipitates of radiolabeled detergent extracts of acrosome-reacted spermatozoa analyzed by SDS-PAGE exhibited two major carbohydrate-containing peaks, one with a molecular weight of approximately 42,000 D and one of 6000 D. The latter may be a glycolipid, since it was immunoprecipitated from the organic phase of chloroform-methanol and *n*-butanol extracts. This study demonstrated the presence of multiple autoantigenic specificities in both plasma membrane and acrosome-reacted spermatozoa and also revealed glycolipid autoantigens in spermatozoa. Finally, the chemical composition of some "immunologically" pure antigens isolated from guinea pig testes and spermatozoa has been correlated with their antigenic behavior (48). The antigens were a spermatozoal glycoprotein, hyaluronidase, acid mucopolysaccharides, testis glycoprotein, and soluble collagen. The spermatozoal glycoprotein had the highest immunologic potency and was a T- and B-cell-dependent antigen, capable of inducing humoral and delayed-type hypersensitivity (DTH) responses as well as moderate inflammatory infiltration and aspermatogenesis.

In conclusion, numerous antigens specific to testis and/or spermatozoa have been purified and isolated by increasingly sophisticated procedures. In many cases, there seem to be striking similarities between products purified by different investigators, and only comparative studies will be able to ascertain whether such preparations are indeed similar. However, it already appears that the number of antigenic moieties found in the testis is quite large and that different epitopes may generate different immune responses and histopathological lesions. From this point of view, much can be learned from the sophisticated studies of Myles and Primakoff. These investigators have obtained a large number of stable hybridomas producing antibodies to surface antigens of guinea pig spermatozoa (49). At least 12 distinct surface antigens that bind monoclonal antibodies in one of the localized regions have been recognized: 5 antigens of the anterior head, 3 of the posterior head, 2 of the whole head, 1 of the posterior tail, and 1 of the whole tail. Some of the antigens have been identified as proteins, with molecular weights ranging from 16,000 to 89,000. It has been shown using the technique of fluorescence redistribution after photobleaching that some of the antigens diffuse rapidly and completely within their surface domains (50). The localizations of these antigens are dynamic and can be altered during changes in the functional state of the spermatozoa (51). One antigen of the posterior head surface has a required function in the binding of spermatozoa to the zona pellucida of the egg, and monoclonal antibodies to this antigen affect its active site (52). Quite recent investigations by the same group have shown that the sperm cell regulates the amount of this antigen on its surface by sequestering about two-thirds of the protein on an intracellular membrane and subsequently exposing this population on the cell surface by an exocytotic event (53). This may be a general mechanism for regulating cell surface composition when a rapid increase in the amount of a cell surface protein is required. It would be interesting to analyze whether any of these antigens are involved in autoimmune responses and disease, both in the guinea pig and in humans.

2. Humoral Responses

As mentioned in the previous section, various components of spermatozoa are effective immunogens in guinea pigs, which is not surprising, since the production of "spermatoxins" by immunized guinea pigs was first reported at the beginning of this century (10,54). Later, Freund et al. (55) noticed that sperm-immobilizing antibodies, complement-fixing antibodies, and antibodies inhibiting hyaluronidase were present in sera of immunized animals, with a positive correlation between titers of complement-fixing antibodies and aspermatogenesis. Similarly, other investigators detected complement-fixing and sperm-immobilizing antibodies in the sera of guinea pigs immunized with testis homogenate and CFA or spermatozoa and CFA (56,57). Sera from immunized animals stained the acrosome of spermatozoa when tested by indirect immunofluorescence (57). Circulating sperm-immobilizing antibodies were detected in guinea pigs immunized with a phenol-extracted, papain-digested preparation of aspermatogenic antigen from autoclaved guinea pig testes (37). Indirect immunofluorescence on cryostat sections of testis showed that sera of immunized guinea pigs stained the cytoplasm of cells in the central areas of the tubules, probably the secondary spermatocytes, spermatids, and spermatozoa. When individual spermatozoa were examined under high power, only the acrosome stained positively. Antisera to the T antigen, present on the whole surface of the spermatozoal cytoplasmic membrane, can induce important and significant complement-mediated lesions to guinea pig spermatozoa, as follows: 90% of spermatozoa are maximally injured, first showing membrane lesions, then acrosomal damage (notches, bulges, and opacity), and finally acrosomal loss (58). Interestingly, other studies utilizing complement fixation have failed to detect antibodies to spermatozoa (59,60), but those negative results were most likely caused by the different antigens used.

Humoral responses to spermatozoa were also observed in vasectomized guinea pigs. Low-titered sperm-immobilizing antibodies, as well as an immediate skin reaction to sperm antigens, were observed in 100% of animals at 1-2 months following vasectomy, 70% at 3-4 months, and 20% after 5-6 months. Later studies showed that 48% of vasectomized guinea pigs had antibodies to spermatozoa detectable by indirect immunofluorescence (61). In these studies, there was always a question about the role of autoantibodies to spermatozoa in guinea pigs, especially since their presence in the serum does not usually correlate with the histopathological lesions of EAO (however, see Sec. I.B.7). Recent investigations have shown that autoantibodies to spermatozoa, isolated from the serum of vasectomized guinea pigs, had profound inhibitory effects on sperm-to-sperm adhesion, the acrosome reaction, sperm-zona binding, and sperm-ovum fusion (62).

3. Delayed-type Hypersensitivity Responses

The guinea pig is by definition the best animal species for studies of DTH. Thus, it is quite interesting to review studies performed in these animals on DTH reactions to testis and/or spermatozoa.

Waksman (59) found mild positive skin tests in guinea pigs with EAO, challenged with testis antigens. Similarly, the intradermal injection of sperm antigen in sensitized guinea pigs produced strong reactions, consisting erythema and induration, that had the appearance of a tuberculin reaction of moderate intensity

(57). Other investigators have found that delayed hypersensitivity to testis antigens correlated rather well with the later development of lesions, except in animals immunized with papain-treated testis antigens, in which skin-negative animals had testis lesions. Delayed hypersensitivity reactions were detected after immunization with a water-soluble papain-resistant fraction obtained by phenol extraction of autoclaved guinea pig testis (60). Kinetic studies were performed comparing the development of DTH reactions with those of circulating antisperm antibodies and histopathological lesions (63). Positive skin tests to sperm antigens were first observed on day 5 after immunization, at which time immunoglobulins could be demonstrated on testis cells by immunofluorescence. Serum antibodies could not be demonstrated until days 7-9, and histological lesions were first observed on day 10. In this study it was also observed that delayed hypersensitivity alone is not sufficient to produce testis lesions and, similarly, circulating antibody alone does not produce lesions, which suggested that both are necessary in the pathogenesis of experimental allergic orchitis in guinea pigs.

Cells from the peritoneal exudate of immunized guinea pigs were inhibited in their migration when cultured in the presence of testis antigens (64). This occurred at 7 days after immunization, i.e., at the time when the first signs of aspermatogenesis occurred in 25% of seminiferous tubules. DTH-type skin reactions became positive only by day 19 when more extensive testis lesions were found in approximately 80% of seminiferous tubules. Positive skin tests were later demonstrated in most guinea pigs immunized with a testis glycoprotein, but negative tests were found in most animals immunized with other testis antigens (hyaluronidase and collagen) (48). Marcus et al. (65) demonstrated DTH to spermatozoa in guinea pigs immunized with either human or guinea pig spermatozoa in CFA. It was found that DTH reactions (measured by production of macrophage migration inhibitory factor (MIF) and sperm cytotoxicity) were directed not only to the sensitizing antigen but also showed cross reactivity.

Thus, the in vitro migration of peritoneal exudate cells from guinea pigs immunized with human spermatozoa was inhibited by guinea pig spermatozoa. These findings suggest that spermatozoa may have tissue-specific antigens cross-reacting between species. They also observed (66) that sensitized lymph node cells from guinea pigs with EAO were able to kill target monolayers in the presence of specific antigen, i.e., were capable of releasing lymphotoxin. Cultures of lymphocytes from guinea pigs immunized with testis homogenates or spermatozoal antigens in CFA have been found to release MIF (67-69). The highest MIF activity was found in supernatants of lymphocytes stimulated with a large dose of testis antigens; however, MIF was also released by lymphocytes cultured in medium without antigen.

It has been shown that female guinea pigs, immunized with spermatozoa in CFA, had DTH skin responses 1 week after immunization (70). In male guinea pigs the skin response varied with the course of EAO, reaching a maximum immediately after the testis lesion was most severe and as histological recovery was beginning. Skin tests on vasectomized guinea pigs were negative at 8 months. It was also found (71) that leukocytes from immunized guinea pigs had a significant in vitro stimulation in the presence of a heat-treated extract of spermatozoa. Vasectomized guinea pigs did not show any such stimulation. Similarly, immunized guinea pigs had positive skin tests, but vasectomized animals were negative. Further studies (72) showed that male guinea pigs immunized with testis antigens in CFA had reduced skin and in vitro responsiveness to these antigens compared with similarly immunized females. Finally, skin reactions to syngeneic testis cells have been observed in inbred guinea pigs inoculated in one of their testis with *Listeria monocytogenes* and in inbred guinea pigs immunized with spermatozoa without the use of adjuvants (73–75). The histological examination of the skin test sites showed basophil and mononuclear infiltration, suggesting that the reactions observed may be of the Jones-Mote type.

4. Histopathology

The first descriptions of the histopathology of EAO were obtained from experiments in guinea pigs. Interestingly, they also provided one of the first controversies in testis autoimmunity; i.e., the nature of the lesions observed in these animals was discussed at length by those investigators who believed that aspermatogenesis was the primary lesion observed in immunized guinea pigs and those who stated that inflammatory lesions were actually the primary event. With the passing of time, and under the influence of other experimental models, such as allergic encephalomyelitis, thyroiditis, and adrenalitis, most immunologists have accepted the concept that inflammation is the primary, if not the most important change in testis autoimmunity. In reality, this may not be completely correct, since we know that autoimmune diseases may be mediated by a number of mechanisms, not all of them of an inflammatory nature. Thus, it should not be difficult to recognize aspermatogenesis, thickening of basement membranes, and interstitial fibrosis as immunologically mediated events.

Indeed, Voisin et al. (19), in their description of the histopathology observed in guinea pigs immunized with testis antigens, reported the development of orchiepididymitis together with aspermatogenesis and then defined the condition as autoimmune aspermatogenic orchitis, i.e., a combination of different lesions. Later, changes characterized by degeneration and necrosis of germinal cells, resulting in aspermatogenesis, were described (55). The testicular lesions were usually not associated with inflammation. In some of the testes, accumulations of large mononuclear cells, plasma cells, lymphocytes, and fibroblasts were found in the intertubular spaces, especially around very damaged tubules, but this cellular reaction seemed to follow rather than precede the aspermatogenesis. Several other investigators concurred with these observations and stressed the importance of aspermatogenesis as the primary lesion. It was found that aspermatogenesis (without inflammatory lesions) can be induced in guinea pigs by the injection of testis homogenate *without* prior incorporation into CFA (20). Lesions tended to be patchy and involved only one or several tubules. These results were obtained by injections repeated over a long period of time, i.e., 6 injections per week for a total of up to 95 injections. It was also noted that separate injections of testis antigen and CFA also elicited aspermatogenesis, as long as both were administered on the same side of the nuchal midline. Aspermatogenesis was also induced in adult guinea pigs that had been injected with testicular antigen and adjuvant in neonatal stages (20). After a long time and a variable latent period of apparently normal testicular development, severe testicular damage was found between 4 and 6 months of age. These animals showed sloughing of germinal cells, accumulation of cellular debris in the lumen of seminiferous tubules and rete testis, vacuolation of spermatocytes, separation of deeper cellular strata from the basement layer, and ultimate loss of all cells (excluding Sertoli cells). Such lesions were localized and regional or widespread. "Germ cell lesions constituted the primary tissue reaction in these experimental animals and seemed in no way dependent upon or casually related to focal or widespread testis inflammation. Interstitial inflammatory reactions were indeed conspicuous for their absence." Other investigators examined the ejaculate of immunized guinea pigs and found that almost half the immunized animals became azoospermic after a single injection, but some required two injections of testis antigens (76). Within 2-3 weeks after sensitization, the ejaculate showed an increasing number of leukocytes (both mononuclear and polymorphonuclear). At 3-6 weeks following immunization, large numbers of exfoliated germinal elements were present in the ejaculate. The period of azoospermia lasted approximately 5.2 months, after which time spermatozoa reappeared in the ejaculate. All guinea pigs immunized with autoclaved testis antigens in CFA were found to have testicular lesions, with inflammatory infiltration present in approximately 50% (37). Approximately 14 days after immunization, multinucleated giant cells (no macrophages, but perhaps the result of failure of division of germinal cells) were present within the seminiferous tubules and cellular infiltration was localized in isolated areas. The early changes appeared to be coagulation of the cells of the inner two-thirds of each seminiferous tubule, followed by a loss of these cells, with increasing interstitial cell reaction of macrophages, lymphocytes, fibroblasts, and, very occasionally, plasma cells. Epididymides, with a few exceptions, remained unaffected. After 21 days, there was almost complete loss of germinal cells in the tubules and infiltration was present in some testes but absent in others. At 28 days there was extensive atrophy of the seminiferous tubules, with variable infiltration; by 48 days tubules were empty, without infiltration. Regeneration, with signs of spermatogenesis, was seen by 133 days, followed by complete regeneration with active spermatogenesis by 421 days. When papain-treated testis extract was used together with CFA, no giant cells, but desquamation of germinal cells with gradual loss of tubular cells was seen. No reactions were noted in the interstitial tissue. In a later study, similar findings were observed; i.e., there was extensive atrophy of the seminiferous tubules with only one layer of basal cells remaining in the majority of the tubules. Cellular infiltration was sometimes present and sometimes absent. The early lesions of EAO in guinea pigs were further investigated, and it was found that testes and epididymides of immunized guinea pigs were normal for the first 4 days after immunization (77). On day 5, there was pavementing of polymorphonuclear leukocytes (PMN) in the blood vessels of the caput epididymis where it adjoins the testis. On day 6, scattered lymphocyte infiltration was noted in the fat around the caput epididymis. On day 9 there was plugging of the tubules in the caput epididymis with PMN, and the interstitial tissue around them was crowded with infiltrating cells, mainly lymphocytes and macrophages. The reaction in the caput was thought to have the appearance of an Arthus reaction. By day 11, PMN were also seen in the rete testis and testis lesions (loss of germ cells) began to appear. It has also been reported that the ultrastructural lesions initially observed in the testes of immunized guinea pigs consist in alteration of the acrosomes of spermatozoa (78). The testis examined 21 days after immunization showed no mature normal cells in the seminiferous tubules, although a massive infiltration of mononuclear cells was present outside the tubules, but not within the seminiferous tubules. These results suggested that cellular infiltration of the testis is a secondary phenomenon and that primary damage can be seen in the complete absence of such infiltration in any part of the testis or epididymis.

On the other hand, Waksman (59) emphasized his findings of early foci of cellular infiltration in the epididymis, rete testis, and adjacent loose connective tissue. Aspermatogenesis occurred later and was never seen in the absence of inflammation, whereas inflammation occurred when there was no evidence of tubular damage. In view of these findings, Waksman suggested the term "orchitis" rather than "aspermatogenesis" to define the disorder experimentally induced in guinea pigs by the immunization with testicular antigens in adjuvant. He suggested that testis damage is the result of local injury mediated by specific sensitized cells, even though he admitted that cells penetrating the basement membrane of the tubules and making direct contact with the germinal epithelium are rarely seen. Atrophy was considered a secondary disturbance due to swelling and circulatory interference. When the kinetics of the histopathological lesions were examined, inflammatory lesions were seen as early as 7-12 days after immunization. A focal interstitial inflammation occurred most frequently in the epididymis, less often in the rete testis, and still less frequently in the testis. The inflammatory infiltrate consisted predominantly of lymphocytes and macrophages, with a lesser and variable number of PMN. There was direct invasion of epididymis tubules, rete testis tubules, and seminiferous tubules by macrophages and PMN. Beginning destruction of germinal epithelium was observed where the tubules had been invaded. After 11-19 days from immunization, histiocytes, PMN, lymphocytes, and plasma cells were more abundant, mostly in the epididymis. There was general hypospermatogenesis that did not appear dependent on the invasion of tubules by inflammatory cells and occurred in parts of the testis where there was no evidence of inflammation. After 26-36 days, there was complete aspermatogenesis and sometimes fibrosis. A histopathological study of 100 outbred guinea pigs immunized with testis antigens prepared by ammonium sulfate precipitation according to the method of Freund showed two different types of lesions (79): one was characterized by mononuclear cell infiltration around the seminiferous tubules; the other consisted in an accumulation of PMN in the vas deferens, epididymis, ductuli efferentes, rete testis, and straight tubules. Testes obtained 5-9 days after immunization were normal. Between 11 and 21 days, infiltrates of monocytes and lymphocytes were noted between the seminiferous tubules, sometimes infiltrating through the basement membrane. The germ cells within tubules surrounded by infiltrates exhibited degeneration. After 3 weeks most testes showed aspermatogenesis with scarce inflammatory infiltration. The authors concluded that in approximately 10 days the histopathologic picture could change from one of predominant mononuclear cell infiltration to one of predominant tubular degeneration. The transitory and focal nature of the mononuclear infiltrate may explain why this phenomenon had not been observed consistently by other investigators. It has been observed that early and late spermatids disappeared 7-9 days after immunization of guinea pigs, and after 14 days almost all spermatogenic cells disappeared (80). Inflammatory cell infiltration appeared only after more than 10 days, i.e., after the spermatozoal lesions occurred. Ultrastructural studies showed that in early stages acrosomes and nuclei of spermatids were irregular in shape and tail filaments disorganized. At 14 days, when almost complete aspermatogenesis had developed, the cytoplasm of Sertoli cells contained many dense bodies and myelin figures as well as large vacuoles. The basal lamina showed protrusions with knobs, containing electron-opaque material. Rarely, mononuclear cells were seen in the cytoplasm of Sertoli cells, after more than 10 days from immunization. Finally, in contrast with the situation occurring in experimental thyroiditis and encephalomyelitis, there seems to be no difference between guinea pigs of strains 2 and 13 as far as the development of testis lesions is concerned (81). Guinea pigs of both strains presented lesions of germ cells as well as cellular infiltrates, consisting of mononuclear cells in the testis and PMN and mononuclear cells in the epididymis. There was no difference in the lesions observed after immunization with syngeneic or nonsyngeneic spermatozoa. Similar testis lesions were observed in strain 2 and 13 guinea pigs immunized with antigen S, and animals of both strains immunized with antigen T presented less intense histopathological changes, especially cellular infiltration. Strain 13 guinea pigs immunized with antigen P showed severe testis and epididymal lesions, and strain 2 guinea pigs exhibited discrete lesions, similar to those observed in initial stages of EAO, i.e., slight germinal exfoliation and minimal or absent cellular infiltration.

A study of the blood-testis barrier of guinea pigs immunized with testis antigens in CFA concluded that the adjuvant causes a loosening of the Sertoli cell junctions, a condition that could enhance exchanges between two antigenically different compartments (82). Light and electron microscopy, freeze etching, and cytochemical techniques showed that, in early stages, Sertoli cell junctions were normal in the area close to the basement membrane, but distended gaps were present between the facing membranes of adjacent Sertoli cells toward the adluminal compartment. Tracer studies using horseradish peroxidase demonstrated that the marker permeated the myoid cells of a greater proportion of tubules in immunized guinea pigs than in control animals. Within the seminiferous epithelium there was a limited passage of the marker toward the lumina of the tubules, but the tracer was always excluded from the adluminal compartment by the tight junctions of the Sertoli cells. Similar events may result from the administration of chemicals, such as α-chlorohydrin and cadmium (83).

Changes in the testis and epididymis of vasectomized guinea pigs have been observed within 5 weeks of surgery, when the seminiferous tubules showed marked degeneration and a reduction of spermatids (84). No spermatids were present 2 months after vasectomy in the tubules, some of which had little germinal tissue left. After 4-6 months, there was desquamation of seminiferous epithelium with accumulation of macrophages inside the seminiferous tubules and rete testis. Sloughed spermatids were found in the epididymal lumen. Atrophy of the germinal epithelium was observed between 12 and 24 months after surgery in 32% and orchitis with interstitial mononuclear cell infiltration in

16% of the animals. Vasectomized guinea pigs were shown to have patchy hypospermatogenesis and intraductal accumulation of macrophages during the first 4 months after vasectomy (61). It is suggested that these early lesions were not immunologically mediated but that lesions resembling EAO, visible 12-24 months after surgery, may have an immunologic mechanism. In a later study of inbred strain 13 guinea pigs, it was noted that 44% of animals, 16 months after vasectomy, had allergic orchitis, characterized by multifocal invasion of the seminiferous tubules by clusters of lymphoid cells and macrophages (85). Typical macrophagic-lymphocytic lesions were shown invading through the boundary tissue into the lumen of the seminiferous tubules. Similar lesions were found in normal guinea pigs, recipients of peritoneal exudate cells from vasectomized donors.

5. Immunohistopathology

Immunoglobulins have been found to be present in the testis of immunized guinea pigs 4-5 days after immunization with testis autoclavate in CFA (77). Nagano and Okumura (80) noted that, 14 days after active immunization of guinea pigs with testis antigen in CFA, guinea pig immunoglobulins were localized in the acrosome of epididymal spermatozoa. However, no immune deposits have been found in the testes of vasectomized guinea pigs (85).

6. Immunogenetics

One of the first mentions of possible immunogenetic influences on testis autoimmunity is found in a paper by Bishop and Carlson (38), who noted that "different strains of guinea pigs vary in their susceptibility to induced testicular lesions; Wright Strain 13, for example, is more responsive than is the equally inbred Strain 2." This lead was followed a few years later by other investigators, who induced autoimmune aspermatogenesis in strain 13 guinea pigs by immunization with syngeneic testis homogenate in CFA (86). It was later confirmed that strain 2 and 13 guinea pigs differ in their humoral immunity to some spermatozoal antigens (81).

Spermotoxic antibodies (directed against antigen T) are found in the serum of guinea pigs from both strains, immunized with syngeneic or allogeneic spermatozoa. On the other hand, stronger humoral immune responses to antigen S are always observed in strain 2 animals. No major differences were observed between guinea pigs of the two inbred strains regarding DTH skin responses or the development of orchitis (81). Similar testis lesions were observed after immunization with antigen S and less intense lesions after immunization with antigen T. The only difference was observed in animals immunized with antigen P, with strain 13 guinea pigs showing severe testis and epididymal lesions, and strain 2 animals exhibiting discrete lesions, i.e., slight germinal exfoliation and minimal or absent inflammatory infiltration.

Interestingly, vasectomized strain 13 guinea pigs behave as high responders to spermatozoal antigens as demonstrated by their autoantibody production against surface antigens or spermatozoa and spermatids (87). Vasectomized strain 2 and PLL *lr* (low responders to poly-L-lysine) guinea pigs are intermediate responders, but PLL *hr* (high responders to poly-L-lysine) are nonresponders. Immunogenetic investigations have provided strong evidence that autoantibody responses to spermatozoal surface antigens in vasectomized guinea pigs are controlled by a single dominant autosomal or X-linked gene.

7. Pathogenesis

As recently reviewed (31), the identification of the mechanism(s) involved in testis damage is based on indirect and direct evidence. Both humoral and DTH autoimmune responses to spermatozoa have been found in guinea pigs with EAO, but most studies have provided stronger (albeit indirect) evidence in favor of a role of cell-mediated immunity (31,88). Over the years, passive transfer experiments have given more direct proof for a cell-mediated mechanism of disease, usually demonstrating that EAO can be transferred not by serum or antibodies, but by cells. We do not attempt here to review the earlier transfer experiments, which usually can be criticized for one or more of the following reasons:

(1) the antigen(s) used for immunization of guinea pigs were not well characterized; (2) cells were transferred into outbred, histo-incompatible animals; and (3) the adoptively transferred cells were unseparated mixtures, comprising T and B lymphocytes as well as macrophages.

More recent investigations have tried to obviate these problems. For example, Carlo et al. (89) successfully transferred EAO to strain 13 guinea pigs with peritoneal exudate and lymph node cells from syngeneic donors immunized with a purified glycoprotein (GP1) isolated from the acrosome of spermatozoa. Attempts to transfer EAO with serum from hyperimmunized guinea pigs (to a total of 16 ml) were not successful. In the same year, Toullet and Voisin (90) reported that passive transfer of hyperimmune serum or immunoglobulins produced EAO in guinea pigs. Anti-P and anti-T (but not anti-S) sera effectively transferred EAO to recipients, with an incidence of 60% for the first type of antibodies and 40% for the second. In both cases, the local lesions were aggravated by prior treatment of recipients with CFA. The same group of investigators have adoptively transferred EAO to syngeneic recipient guinea pigs (91). Donors of strains 2 and 13 were sensitized with a variety of spermatozoal autoantigens (whole spermatozoa and antigens S, P, and T). Lymphoid cells were adoptively transferred by intravenous injection, and recipients were sacrificed 3 weeks after transfer. The lesions observed in testis and epididymis were similar but less severe than those observed in the donors. The incidence and severity of the histopathologic changes were dependent on the type of inducing antigen (S, T, and P in order of decreasing efficiency), the length of immunization of the donors (increasingly severe lesions with periods of up to 4 weeks), and the presence of complementary treatment of recipients with CFA.

Other adoptive transfer experiments based on *local*, not systemic transfer of cells have shown that sensitized T lymphocytes can mediate antigen-specific, macrophagic "invasive" lesions like those observed in EAO (31,92,93). On the other hand, there is also recent evidence that adoptive transfer of EAO requires the presence of B cells (94). The intratesticular injection of purified

T cells from syngeneic strain 13 guinea pigs immunized with testis antigens in CFA produced only minimal lesions or none. More severe lesions were obtained with the addition of nonimmune macrophages or immune B cells or even nonimmune B cells. When various combinations of T and B cells were transferred, the number of B cells correlated with the severity of the lesions. Immune B-cell populations, either alone or combined with small numbers of immune T cells or macrophages, were capable of eliciting lesions in the recipients.

These results, which otherwise might appear rather confusing, are better interpreted in the light of Voisin's suggestions for the pathogenesis of EAO, i.e., that for each autoantigen there may be a different mechanism of damage (91). In the case of antigen P, immune complexes initiate the disease by a mechanism similar to that observed in the Arthus reaction. Therefore, anti-P immune serum is far more pathogenic in passive transfers than corresponding sensitized lymphoid cells. In the case of antigen S, cytotoxic cells and lymphokines are probably at the origin of tissue damage; thus lymphoid cells sensitized against S are far more efficient in transfers than immune sera. With antigen T, both sensitized cells and antibodies are directly active, and as a result transfers of either cells or antibodies are successful. Finally, the existence of a synergistic association between cells and antibodies must always be considered.

8. Comments

A superficial reading of the voluminous literature on guinea pig models of testis autoimmunity leaves us with a strong feeling of confusion, because of too many conflicting results. In such circumstances, it is not surprising that many immunologists have preferred to select certain interpretations supporting their own individual bias. After all, this is a phenomenon characteristic of the early stage of development of any science, when one of the preparadigm schools "becaue of its own characteristic beliefs and preconceptions" emphasizes "only some special part of the too sizable and inchoate pool of information" (95). Examples of this phenomenon are seen in the interpretation of the histopathological findings of guinea pig EAO, with aspermatogenesis considered the result of inflammation, not an independent lesion, and the conclusion that the testis damage is caused by effector T cells. Such a conclusion would be perfectly acceptable if other studies had not suggested a more complex reality. Guinea pig models of testis autoimmunity have shown that guinea pig spermatozoa contain a large variety of well-defined antigens, many of which are capable of inducing lesions characterized by inflammatory infiltration and aspermatogenesis. Some of these autoantigens can elicit immune responses at the humoral level, others induce DTH responses, and others can generate both humoral and cellular responses. Thus, the major lesson of the guinea pig models is that several mechanisms, both humoral and cellular, are at the basis of the pathogenesis of EAO and vary depending on the autoantigens involved. Such a paradigm is quite useful for a more balanced understanding of testis autoimmunity and perhaps autoimmunity in general.

At this point we should also ask whether guinea pig models of testis autoimmunity can be utilized for additional studies. It is obvious that immunogenetic investigations in this species have limited value because of the small number of inbred strains available and the lack of congenic and recombinant strains. Similarly, additional studies of "classic" EAO seem redundant. On the other hand, more sophisticated analysis of those models caused by infections and chemicals is warranted. Otherwise, one must reluctantly admit that guinea pig models of testis autoimmunity are not likely to provide new and relevant information.

C. Rabbit Models

Rabbits have been extensively utilized in classic immunologic experiments because of their excellent humoral responses to a variety of antigens (including autoantigens) and the relative ease by which immune complexes may be produced. Therefore, it is quite surprising that immune responses to testis-specific antigens and localized tissue damage to the testis have been rather difficult to obtain in this species.

The production of antirabbit "spermatotoxins" in rabbits was reported by several investigators in the early 1920s (96). However, later studies suggested that autoantibodies to spermatozoa or testis-specific antigens could *not* be induced in rabbits after immunization with rabbit spermatozoa in CFA (97,98). Similarly, Swanson and Hafs (99) did not observe any production of antibodies to spermatozoa in vasectomized rabbits. Even more difficult proved to be the induction of the histopathological changes of classic EAO by immunization with testicular antigens and adjuvant. Various investigators reported that testis lesions of the type observed in other animal species were not obtainable in rabbits after the usual immunization regimens for EAO (97,98). The negative results obtained were attributed to lack of antigenicity of rabbit spermatozoa, although they were most likely due to the methodology used or the time frame of the experimental protocols. Indeed, at the same time, autoimmune responses to spermatozoa were obtained by Bratanov et al. (100,101) in rabbits that had been vasectomized or immunized with suspensions of their own spermatozoa. Immunization with seminal plasma or testis cryoinjury was also found to induce autoantibodies to spermatozoa (102-104). Similarly, testicular lesions were obtained by less conventional immunization protocols. For example, Eyquem and Krieg (105) obtained orchitis in the right testis of rabbits injected with complete Freund's adjuvant in the left testis. This so-called sympathetic orchitis was thought to be of an autoimmune nature. Freezing one testis also produced a picture resembling EAO in the contralateral organ (103,104). Finally, the immunization of rabbits with chemically modified seminal plasma resulted in inflammatory damage to the testes (102).

The question of whether rabbits are capable of responding to their own testis antigens has been answered by our experiments on vasectomized rabbits. These animals produced autoantibodies to spermatozoa, detectable by a variety of procedures, and underwent a pathological process in their testes characterized by a reduplication of basement membranes and deposition of immune complexes, with a pattern similar to that of membranous glomerulonephritis. We have therefore termed it "membranous orchitis" (106). These findings have renewed interest in a rabbit model of EAO, and recently Tung and Woodroffe (107) have had successful results by immunization with partially purified testicular antigens in CFA. They have noted that both heterologous and homologous testis antigens are capable of inducing this condition, but with differences that relate both to humoral antibody production as well as the immunohistopathology and histopathology. In general, these authors have noted that the amounts of antigens required to induce EAO in the rabbit are much higher (up to 10 times) than those used for the induction of EAO in the guinea pig. Their observation suggests that the negative results obtained in earlier studies may have been due to inadequate antigen dosage or too short immunization protocols.

1. Testis-Specific Antigens

Initial studies on the induction of autoimmunity to testis and EAO in rabbits utilized crude homogenates of testis, seminal plasma proteins, or seminal plasma proteins coupled to diazonium derivatives (97,98,102). Tung and Woodruffe (107) prepared a partially purified testicular antigen (TCA) following the technique outlined by Jackson et al. (42). Rabbit or guinea pig testis was homogenized in chloroform-methanol and extracted in acetone, followed by solubilization in trichloroacetic acid. However, even this preparation was not well characterized. Progress in identification of testis-specific antigens has been obtained by the studies of O'Rand and Porter (108,109). These investigators have purified a rabbit sperm membrane autoantigen (RAS-1) and determined its amino acid and carbohydrate composition. RSA-1 is specific for the testis and in particular spermatocytes, round spermatids, and epididymal and ejaculated spermatozoa but is not present in Sertoli cells, Leydig cells, and spermatogonia. Preliminary results with monoclonal antibodies indicate that the antigen is also not present in normal rabbit liver, ovary, heart, spleen, and kidney. Antisera specific for RSA-1 are capable of inhibiting fertilization in rabbits. This autoantigen is located in the spermatozoal plasma membrane and blocks the sperm cytotoxic (immobilizing) activity of autoantisera. RSA-1 is a sialoglycoprotein, approximately 40% carbohydrate and containing 0.2 μg sialic acid per microgram protein. Its molecular weight was estimated at approximately 13,000 D. A second rabbit sperm autoantigen (RSA-2) of slightly lower molecular weight (approximately 11,000 D) has also been isolated by the same investigators (109). A third antigen has been purified from deoxycholate-solubilized rabbit testis and spermatozoa using an immunosorbent column containing IgG from a monoclonal antibody that inhibits fertility (110,111). Elution by stepwise increases in pH provided a fraction of pH 11.4 that showed a single band of 63 kD in SDS-PAGE analysis. The antigen molecule is composed of two subunits and contains 21% carbohydrate.

2. Humoral Responses

As previously mentioned, the purification and identification of rabbit testis-specific antigens is still in a rather preliminary stage. The complete spectrum of autoantigens specific to spermatozoa or other cells of the testis is still unknown; therefore, in reviewing rabbit autoimmune responses to testis we perforce use the terms "testis antigens" and/or "spermatozoal antigens." The term "testis antigens" refers to those experiments in which animals are immunized with crude or semicrude suspensions of testis and sera were tested with the same. The term "spermatozoal antigens" refers to those experiments where animals were immunized with spermatozoa and/or sera were tested using suspensions of spermatozoa. In the few cases where purified and characterized antigens were employed, reference will be made by the specific names and procedures used.

Rabbits immunized with spermatozoa or testis antigens produce autoantibodies that can be detected in the circulation by various procedures. Early studies failed to demonstrate antibodies to spermatozoa in the sera of rabbits immunized with rabbit spermatozoa in CFA (97,98). Similarly, no changes were found in the level of complement-fixing antibodies to spermatozoa after vasectomy in rabbits (99). These negative results may be explained by the observation the "normal rabbit serum fixes complement in the presence of rabbit spermatozoa," which made the complement fixation procedure utilized in those studies quite unreliable. However, other tests also gave negative results.

Bratanov et al. (100) were the first to report the presence of spermagglutinins and precipitating antibodies to spermatozoa in the sera of rabbits that had undergone unilateral and bilateral vasoligation, with titers similar to those of rabbits experimentally immunized with spermatozoa. No antibodies to spermatozoa were detectable in the sera of the same animals before surgery or immunization. Later studies showed that the immunization of rabbits with seminal plasma resulted in the production of autoantibodies reacting with rabbit seminal plasma, testis antigens, and spermatozoa (102). Repeated cryoinjury to the testis of rabbits produced antibodies to testis, which reacted with isologous as well as autologous testis extracts (103). These observations were only partially confirmed by other investigators, who detected circulating sperm-agglutinating antibodies in 2 of 13 rabbits that had undergone testis cryoinjury (104).

In our laboratory, we have investigated a large group of bilaterally vasectomized rabbits and found that 14-18 months after surgery 58% of these animals had developed circulating antibodies to spermatozoa or testis antigens, detectable by various procedures (112). Passive hemagglutination and complement fixation using a crude extract of rabbit testis detected circulating antibodies in 30 and 50%, respectively, of vasectomized rabbit sera. A smaller percentage of rabbits (11%) reacted with the same testis extract in agar gel diffusion. Indirect immunofluorescence on cryostat sections of rabbit testis or on sperm smears revealed circulating antibodies in 33 and 50%, respectively, of the same sera. The incidence of circulating antibodies to spermatozoa increases with time and reaches its peak by 18 months after vasectomy. These findings have been confirmed in our laboratory on a larger number of vasectomized rabbits (Bigazzi et al., in preparation) and also by Alexander and Tung (113,114), who, in two groups of vasectomized rabbits, have detected sperm antibodies by immunofluorescence and sperm immobilization with a total incidence of 30% at 6 months and 97% at 8 months after surgery. Interestingly, Tung and Woodruffe (107), in their recent study of EAO in the rabbit, have noticed that circulating antibodies to rabbit spermatozoa appeared rather late (day 60) in rabbits immunized with rabbit testis antigens but were found quite early (day 10) in rabbits immunized with guinea pig testis antigens. Finally, high levels of circulating immune complexes have been detected in vasectomized and immunized rabbits (115).

3. Delayed-type Hypersensitivity Responses

As usual in reproductive immunology, there is a scarcity of data on delayed-type hypersensitivity responses to spermatozoal antigens of rabbits. Technical problems are the main reason for this lack of experimental findings, first and foremost among them the lack of purified antigens that could be used in the in vitro procedures currently utilized for the demonstration of DTH responses.

The majority of rabbits immunized with seminal plasma had positive DTH skin reactions to extracts of accessory glands or testis (102). In a later study on a small number of animals, cell-mediated immunity to spermatozoa has been detected by migration inhibition of peripheral blood leukocytes in vasectomized rabbits 6, 12, and 18 months after surgery (116).

4. Immunohistopathology

In the testes of vasectomized rabbits we have detected granular deposits of immunoglobulins and complement components along the seminiferous tubules (106). Rabbit immunoglobulins eluted from these deposits were found to contain antibodies to acrosomal antigens of spermatozoa, and small granular deposits of acrosomal antigens were detected along the basement membrane of the seminiferous tubules, with a pattern similar to that of immunoglobulins and complement. In addition, a small number of vasectomized rabbits also had granular deposits of immunoglobulins and complement in the glomeruli of their kidneys. Immunoglobulins eluted from kidney homogenates did contain antibodies to acrosomal antigens of spermatozoa, but such antigens were not revealed by immunofluorescence in the kidney glomeruli. A rabbit spermatozoal membrane autoantigen was later isolated, purified, and characterized from the kidneys of bilaterally vasectomized rabbits (117). First, immune complexes were isolated from kidneys using an anti-immunoglobulin affinity chromatography column, then the sperm antigen was isolated using an antisperm antibody column. Finally, our immunohistopathological observations were confirmed by Alexander and Tung (113), who demonstrated immune deposits in the testes and kidneys from 63 and 32% of vasectomized rabbits, respectively.

5. Histopathology

A wide range of histopathological changes have been observed in the testes of rabbits with autoimmune responses to spermatozoa. These changes may be similar to those of classic EAO, as seen in the guinea pig, or may be completely different, i.e., with a scarce inflammatory component and a heavy proliferation of connective tissue elements, as observed in vasectomized rabbits.

Early studies of rabbits immunized with rabbit spermatozoa failed to demonstrate any lesions in the testis (97,98). On the other hand, spermatogenic arrest or alterations of spermatogenesis were observed in rabbits immunized with seminal plasma, with scarce signs of inflammation (interstitial infiltration and thickening of basement membranes in a few rabbits) (102). Multiple in situ freezing insults to rabbit testis were found to cause atrophy of the seminiferous tubules as well as interstitial edema and lymphocytic infiltration, similar to those observed in guinea pig EAO, in the contralateral testis (103). A single, focal cryoinjury to the testis was followed by a moderately severe inflammatory reaction, with infiltration of the testis by macrophages, lymphocytes, and eosinophils (104). This lesion terminated within 1 month with fibrous replacement of the necrotic tissue and functional restitution of the gonad. The same cryoinjury in rabbits sensitized by the progressive destruction of the contralateral testis resulted in an intense inflammatory reaction, characterized by the early presence of lymphocytic perivascular cuffs and macrophages, followed by the development of giant cells, infiltration with plasma cells, epithelioid cells, and caseous necrosis. Similarly, Tung and Woodroffe (107) found that a large percentage of rabbits immunized with rabbit testis in CFA develop diffuse orchitis and/or aspermatogenesis, usually quite early (day 10). On the other hand, rabbits immunized with guinea pig testis develop orchitis and/or aspermatogenesis to a degree related to the number of immunizations (diffuse extent in hyperimmunized animals).

Testis lesions in vasectomized rabbits vary according to the time of observation and the immune status of the animal. Flickinger (118) observed that 6-9 months after vasectomy (i.e., at a time when the autoimmune response to spermatozoa has not yet reached its peak), rabbits exhibited alterations of the seminiferous epithelium, with multinucleated spermatids or lack of spermatids and phagocytosis of germ cells in the lumen of seminiferous tubules. Patchy regions of disrupted germinal epithelium or complete atrophy of rabbit testes were found 1½ years after vasectomy (119). Tumboh-Oeri and Roberts (116) found aspermatogenesis accompanied by inter- and intratubular mononuclear infiltration in their vasectomized rabbits. More recently, it has been noted that 73% of vasectomized rabbits show some degree of disruption of the germinal epithelium (120). In contrast, other investigators have reported no ultrastructural changes in the seminiferous tubules of six vasectomized rabbits at 18 months postsurgery, stressing that both the basal lamina and the germinal epithelium appeared normal (121). Most of these studies on vasectomized rabbits lacked an investigation of the autoimmune status of the animals, with particular attention to circulating antibodies to spermatozoa and testis immunopathology.

Such a correlative study was performed in our laboratory during our initial investigations of vasectomy in rabbits (106). Rabbits with circulating antibodies to spermatozoa and immune deposits in their testes were found by light and electron microscopy to have interesting lesions in their testes. Light microscopy showed thickening of basement membranes in the seminiferous tubules, vacuolization of the basal portion of the tubules, and partial or total disappearance of germinal cells in some tubules. Classic inflammatory components (either PMN or lymphocytes) were quite scarce. The most characteristic ultrastructural findings were the presence of electron-opaque material in the basement membranes and the development of "spikes" directed toward the epithelium. The electron-opaque deposits, often surrounded by newly formed layers of basement membranes, were localized either within the spikes or between the collagenous layers of the basement membrane. Degenerative changes of spermatids were present, with widening of the subacrosomal space, vacuolization, fusion of sperm nuclei with swelling, fragmentation, loss of plasma membranes, and acrosomal material. Small numbers of macrophages and lymphocytes, together with a few polymorphonuclear leukocytes, were present in the collagenous part of the basement membrane and surrounded parts of the basement membrane itself, the electron-opaque deposits, and/or the spikes. In addition, light and electron microscopy studies of kidneys from vasectomized rabbits that had renal immune deposits showed increased amounts of mesangial matrix, mild mesangial proliferation, and electron-opaque deposits in the mesangium. Later investigations on another group of vasectomized rabbits with similar immune deposits in their kidneys have shown definite signs of glomerulonephritis (Bigazzi et al., in preparation).

6. Pathogenesis

The mechanisms of damage in rabbit EAO are still unclear, one of the major reasons being the lack of adoptive transfer studies in inbred animals. Admittedly, there are a few inbred or partially inbred strains of rabbits and the major histocompatibility complex (RLA) of this species has been defined (122), but because of the number of animals required and the expense involved, passive transfer experiments have not been undertaken. We are left therefore with speculations regarding the possible role of humoral versus cellular immunity in this species. It seems that in situ immune complex orchitis may be the major mechanism of damage in the membranous orchitis observed in vasectomized rabbits. Similarly, EAO induced in rabbits by immunization with heterologous (guinea pig) testis antigens may be caused by in situ immune complex formation. On the other hand, rabbits immunized with homologous testis antigens do not develop immune deposits in their testes, and therefore, EAO may be obtained in these animals through other mechanisms, e.g., DTH reactions.

The variety of mechanisms that may be involved in producing testis damage in rabbit EAO is most likely another example of the consequence of immunization with different antigens, as demonstrated by Voisin in guinea pigs. Thus, rabbits that have been vasectomized or immunized with heterologous testis antigens may respond to epitopes that induce strong antibody responses and immune complex formation, but the animals immunized with homologous antigens may react to different epitopes that induce DTH or ADCC reactions.

7. Comments

The study of rabbit models of testis autoimmunity has provided a major lesson regarding the heterogeneity of the lesions of EAO. As in other models of autoimmunity, it has been clearly demonstrated in rabbits that testis autoimmunity does not necessarily and exclusively result in inflammatory damage but can express itself in changes of basement membranes and other components of the target organ. Thus, the histopathology of EAO need not be stereotyped as only inflammation and aspermatogenesis. One wonders whether other, more subtle functional lesions have escaped our attention. For example, the testis might be affected as the result of autoimmune-mediated stimulation or inhibition of cell receptors, a possibility that to our knowledge has thus far been ignored.

Is there a future for studies of testis autoimmunity in rabbits? Reluctantly, we have to admit that this species, like the guinea pig, may have reached the limits of its usefulness. There are few strains of inbred rabbits available, studies of rabbit MHC are not being continued (122), and both purchase and maintenance costs for these animals are much higher than those of mice and rats. Therefore, except for those instances in which size may be of importance (e.g., perfusion studies for demonstration of changes in blood-testis barrier and purification of spermatozoal antigens) it is unlikely that much more will be learned from further studies of testis autoimmunity in rabbits.

D. Rat Models

Experimental models of autoimmunity in rats are becoming increasingly popular. The availability of over 100 inbred strains, well characterized from the point of view of their MHC and the production of some MHC congenic lines, in addition to a few intra-MHC recombinants (122), and the recent development of monoclonal antibodies to markers of lymphocytes (including subpopulations of T cells) and macrophages are all definite advantages that render rats much more desirable than other species, such as rabbits and guinea pigs.

1. Testis-Specific Antigens

Studies of rat testis-specific antigens have not yet reached the sophistication of investigations of similar antigens in guinea pigs. Immunization protocols have utilized suspensions of rat testis, prepared following Freund's procedure for guinea pig testis antigens, or suspensions of dissociated testis cells or spermatozoa (123). At least three organ-specific antigens, contributed mainly by cells of the seminiferous tubules, have been obtained from rat testes (124). Similarly, three different testis antigens have been detected in Sprague-Dawley rats (125). One of these antigens was present in the testis of animals 30 days old, even though no spermatozoa were visible, and was also found in adult testis and spermatozoa, together with two additional antigens. Argentinian investigators have purified a preparation rich in seminiferous tubule basement membrane, obtained by a multistep procedure aimed at eliminating blood, proteoglycans, and cells present in the tissue (126–128). This preparation and a noncollagen fraction, purified by collagenase and trypsin digestion, were found to be antigenic.

Quite interesting are more recent studies of class I and II antigens on cells of the testis. Using Sprague-Dawley rats and antisera produced in rabbits against isolated H-2 and Ia molecules from mice, which reportedly recognize the equivalent rat antigens, Soderstrom et al. (129) have shown that Ia-like antigens are present on all spermatogenic cells, although the relative expression seems to decrease slightly concomitant with the differentiation. The AgB-SD antigens are detected on spermatogonia, leptotene, and zygotene spermatocytes but not on later developmental stages. However, Head and Billingham (130) have observed that testes of normal inbred rats (DA and F344) contain substantial numbers of Ia^+ cells throughout the interstitial tissue. These are often single, medium-sized cells, sometimes seen in clusters and especially abundant near blood vessels. The majority lack a dendritic morphology, even though some dendriticlike cells are seen, usually near blood vessels. Sustained numbers of esterase-positive cells (possibly Leydig cells and macrophages) are present in the interstitium. Similar studies on testis cell suspensions have revealed a substantial number of cells that are both Ia^+ and esterase positive. These cells are most likely macrophages, known to be abundant in the testicular interstitium. There are other cells that are Ia^+ and esterase positive and these may be similar to dendritic cells. Thus, the presence of intensely Ia^+ cells in the testicular interstitium, especially those that are esterase negative, is presumptive evidence that local processing of antigen can occur at this site. Rhodamine-conjugated lectins have been used to study the staining pattern of glycoproteins in rat testis and epididymis after ligation of the vas deferens (131). During the observation period no apparent change was noted in the apical part of the seminiferous epithelium. However, after 7 days from surgery, a cell population in the periphery of the seminiferous tubules (close to the tubular basement membranes) showed a nuclear affinity for lectins. This granular nuclear reactions was initially found only with a few lectins, but during further cell degeneration other lectins also become reactive. In the final stages the condensed remnants gave the strongest reaction with concanavalin A (ConA), indicating the possibility that high-mannose cores of the N-glycosylated oligosaccharide chains are exposed at a stage when Sertoli cells are ready to absorb the remnants of these cells. It is possible that some of the glycoprotein antigens of spermatozoal plasma membranes are synthesized prior to the stage (preleptotene) when the spermatogenic cell is transported across the blood-testis barrier formed by the tight junctions between Sertoli cells. Thus, a particular stage of early spermatogenic development may become vulnerable to circulating antibodies or lymphoid cells.

2. Humoral Responses

Several laboratories have demonstrated that rats are capable of humoral immune responses to spermatozoa. In early studies, some investigators observed the production of autoantibodies to spermatozoa in rats and others reported negative results (see Ref. 91). In later investigations, Rumke and Titus (132) immunized inbred Wistar rats with syngeneic spermatozoa and detected sperm-agglutinating antibodies in their sera. A dose-effect relationship was observed, since rats immunized with 1.5-2.3 $\times 10^9$ spermatozoa produced good antibody titers within 7 days, but animals injected with lower doses responded less vigorously or not at all. The same investigators also found sperm-agglutinating antibodies in the circulation of unilaterally vasectomized rats. They noted that 8 of 8 rats, vasectomized but not vasoligated, developed high titers, ranging from 40 to 1280, but only 2 of 7 vasectomized and vasoligated animals had high sperm-agglutinating titers. Gupta et al. (133) also detected circulating antitestis antibodies in the sera of immunized rats. Lewis male rats immunizeded s.c. with syngeneic or allogenic (BN) spermatozoa in CFA developed antibodies to spermatozoa as determined by the Arthus reactions (3-hr foot swelling) and cytotoxic antibody measurements (134). On the other hand, vasectomized and vasoligated inbred Lewis rats had humoral responses to syngeneic spermatozoa (detectable by an Arthus reaction and serum cytotoxicity) but vasectomized and not ligated animals did not have any significant response (135, 136). This difference may be attributed to different surgical procedure, different methods to detect sperm antibodies, and different inbred strains.

In our laboratory, we have demonstrated that vasectomized inbred rats develop antibodies to the acrosome of spermatozoa, detectable by indirect immunofluorescence on methanol-fixed rat sperm smears (137). In an initial study, circulating antibodies to spermatozoa were detected in 80% of Lewis rats, 47% of Brown Norway, 13% of Buffalo, 12% of Wistar-Furth, and 11% of ACI, but no such antibodies were observed in sera from Fischer and Dark Agouti as well as outbred Sprague-Dawley rats. Further studies have confirmed these findings and in addition have demonstrated that antibodies to spermatozoa may develop in up to 100% of Brown Norway rats, depending on the source from which these animals are obtained. August, BDII, and BDIX rats were negative (138). In other laboratories it was found that both vasectomized and control Sprague-Dawley rats all had circulating antibodies to spermatozoa detectable by indirect immunofluorescence on cryostat sections of testis (139), and sperm-agglutinating antibodies were noted in the sera of 100% vasectomized inbred Wistar-Furth (140). The injection of CFA into the epididymis of vasectomized Wistar-Furth rats causes localized granulomas as well as high titers of sperm agglutinins. Another study has correlated the incidence of sperm granulomas and autoantibodies to spermatozoa in vasectomized rats (141). These autoantibodies were found in 71% of Brown Norway, 50% of Lewis, 25% Fischer, and 33% of Sprague-Dawley. Sperm granulomas had the same incidence as autoantibodies in Brown Norway, but not in the other strains. Recently, circulating antibodies to spermatozoa (detectable by indirect immunofluorescence) have been found in 90% of inbred Lewis rats, vasectomized either at prefertile age (2-3 weeks) or at 10-11 weeks of age. No significant difference was found between the two groups of rats (142). Other investigators have found that all vasectomized Lewis rats have developed significant cytotoxic sperm antibody titers by the first week from surgery and have a second peak of response by the fourth week (143). Herr et al. (144) have developed an enzyme-linked immunosorbent assay

(ELISA) for rat antisperm antibodies and have found that 88% of vasectomized Lewis rats develop such antibodies by 7 weeks after surgery. Prevasectomy treatment with cyclosporine may significantly reduce or delay the production of cytotoxic sperm antibodies in Lewis rats (143). Humoral responses to spermatozoa are also induced in rats by other procedures. For example, both circulating and sperm-bound antisperm antibodies were detected in most rats with an experimentally induced testicular torsion (145). Sperm-agglutinating antibodies are also found in approximately 60% of neonatally thymectomized Lewis rats (146). Finally, circulating antibodies to basement membrane antigens were detected in rats immunized with basement membranes from seminiferous tubules in CFA (148).

3. Delayed-type Hypersensitivity Responses

As usual, studies of DTH in rats with EAO are rather sparse. Male Lewis rats immunized with allogeneic (BN) spermatozoa in CFA develop DTH responses (footpad swelling, cell cytotoxicity, and MIF production), but animals immunized under similar conditions with syngeneic spermatozoa did not show any evidence of DTH responses (134). Negative skin tests were also observed in rats immunized with testis antigens (133). On the other hand, rats immunized with solubilized tubular basement membranes in CFA showed production of MIF when their lymphocytes were reacted with basement membrane antigens, but not with testis homogenates (147). Vasectomized (but not vasoligated) inbred Lewis rats showed both in vivo and in vitro manifestations of delayed-type hypersensitivity (148). When tested with syngeneic spermatozoa 3 months following surgery, these animals presented footpad swelling, lymphocyte cytoxicity, and MIF production. Rats that had been vasectomized and vasoligated did not have signs of cell-mediated immunity to spermatozoa.

4. Immunohistopathology

Deposits of IgG were observed in 50% of rats immunized with tubular basement membranes in CFA (147). In our laboratory, deposits of IgG and/or C3 have been detected in the testis and

Table 2 Immunohistopathology of Male Reproductive System in Vasectomized and Control Inbred Rats[a]

		(%) Rats with immune deposits in			
		Testis		Epididymis	
Strain	Treatment	IgG	C3	IgG	C3
BN	Vx	91	74	97	94
	Sham Vx	55	36	100	100
	Untreated	47	27	100	100
BN.AUG	Vx	83	17	67	50
	Sham Vx	33	0	33	0
MAXX	Vx	13	13	0	0
	Sham Vx	0	0	20	20
LEW	Vx	20	20	0	0
	Sham Vx	0	0	0	0

[a]Abbreviations: BN, Brown Norway; AUG, August; LEW, Lewis; Vx, vasectomy.

epididymis of vasectomized Brown Norway rats, but not in the same organs of MAXX or Lewis (LEW) rats (Bigazzi et al., in preparation) (Table 2). However, similar deposits have also been noted in control animals (Table 2).

5. Histopathology

The initial study of EAO in rats was published by Freund et al. (123), who reported that 19 of 29 rats (Wistar and Sherman) immunized with rat testis extract in CFA developed EAO with varying degrees of aspermatogenesis (i.e., from diminished numbers of spermatozoa in the seminiferous tubules to partial or complete devastation of the tubules, with only Sertoli cells and basement membrane remaining). The lesions were not usually associated with inflammation in the intertubular spaces, except in some far-advanced cases that showed focal accumulations of large mononuclear cells and lymphocytes. They concluded that the rat is less susceptible than the guinea pig to the effects of immunization with testis antigens. A discrepancy between circulating sperm agglutinins and histopathological lesions was reported by Rumke and Titus (132), who observed that testes from Wistar rats immunized with spermatozoa without Freund's adjuvant appeared to be normal (in spite of the presence of serum antisperm antibodies), but those of animals immunized with adjuvant had histological signs of degeneration. Testes from vasectomized rats showed signs of degeneration on the side of vasectomy or vasoligation, but the contralateral testis appeared normal. More striking were the results obtained by Levine and Sowinski (149), who immunized Lewis rats with a single injection of isologous rat testis homogenate in CFA and pertussis vaccine. After 14 days, 22 of 36 rats had developed orchitis and/or infarcts in one or both testes. The orchitis was manifested as one or more unilateral or bilateral foci of infiltration with mononuclear cells, beginning around vessels but soon filling the intertubular areas. Seminiferous tubules in the inflamed areas exhibited damage that varied from minimal necrobiotic changes (altered staining of cells, nuclear pyknosis, and loosening of the normal compact organization to the lining cells) to total necrosis (tubules filled with necrotic cells and granular debris). Inflammation and tubular damage were coextensive and were parallel in severity from the central area of greatest involvement to the fringe areas with minimal changes. Some of the larger foci of orchitis had areas of intense edema with masses of polymorphonuclear leukocytes around necrotic tubules. In other rats, focal infiltration by PMN was even more extensive and necrosis affected both tubules and interstitial tissue to the extent of forming subtotal or total infarcts. Epididymides had mononuclear and PMN infiltrates. The kinetics of EAO in these rats showed that little or no orchitis was present 8-11 days after immunization, but lesions were found in two-thirds of rats sacrificed 19-35 days after the usual immunization. After 35 days, focal chronic inflammation was accompanied by widespread parenchymal atrophy. Localized thermal damage to the testis at the time of immunization accelerated the process, and focal orchitis, manifested as a dense infiltration of mononuclear cells in the intertubular spaces, was seen as early as 5-6 days after immunization.

An ultrastructural study of the testis has been performed in Wistar rats immunized with testis homogenate in CFA (150). There was a marked convolution of the limiting membranes surrounding the more severely damaged seminiferous tubules, which exhibited few if any germ cells and appeared to consist almost entirely of Sertoli cells. The ultrastructure of these cells appeared normal, but their cytoplasm contained spherical lipid bodies, highly variable in size, granular, and moderately electron opaque (possibly fragments of phagocytized germ cells), as well as areas of dilated smooth endoplasmic reticulum. The ultrastructural features of the Sertoli cells were consistent with the concept that they are responsible for the degradation and phagocytosis of germinal elements. Increased numbers of lymphocytes were evident throughout the intertubular areas and occasionally within layers of the limiting membrane. There was also an apparent increase in the number of macrophages in the interstitium. Histochemical studies showed increased localization of nonspecific esterase and acid phosphatase associated with lipid bodies of the tubules and in intertubular areas.

Studies in neonatally thymectomized rats (outbred Wistar and inbred Lewis) have revealed that these animals develop complete atrophy of their testes (151). Other investigators have confirmed that approximately 60% of neonatally thymectomized Lewis rats develop orchitis, with mononuclear cell infiltration, granulomata, and giant cells (146). Similar changes were observed by Wekerle and Begemann (152), who noticed that lymphocytes immunized in vitro injected into the testis of syngeneic recipients cause a range of lesions characteristic of EAO, i.e., from desquamation of seminiferous tubules and giant cell formation to focal necrosis. Argentinian investigators (153-155) obtained multifocal damage to the testis in 60% of rats immunized with solubilized tubular basement membranes or after passive transfer of rabbit antibodies to rat testis tubular basement membranes. The damaged areas were characterized by perivascular and peritubular cell infiltrates, changes in the walls of small vessels and seminiferous tubules, and sloughing of germinal epithelium. Ultrastructural studies showed folding and focal thickening and delamination of basement membranes.

Testicular and epididymal hypertrophy have been observed in vasectomized rats, alterations being greater in long-term than in short-term animals (156). However, according to Flickinger (157), the fine structure of the seminiferous epithelium after vasectomy resembles that previously described for normal rats, at least for a period of up to 9 months after surgery. Numerous residual bodies were identified in the cytoplasm of Sertoli cells, but there were no indications of increased uptake of parts of spermatozoa by Sertoli cells after vasectomy. On the other hand, there were alterations in the fine structure of the rat epididymis after vasectomy, possibly reflecting the absorption of parts of spermatozoa by the epithelium of the cauda epididymis (158). Instead, other investigators have observed a spectrum of histopathological findings in the testes of vasectomized Lewis rats, ranging from completely normal seminiferous tubules in some testes to degeneration of up to 79% of these tubules in others (159). Degenerative changes included patchy distribution of reduction in tubule diameter, fusion of spermatids, and loss of germinal elements of seminiferous epithelium. Leakiness of the blood-testis barrier was detected by lanthanum distribution in the most degenerated seminiferous tubules. Barrier leakiness was detected only in vasectomized Lewis, not Sprague-Dawley rats. A higher frequency of stages VII-VIII of the tubular cycle has been found in the testes of vasectomized rats (indicating sperm accumulation) as well as increased diameters of seminiferous tubules and tubular lumen and possible hyperactivity of Leydig cells (160). In our laboratory, we have observed that vasectomized rats have alterations of the seminiferous tubules ranging from loss of spermatozoa to complete loss of germinal epithelium and thickening of basement membranes (Bigazzi et al., in preparation). Such changes occur in 70% of Lewis rats but are also found in animals of other strains. Finally, orchitis has been induced in rats by injection with BCG or chemicals such as α-chlorohydrin (83,161).

6. Immunogenetics

A full-scale immunogenetic study of autoimmune responses to spermatozoa was first performed in our laboratory when we investigated various inbred strains of vasectomized rats (137). That study demonstrated that a large percentage of vasectomized Lewis (LEW) and Brown Norway (BN) rats produce antibodies to acrosomal antigens of spermatozoa, compared with very small numbers of rats from other inbred strains, such as Buffalo, Wistar-Furth, and ACI. In addition, vasectomized rats from other strains, such as Fischer (F344), Dark Agouti (DA), August, BDII, and BDIX are consistently negative for sperm antibodies, even though their spermatozoa possess acrosomal antigens. Therefore, rats of some inbred strains behave as high responders to sperm antigens, but others may be considered mediocre or poor responders. These differences are not easily explained on the basis of a simple correlation between major histocompatibility loci and immune response genes controlling autoimmune responses to sperm antigens. Rats that may be considered good responders, such as the LEW and BN strains, belong to different genotypes—RT1l and RT1n, respectively. On the other hand, two strains of rats belonging to the same MHC differ in their responses; i.e., LEW rats produce anti-acrosomal antibodies and F344 do not. Since other background genes could be obscuring the detection of MHC-linked genes, we have used congenic rats in additional investigations (138). Antisperm antibodies were detectable in the sera of 100% BN and 0% AUG 1 month after vasectomy. Similarly, circulating antibodies were found in 100% BN.AUG and 0% AUG.BN. These data confirm the lack of association between MHC and production of antibodies to acrosomal antigens of spermatozoa. A second important finding of that study was the absence of sperm antibodies in doubly congenic rats carrying both the RT1 genes and the Y chromosome of the BN strain, showing that autoimmune responses to rat spermatozoa are not controlled by genes on the Y chromosome. Finally, the incidence of antisperm antibodies in BN rats (one of the two high responder strains) was found to vary with the source of the animals. At 3 months postvasectomy, only 47% of BN rats purchased from a commercial company were positive for antibodies to spermatozoa, but positive results were obtained in 63, 84, and 100% of BN rats obtained from three other sources. Variations in the incidence of autoantibodies (162) or susceptibility to the induction of EAO (163) have also been observed in sublines of inbred mice. This phenomenon may be due to environmental factors and/or genetic drift.

7. Pathogenesis

First we examine the results of transfer studies, since these may give evidence of the pathogenetic mechanism(s) involved in EAO of rats. Cells from a sterile peritoneal exudate of rats (Holtzman strain, defined by the authors as "inbred but not histocompatible") immunized with testis antigens in adjuvants did transfer testis lesions to normal animals (164). The damage was specific to the testis and limited to the germinal epithelium. In testes removed from rats 7 days after multiple transfer ($2.9\text{-}3.5 \times 10^6$ cells, by intravenous injection, repeated three times during a 5-day period), areas of damaged seminiferous tubules were consistently observed. The extent of damage was variable, and in most cases the area of damaged tubules was peripheral and close to blood vessels. Testis damage was even more apparent 14 days after transfer. Sertoli cells had become vacuolated, and in many instances the only germinal elements remaining in the tubules were the spermatogonia. No inflammatory cells were shown in the illustrations, and no mention of inflammation was made by the authors. In later studies, delayed hypersensitivity reactions to testis antigens were reportedly transferred in vitro with immune RNA from rats with EAO (165). Unfortunately, no other experiments with transfer of lymphocytes from animals with EAO have been reported in this species, in spite of the availability of markers of rat T and B cells and the success of adoptive transfer in other experimental rat models of autoimmune disease. Studies of passive transfer of EAO with antibodies have given contradictory results. The intratesticular injection of rabbit antiserum to rat testis antigens caused localized degeneration of the germinal epithelium (166,167), but similar injections with control sera also resulted in altered spermatogenesis (166). On the other hand, EAO has been successfully transferred in rats by repeated injections of antibodies to antigens of seminiferous tubule basement membranes (153–155).

Interesting experiments have been performed by Wekerle et al. (168-171), who first demonstrated that EAO can be induced in vitro. Normal rat lymphocytes cultured with autologous testis cells were found to form rosettelike aggregates and later undergo blast transformation and proliferation. These in vitro immunized lymphocytes are capable of inhibiting the in vitro growth of testis cell-derived monolayers and induce EAO when injected into the testis of syngeneic recipients. These responses show tissue specificity and are determined by the MHC. The actively responding cells are T lymphocytes, and Sertoli cells may be the cell population capable of stimulating the lymphocytes. The self-reactivity to testis antigens is increased in aged animals and is not due to age-dependent alterations of the relevant autoantigens or changed function of accessory non-T cells, but is rather a property of the T-cell compartment. This may indicate an age-dependent loss of T-lymphocyte self-tolerance, which may play an active role in the generation of autoimmune disease with aging. It was also observed that rat thymic cells (from inbred Lewis-Wistar rats) cocultured with syngeneic Sertoli cells became autosensitized and caused alterations of Sertoli cells in vitro (172). When these thymic cells were injected into the testis of rats, derangement of the seminiferous epithelium was obtained. Finally, it has been demonstrated that thymectomy alone in LEW rats and thymectomy followed by immunization with testicular extract in either F344 or LEW rats increases both the incidence and the severity of EAO (146). It appears that LEW rats are genetically predisposed to the development of EAO, but normally the disease process is under control such that overt manifestations do not occur in the majority of rats. Following thymectomy, this delicate balance is apparently shifted toward an increased reactivity to testis antigens.

Immune privilege in the testis, an intriguing immunologic phenomenon that may have some relevance for a better understanding of the pathogenesis of EAO, has also been investigated in-depth in inbred rats (173,174). Intratesticular skin allografts survived at least several days longer than orthotopic grafts of similar size, whether MHC compatible or MHC incompatible, and failed to induce an alloantibody response in most recipients or to prime for secondary antibody responses on rechallenge, in spite of an efficient lymphatic drainage. The testis interstitial tissue has antigen-processing capability since it is well endowed with cells bearing class II histocompatibility antigens; therefore, local suppressive factors (possibly steroids secreted by Leydig cells or other cellular elements of the seminiferous tubules) may be responsible for immune privilege. Studies of this phenomenon may elucidate the role of the testis environment in the predilection of certain microorganisms for this organ, recurrence of tumors in this site, and possibly the development of autoimmune orchitis.

8. Comments

Several lessons have already been provided by rat models of testis autoimmunity. The influence exercised by genetic factors on autoimmune responses to certain spermatozoal antigens is not surprising, as similar observations have been previously obtained in other animal models of autoimmune disease. What is unique is the lack of association between the production of antibodies to autoantigens of spermatozoa and the MHC, a finding not easily explained by current immunogenetic views. Another interesting observation is the variability in autoimmune responses to spermatozoa between different "sublines" of one inbred strain and between different rats of the same inbred strain. It is possible that these differences may be caused by genetic drift; however, one should not discount the influence of environmental factors, such as microorganisms or chemicals, that are known to influence autoimmune responses (9). Of great interest also are studies of the antigens located within the basement membranes of the seminiferous tubules. Traditionally, investigations of EAO have been limited to antigens of spermatozoa, without considering the numerous other cells and structures of the testis. Instead, more attention should be given, as is commonly done in kidney autoimmunity, to the various autoantigens present within basement membranes, which may be more accessible to antibodies and lymphocytes than the constituents of the adluminal compartment. Finally, rat models have provided intriguing data on the interactions between T lymphocytes and Sertoli cells, indicating both another possibility of autosensitization and another cell target for autoimmune-mediated damage.

In our opinion, we have barely touched the surface of the abundant information that can be gained from the study of rat models of testis autoimmunity. Autoantigens of spermatozoa and Sertoli and Leydig cells, as well as other structures of the testis, should be better defined in this species, taking advantage of the experience gained in investigations of guinea pigs and mice and utilizing the modern hybridoma procedures. Once the numerous epitopes present on cells and structures have been defined, autoimmune responses, both humoral and cellular, should be carefully characterized, together with the histopathology and the immunohistopathology observed in various rat models of testis autoimmunity. At that point, it should also be possible to better define the pathogenesis by adoptive transfers, taking advantage of the powerful help of monoclonal antibodies that identify subsets of rat lymphocytes. In conclusion, the study of rat models of testis autoimmunity should be encouraged as much as possible, since they may provide unique and essential answers to problems of human infertility and population control.

E. Mouse Models

The mouse has become the animal of choice for most studies of basic immunology, especially immunogenetics, since it breeds rapidly, produces large numbers of progeny, and is genetically well characterized (122). Numerous inbred strains, coisogenic and congenic lines, and recombinant inbred strains are available, as well as monoclonal antibodies to surface markers of lymphocytes (T, B, and subpopulations) and macrophages. Thus, it is not surprising that models of testis autoimmunity have recently been developed in this species and it is to be expected that they will be utilized even further in the future.

1. Testis-Specific Autoantigens

In the mouse, a large number of sperm or testis-specific autoantigens are present on spermatocytes, spermatids, and spermatozoa (175-182). In most of these studies, surface antigens of mouse spermatozoa have been characterized by SDS-PAGE and Western blots, often taking advantage of the availability of monoclonal antibodies. Four acrosomal antigens have been described, with molecular weights of 28,000, 69,000, 82,000, and 200,000 D, respectively, and one 68,000 D antigen has been identified on the surface of the tail. At present it is uncertain whether any of these antigens is capable of inducing autoimmune responses and EAO in the mouse.

As recently summarized by Klein (122), the results of studies on the expression of MHC molecules on male germ cells are controversial. By fluorescence activated cell sorter (FACS) analysis, cultured mouse Sertoli cells were found to have detectable H-2 but not Ia antigens (183). Similarly, little or no class I and no class II antigens were detectable on mouse testis cells (184). Interstitial dendritic cells were increased in both testis and epididymis after interferon gamma treatment; however, such treatment did not increase the expression of either class I or II antigens in the seminiferous tubules. To date, the consensus is that if MHC molecules are present on spermatozoa, their quantity is at least 10 times lower than that on lymphocytes (122).

2. Humoral Responses

Mice are capable of humoral immune responses to their own testis antigens, as demonstrated in various models of testis autoimmunity in this species. Circulating antibodies to spermatozoa were detected in 66% of ASW and C57Bl mice immunized with testis antigens in CFA (185) and have later been observed in BALB/c, DBA-1, and C3H mice similarly sensitized with syngeneic spermatozoa (186,187). Interestingly, a recent study has detected serum antibodies to testis cells in immunized BALB/c mice but no antibody-dependent complement-mediated cytotoxicity or antibody-dependent cell-mediated cytotoxicity (188). Spermagglutinins have been detected in the sera of bilaterally vasectomized CFW mice (189), and antibodies to protamine of mouse spermatozoa were found in vasectomized CBA/Crc mice, cross-reacting with the protamine of human spermatozoa (190). In our laboratory, we have detected circulating antibodies to acrosomal antigens in 26% of vasectomized mice (191) (see Sec. I.E.6). Circulating antisperm antibodies were observed as early as 1 month postvasectomy in (C57Bl/6 × DBA/2)F1 hybrid mice (192). Antisperm antibody titers increased with time and were highest in animals that had been vasectomized for over 2 years. Unilaterally vasectomized DBA/1J mice produce antisperm antibodies and are infertile (193). Interestingly, the development of antisperm antibodies in vasectomized mice can be prevented by the perfusion of heterologous antisperm serum (194). Finally, humoral immune responses have been demonstrated in another model of testis autoimmunity. After neonatal thymectomy, 42% of (C57Bl/6 × A/J)F_1 hybrid mice as well as 34% A/J, 19% SWR/J, and 17% C57Bl/10J had circulating autoantibodies to spermatozoa (195,196).

Recently, more sophisticated and sensitive procedures have been developed to demonstrate antisperm antibodies in mice. An ELISA has been used for the detection of such antibodies in the serum of immunized outbred mice (197), and circulating antisperm antibodies to spermatozoa have also been demonstrated by Western blotting, a technique that separates sperm antigens according to molecular weight and reveals reactive antibodies to different sperm antigens (187). Finally, modern techniques of hybridoma production have been applied to studies of humoral immunity and sperm antigens in mice. Monoclonal antibodies have been obtained from vasectomized (C57Bl/6 × DBA/2)F1 hybrid mice (181). Of these antibodies, four recognize topographically restricted sperm-specific antigenic determinants that appear in the germinal epithelium as spermatogenesis progresses. A single clone reacts with the nuclei of somatic and testicular germ cells, but not the nuclei of sperm.

3. Delayed-type Hypersensitivity Responses

There are very few studies devoted to delayed hypersensitivity in mice. As an exception, Pokorna et al. (198) found a correlation between the histological damage of EAO and the presence of MIF. Lymphocytes obtained from mice with EAO showed a significantly enhanced response in a mixed culture with syngeneic testicular cells. Cytotoxic lymphocyte activity has recently been observed in BALB/c mice with EAO (188). In addition, it has been demonstrated that A-strain mice vasectomized without vasoligation develop DTH responses to syngeneic spermatozoa, as detected by MIF and leukocyte adherence inhibition assays (199). Such responses do not occur in mice that have been vasectomized and vasoligated.

It should also be noted that Anderson and Tarter (200) found that mouse seminal plasma exerts potent immunosuppressive effects in vivo, suppressing both primary and secondary humoral immune responses in mice to low immunizing doses of antigens, such as bovine serum albumin or washed epididymal spermatozoa. When mouse seminal plasma and its individual components were tested in vitro, it was also found that they suppressed mitogen-induced lymphocyte transformation.

4. Immunohistopathology

There are few published studies of the immunohistopathology of mice with EAO. Granular deposits of mouse C3 were found within thickened basement membranes surrounding seminiferous tubules of BALB/c mice immunized with homologous testis antigens in CFA (201). In a few of these animals, granular deposits of mouse IgG were found in pericellular or perinuclear locations inside the seminiferous tubules, an unusual immunohistochemical finding. On the other hand, deposits of mouse IgG were found both in the basement membranes and within the seminiferous tubules of a few long-term vasectomized (C57Bl/6 × DBA/2)F1 hybrid mice (192). In our laboratory we have observed that the testes and epididymis of most vasectomized mice did not contain immune deposits, even though a few animals were positive at these levels (Bigazzi et al., in preparation). Finally, granual deposits of immunoglobulins and complement have been noted along the basement membrane of the seminiferous tubules of the testis and the epididymal ducts in mice with EAO induced by neonatal thymectomy (195).

5. Histopathology

Hargis et al. (202) were the first to obtain profound aspermatogenesis in all mice immunized with a mixture of testicular tissue and *Bordetella pertussis* vaccine. EAO in mice was characterized by disappearance of mature spermatozoa, formation of multinucleated giant cells in the seminiferous tubules, and infiltration of lymphocytes in the stroma (195). Epididymitis was observed prior to the development of EAO. Sato et al. (203) induced EAO in (C57Bl/6J × A/J)F1 hybrid mice and observed that in the initial stage there was occasional focal degeneration and desquamation of both spermatogonia and Sertoli cells within limited parts of the seminiferous tubules, in the peripheral region of the testis. No inflammatory change was present. Subsequently, marked infiltration of lymphocytes, monocytes, and polymorphonuclear leukocytes was found not only in the testis but also in the rete testis and epididymis. In later stages, the inflammation subsided but the testes became atrophic owing to progression of spermatogenic arrest. Many tubules were lined only with monolayers of Sertoli cells, surrounded by hyperplastic Leydig cells in the interstitium. Kohno et al. (201) induced EAO in BALB/c mice and found that animals had lesions in the testis (100%), rete testis (37%), cauda epididymis (21%), and vas deferens (37%). Early lesions in the seminiferous tubules were characterized by peritubular and/or intratubular accumulation of eosinophils, neutrophils, lymphocytes, and macrophages, later followed by aspermatogenesis. Late lesions included massive necrosis and extensive fibrosis of the seminiferous tubules. Disruption of the blood-testis barrier was suggested by the deposition of mouse immunoglobulins in the germinal epithelium and the presence of granular deposits of mouse C3 in the basement membrane of the seminiferous tubules. Loss of integrity of the blood-testis barrier was confirmed by the penetration of perfused lanthanum inside the seminiferous tubules. Disturbances in spermatogenesis (but no inflammation) were observed in BALB/c mice after intratesticular injection of monoclonal antibodies against Sertoli cells or basement membranes of seminiferous tubules (204).

The EAO obtained after neonatal thymectomy has been compared with that caused by vasectomy (196). In the first, there was degeneration and desquamation of the germinal epithelium and variable interstitial infiltration with lymphocytes, plasma cells, and macrophages. In postvasectomy EAO the damage was less severe and lymphoid infiltration never seen. On the other hand, it has also been reported that spermatogenesis was impaired in long-term vasectomized mice: orchitis lesions characterized by immune deposits and lymphocytic infiltration were found in 3 of 14 mice compared with none of the controls (192).

6. Immunogenetics

One of the first immunogenetic studies of EAO was performed by Pokorna et al. (185), who observed that more or less pronounced damage to spermatogenesis results from immunization with testicular antigens in all mice from three different inbred strains, C57Bl/Ks, C57Bl/Sn, and ASW. A similar investigation utilized two different strains of mice, one susceptible (BSVS) and the other resistant (BRVR) to the virus of St. Louis encephalitis, *Salmonella typhimurium*, and experimental allergic encephalitis (205-207). EAO developed only in BSVS mice treated with BSVS antigen, but not in BSVS mice immunized with BRVR antigen or BRVR immunized with BRVR antigen (there was not report on immunization of BRVR with BSVS). All groups showed stimulation of reticuloendothelial system activity, which appeared highest in the mice that developed EAO, but the difference was not statistically significant.

Following this lead, we investigated the immunologic effects of vasectomy in BRVR and BSVS mice, on the assumption that the former might be "poor responders" and the latter "good responders." However, none of the mice of either strain developed antibodies to spermatozoa in a period of 15 months following vasectomy. We then investigated mice of seven different inbred strains (191). Overall, we found that 26% of vasectomized mice developed antibodies to acrosomal antigens of spermatozoa, detected at 7 and 10 months after surgery. This response was actually restricted to three of the seven strains, i.e., C57L/J (78%), DBA/1J (67%), and C57Bl/6 (30%). This was one of the first immunogenetic studies of autoimmune responses to spermatozoa in inbred mice of various strains, defining good and poor responder animals. Later investigations in our laboratory have shown that BALB/cJ mice are also good responders (75% positivity for antibodies to spermatozoa), and other strains are intermediate or low responders (Table 3). Circulating antibodies to spermatozoa have been detected in 89% of congenic CH3W3 mice, 50% of B10s, 38% of B6H2K, and 20% of B6(TL+) (Bigazzi et al., in preparation). Similar studies in different inbred strains of mice have shown a correlation between postthymectomy and postvasectomy EAO; i.e., good responder strains in one model are also good responders in the other (196). Kille et al. (208) investigated the response of female mice of various inbred strains to the sperm-specific isozyme of murine lactate dehydrogenase (LDH-C4) and found high-responder strains (SWR, SJL, BALB/c, and C3H/He) as well as intermediate to low responders (A, CBA, DBA/2, DBA/1, and C57Bl/6). These responses are not associated with the H-2 complex.

Bernard et al. (109) induced experimental autoimmune orchitis in inbred strains of mice by injection of mouse testis homogenate in complete Freund's adjuvant and pertussis vaccine. They observed marked strain variations in susceptibility to EAO, suggesting that genetic factors may be involved. Most SJL/J, BALB/c, NZC, and A.SW mice developed severe lesions of EAO (good responders), but the severity of orchitis was less in DBA/CaH and C57Bl/6 mice. Immunized nude BALB/c did not develop EAO. Susceptibility to EAO was found linked to the MHC in BALB/c and C57Bl/10 mice and mapped to genes encoded within the H-

Table 3 Circulating Antibodies to Spermatozoa in Vasectomized Mice of Various Inbred Strains

Strain	H-2 haplotype	Mice with antibodies (%)
C57L/J	b	78
BALB/cJ	d	75
DBA/1J	q	67
C57Bl/6J	b	30
DBA/2J	d	30
SWR/J	q	10
C57Bl/KsJ	d	10
CBA/J	k	10
C57Bl/10J	b	0
A/WySn	a	0
BUB/BnJ	q	0

2Dd region (210). It was also found that susceptibility to the induction of murine EAO was associated with the locus controlling *B. pertussis*-induced sensitivity to histamine (211). Finally, Teuscher et al. (163) observed that there are marked differences in susceptibility to EAO induction between BALB/c substrains and that BALB/c mice can be grouped into substrains of high susceptibility, intermediate susceptibility, and resistance. They suggested that these differences may be the result of genetic drift and/or mutations involving one or all of the loci controlling susceptibility to EAO.

7. Pathogenesis

Passive transfer experiments have shown that EAO can be transferred in mice with both immune sera and lymphocytes. For example, Pokorna (212) induced EAO in inbred C57Bl/10 mice by passive transfer of both immune serum and noncellular material prepared from lymphocytes of mice with EAO. Later investigation showed that lymphoid cells from the spleen and peripheral lymph nodes of immunized BALB/c mice were capable of adoptively transferring EAO to naive BALB/c *nu/nu* mice, injected intravenously with pertussis vaccine (209). On the other hand, serum from the same immunized mice (probably containing antibodies to spermatozoa) did not transfer EAO. Treatment of immune lymphoid cells with antibodies to Thy-1.2 and complement markedly reduced but did not completely abolish the capacity of those cells to adoptively transfer EAO, leading to the conclusion that possibly both T cells and antibodies are necessary in the effector stages of this experimental disease. Other investigators have demonstrated that delayed-type hypersensitivity reactions to syngeneic testicular cells can be transferred using peritoneal exudate cells from immunized donors pretreated with cyclophosphamide (213). In more sophisticated adoptive transfer experiments, almost half the recipient mice injected with spleen cell suspensions depleted of specific Lyt subsets developed orchitis (214). Cells that had been pretreated with antibodies to Lyt-1.2 plus complement or antibodies to Lyt-1.2 and Lyt-2.2 plus complement prior to transfer induced EAO in 41 and 40% of the recipients, respectively, indicating the possible role of Lyt-negative T lymphocytes in the induction of this condition. At the same time, other investigators observed that the combined local injection of two monoclonal antibodies, one against Sertoli cells and the other against the basal lamina of seminiferous tubules, caused alterations of spermatogenesis without inflammatory cell infiltration (204). Therefore, on the basis of the limited evidence available, testis damage in the mouse can be mediated by antibodies and/or lymphocytes sensitized against testis antigens. These results are not contradicted by Bernard's finding that nude mice do not develop EAO (109), since the absence of thymus-derived cells is bound to have a negative effect on the induction phase of testis autoimmunity. Interestingly, Japanese investigators (195) have reported that EAO develops in (C56Bl × J/1)F1 mice 3-4 months after neonatal thymectomy, without the need for an experimental immunization with testicular antigens. The time of neonatal thymectomy was critical; i.e., the procedure was effective when performed on day 3 after birth, but not on day 0 or day 7. Circulating autoantibodies against spermatozoa were found in 42% of animals. Finally, experimental allergic orchitis has been induced in cyclophosphamide-pretreated C3H/He mice by immunization with viable testicular cells without any adjuvants (215). Pathological changes, such as hypospermatogenesis and mild cellular interstitial infiltration, were observed in most of these mice, as well as delayed hypersensitivity responses to testicular antigens and circulating antisperm antibodies. These observations may all indicate that a suppressor cell population normally interferes with the induction of testis autoimmunity in mice and that its removal, either by neonatal thymectomy or cyclophosphamide pretreatment, facilitates the occurrence of EAO.

8. Comments

Mouse models of testis autoimmunity show great promise. In recent years numerous spermatozoal antigens of mice have been characterized and the immunogenetics of autoimmune responses to antigens of the testis in this species have been well delineated. Much work remains to be done. First, further characterization of the numerous spermatozoal antigens is needed, with particular attention given to their autoantigenic epitopes and their role in EAO. Second, additional studies of those models not induced by combinations of adjuvants are necessary. In particular, a careful analysis of the role of the thymus in EAO is warranted, considering this organ not just as a site for cell maturation but as a microenvironment with endocrine capabilities. Additional mechanistic studies of the cellular events involved in sensitization to testis autoantigens are also required.

The advantages of mice for immunologic research are well known, and investigators of reproductive immunology are finally taking advantage of them. The availability of numerous markers of subsets of T and B lymphocytes, as well as a variety of inbred mouse strains and congenic and recombinant animals will allow an in-depth investigation of testis autoimmunity in this species. In addition, cell hybridization studies and the possibility of T-cell cloning will open the field of testis autoimmunity to more sophisticated research at the cellular and molecular levels.

F. Models in Other Species

Autoimmune responses to spermatozoa and/or autoimmune orchitis have been experimentally induced in animals of various other species, such as bulls, rams, quails, and salmons (216-218). For example, bulls immunized with testis antigens in CFA developed antibodies to spermatozoa, positive DTH skin reactions and aspermatogenesis. Tubules showed thickening of basement membranes, and the interstitium was infiltrated with lymphocytes. No immune deposits were observed in tubules. These studies do not add much to what has been previously observed in guinea pigs or mice, for example, and to date it seems quite obvious that any animal species with a sufficiently developed immune system is capable of autoimmune responses to germ cells. However, studies in primates may provide indications more directly correlated with the situation in humans. Thus, we briefly review the work that has been performed in monkeys as well as a unique study in which human volunteers were experimentally immunized with testis antigens.

1. Humoral Immune Responses

No in-depth studies of testis-specific antigens have been performed in monkeys, and most of the serological experiments that we review here utilized crude testis homogenates, suspensions of spermatozoa, or sperm smears.

To our knowledge, there is only one study reporting the experimental induction of autoimmunity in human volunteers (219). Patients with prostatic carcinoma were immunized with autologous or homologous testis antigens in CFA. It was observed that transient low-titer antibodies to spermatozoa appear 2–8 weeks after sensitization. Indirect immunofluorescence on testis sections showed that the antisperm antibodies reacted with germinal cells, presumably spermatids and spermatozoa.

The first investigators to induce autoimmunity to testis in rhesus monkeys were Andrada et al. (220), who utilized either autologous (obtained by hemicastration) or isologous testis antigens. Antibodies to spermatozoa were detected in the sera of animals that had been castrated during the immunization period. No additional studies in this species were reported, until those of Alexander (221) in vasectomized monkeys. Antibodies to spermatozoa were detected in the serum of vasectomized monkeys, with percentages varying from 20% for sperm-agglutinating antibodies and 27% for sperm-immobilizing antibodies in animals 2-5 years postvasectomy to 9% for sperm-agglutinating and 27% for sperm-immobilizing antibodies in monkeys 5-10 years after surgery. In rhesus monkeys the levels of circulating sperm-agglutinating antibodies rise and increase with time after vasectomy. These initial findings have been confirmed and extended in later studies of various groups of vasectomized animals (222,223). Alexander and Tung (224) summarized the results obtained in a total of 58 vasectomized rhesus monkeys. Antibodies to spermatozoa developed in all monkeys within 17 days of surgery. However, antibody levels decreased rapidly so that 3-4 months after surgery approximately only 50% of the animals were producing autoantibodies to spermatozoa. In animals vasectomized 6 months or longer, sperm-immobilizing antibodies were present in 43% and sperm-agglutinating antibodies were detected in 32%. Antibodies to spermatozoa detectable by indirect immunofluorescence were found in 53%, with the most common those against the acrosome (90%). Less frequent were those to the postacrosomal area (45%), equatorial region (32%), and the tail (16%). Only 14% of the animals had all three kinds of antisperm antibodies, i.e., spermagglutinating, sperm immobilizing, and detectable by indirect immunofluorescence. Alexander and Tung have stated that animals without circulating antibodies may be in antigen excess and have immune complexes in their sera. It is also possible that these animals had ceased producing such antibodies. The same investigators (225) examined a total of 25 long-term vasectomized monkeys. Antisperm antibodies were found in the sera from 60% of vasectomized animals, but all of 13 age-matched controls were negative. Another study of vasectomized monkeys (226) found no significant changes in antisperm antibodies, a result difficult to interpret and possibly due to differences in techniques. Finally, the administration of dexamethasone at the time of vasectomy prevents the formation of antibodies to spermatozoa in cynomolgus monkeys, suggesting that sensitization to testis antigens occurs at the time of surgery (227).

2. Delayed-type Hypersensitivity Response

Volunteer patients with prostatic carcinoma, immunized with testis and CFA, showed DTH skin tests to sonicated spermatozoa (219). Decreased lymphocyte responses to phytohemagglutinin (PHA) stimulation (but not to ConA or pokeweed mitogen, PWM) and lack of skin test responsiveness to various antigens, such as *Candida albicans*, have been noted in vasectomized monkeys (224, 228).

3. Immunohistopathology

Alexander (221), in her initial study of vasectomized monkeys, reported that the efferent duct of one animal showed green-yellow fluorescence at the basement membrane level. Granular deposits of immunoglobulins and C3 were later found in the basement membranes of seminiferous tubules, rete testis, and epididymis of most vasectomized monkeys (225). In the same study, granular immune deposits were also observed in the efferent ducts, but not along the seminiferous tubules, of control monkeys.

4. Histopathology

Biopsy specimens from volunteer patients with prostatic carcinoma, immunized with testis antigens in CFA, showed changes of an inflammatory nature 20-40 days after sensitization (219). Polymorphonuclear leukocytes, as well as discrete accumulations of mononuclear cells, were observed around vessels. The seminiferous tubules showed a normal or slightly thickened basement membrane and progressive sloughing of germinal cells. Similar findings were observed in testes removed by castration 60-90 days after immunization. Conspicuous testis lesions, consisting of congestion and edema accompanied by sloughing of germinal cells, were observed in immunized monkeys (220). Moderate lymphocytic infiltration was present in only one animal.

Alexander (221) examined testes from vasectomized monkeys and found an increase in the diameter of the ductuli efferentes, which also showed a thickened basal lamina, There were also changes in the epididymis, particularly in the ductuli efferentes. Thickening of the basal lamina of the efferent ducts has also been noticed, but the morphology of the testis appeared normal, with intact spermatogenesis (222). Orchitis, aspermatogenesis, or both were later found in 92% of vasectomized animals (225). Orchitis, i.e., mononuclear cell infiltrates in the interstitial spaces, diffuse, patchy, or focal, was observed in 56% of animals, aspermatogenesis was noted in 85%, and epididymal changes were noted in 52%.

An additional finding, which has created much interest as well as concern, was reported by Alexander and Clarkson (229), who noted an increased severity of atherosclerosis in vasectomized monkeys (both *Macaca mulatta* and *Macaca fascicularis*) fed an atherogenic diet. It was suggested that the immune response to spermatozoa may exacerbate the atherosclerotic process. Atherosclerotic plaques were noted more frequently in the thoracic aorta and iliac arteries of vasectomized monkeys, and when the extension of the lesions was analyzed there was a striking increase in atherosclerosis of the abdominal aorta. It was also reported (230) that rhesus monkeys vasectomized for 9-14 years and fed monkey chow rather than an atherogenic diet also had more extensive and severe atherosclerosis than did controls of the same age. Interestingly, there was more extensive atherosclerosis in those animals that did not have free circulating antibodies against spermatozoa, a finding that was interpreted at that time as indicating that such animals were in sperm antigen excess and therefore had a higher concentration of immune complexes. However, there was no solid evidence of immune deposits (not to mention immune complexes) associated with the atherosclerotic lesions and one might actually assume that those animals were not producing antibodies against spermatozoa and that the atherosclerotic lesions were mediated by other, nonimmunologic mechanisms. Later studies have shown that "normal," untreated monkeys have high levels of circulating immune complexes (231), and that with a slight hyperlipoprotinemia vasectomy seems to result in a small protective effects against atherosclerosis (232). It is very difficult to interpret these findings in primates, especially since various studies of vasectomized men have shown no increase in atherosclerotic heart disease (see Chap. 5). Other investigators have found no difference in the occurrence of atherosclerotic plaques between vasectomized and control monkeys on an atherogenic diet, in spite of the development of antisperm antibodies in the vasectomized animals (233). It is hoped that future investigations will provide an explanation for this controversy.

5. Pathogenesis

At this point in time, it is quite difficult to speculate on the mechanisms of testis damage in monkeys with autoimmune responses to testis antigens induced by immunization or vasectomy. As usual, one can invoke both humoral and cell-mediated mechanisms, as well as combinations thereof.

6. Comments

Models of autoimmunity in primates are of obvious value because of their phylogenetic closeness to humans. However, the use of primates in studies of autoimmunity has been limited, most likely because of the high costs involved. Monkeys have been used to develop various experimental models of autoimmune disease, to search for spontaneous disorders similar to human autoimmune conditions, to demonstrate the potential autoimmunogenic effects of drugs, and as a source of autoantigens to reveal autoimmunization in humans (234). Thus far, the results obtained from the few studies of testis autoimmunity in monkeys have not been strikingly different from those observed in other species and have not provided additional insight. Yet it is important that such investigations be pursued, perhaps after primates have been better characterized from the point of view of MHC, lymphocyte markers, and other immune reagents.

II. NATURAL MODELS OF TESTIS AUTOIMMUNITY

In the past, immunologists have used the adjective "spontaneous" to define those animal models of autoimmunity that arise without apparent external cause, i.e., not induced by experimental manipulations, such as immunization or surgery (4,235). Surprisingly, the same term has also been applied to models obtained after neonatal thymectomy and x-irradiation (236,237). To avoid confusion, we use the term "natural" rather than "spontaneous" to indicate those models of autoimmunity that are not experimentally manipulated but produced by nature. To date, the best investigated natural models have been the lupus like conditions observed in various strains of mice (often referred to as murine lupus) and the thyroiditis that spontaneously develops in chicken and rats (4,6,7, 235). Less investigated are natural animal models of infertility occurring on an autoimmune basis. Obviously, there are considerable difficulties in maintaining colonies of animals that spontaneously develop autoimmune infertility. However, such a condition has been observed in a variety of animal species, such as mink, mice, beagles, and monkeys, and its study may prove of great help in understanding autoimmune responses to testis antigens and autoimmune disease of the male genital system.

A. Black Mink Model

The process of breeding mink with fine black fur has apparently selected for the phenotype of male infertility, resulting in a colony wherein approximately 20-30% of the males are infertile. Some mink are infertile quite early (soon after puberty); others become infertile at a later stage, after a period of proven fertility. Immunologic investigations performed in the laboratory of Tung have provided valuable information on autoimmune responses to spermatozoa, testis immunopathology, and histopathology of these animals, demonstrating that the infertile black mink is a natural model of testis autoimmunity (238,239).

1. Humoral Immune Responses

Indirect immunofluorescence on methanol-fixed mink spermatozoa revealed the presence of circulating antibodies, reactive with acrosomal material, in infertile black mink. The prevalence of these antibodies was 85% in mink with early infertility (mean antibody titer 20), 97% in late infertility (mean antibody titer 85), 82% in mink without orchitis (very low titer), and 100% in animals with orchitis (mean antibody titer 150). Thus, the mean antibody levels of animals with orchitis were significantly higher than those of animals without orchitis. Interestingly, antibodies to spermatozoa were also detected in the sera of 72% of a control group composed of fertile black mink. When these controls were divided according to coat color, it was found that black mink and pastel mink (genetically related to black mink) had the highest (100%) prevalence of antisperm antibodies, with comparable mean antibody titers (90), and opal and violet mink had lower prevalence and titers. Circulating antisperm antibodies were also detected in 29% of control females, mostly black and pastel. Indirect immunofluorescence on fixed smears revealed only antibodies to the acrosome, not other components of spermatozoa. However, antibodies to epitopes of the cell surface may not have been detected because of the limitations of the procedure. At present, there are no published reports characterizing the antigens involved in autoimmune responses of infertile mink and no studies of delayed-type hypersensitivity in this model.

2. Immunohistopathology

Heavy granular deposits of IgG and/or C3 were found in the basal lamina of the seminiferous tubules in 71% of mink with late infertility. Immunoglobulins eluted from these deposits contained antibodies to the acrosome of mink spermatozoa. Spermatozoal antigens were not detected in the immune deposits. It is of interest that none of the mink with early infertility had immune deposits in their testes.

3. Histopathology

Patchy and diffuse orchitis was found almost exclusively in animals with late infertility (47%), which showed heavy infiltration with lymphocytes, monocytes, plasma cells, and polymorphonuclear leukocytes around and inside the seminiferous tubules, which were devoid of germ cells, replaced by numerous macrophages. Smaller percentages of these animals showed focal or interstitial orchitis. Aspermatogenesis in the absence of orchitis or immune deposits in the testes was noted only in 15% of these mink.

On the other hand, black mink with early infertility presented quite a different picture; i.e., orchitis was much less prevalent (focal in 18% and interstitial in 13%), and aspermatogenesis alone was found in 62% of animals. Thus, the different kinetics of infertility in black mink are also reflected in the histopathology of their testes and suggest possible differences in etiology and pathogenesis.

4. Pathogenesis

It would be premature to draw any conclusions about the mechanisms of testis damage in infertile black mink. The condition seems quite heterogeneous, as shown by the timing of its development and the differences in histopathology and immunohistopathology. Tung has suggested that animals with early infertility (defined as "primary") may have a genetically determined abnormal development of the testis, perhaps mediated by hormonal disturbances. On the other hand, mink with late infertility (defined as "secondary") may develop an autoimmune orchitis, possibly mediated by in situ immune complex formation. The cause of the infertility, both early and late, is obviously unknown, but in both instances may be related to genes associated with the black coat color. There are many points that still need elucidation, such as the relationship between early and late infertility, the role of delayed-type hypersensitivity in mink infertility, and the status of the blood-testis barrier in fertile and infertile black mink. We look forward to further investigations of this interesting natural model of infertility.

B. Tailless Mouse Model

A natural model of testis autoimmunity was observed in a line of backcross mice developed in the laboratory of Bennet (240). Almost all tailless (T/tw 18) male mice and the great majority of tailless females are completely sterile. Since sterility is observed in both male and female mice, the genetic effects are obviously not limited to spermatogenesis. However, it is of interest that inflammatory lesions of the testis have been observed in sterile male mice.

1. Histopathology

Observations by light microscopy have shown that 40% of sterile tailless males had orchitis in one or both testes, and the remaining 60% had testes of normal histological appearance. The affected testes contained clusters of mononuclear cells in the interstitial tissue, mostly small to medium-sized lymphocytes with occasional plasma cells. Aspermatogenesis was observed in areas of lymphocytic infiltration, with germ cells absent or present in abnormally low numbers. Ultrastructural studies confirmed these observations. Lymphocytes were lodged between cytoplasmic processes of the adventitial cells, which normally form an uninterrupted layer between germinal epithelium and extratubular space. Basement membranes of seminiferous tubules were frequently disorganized, with dense lamellae of amorphous material and an extensive network of collagenous fibrils. Occasionally, lymphocytes were seen to protrude through gaps in the layer of adventitial cells, but only rarely were they observed within the germinal epithelium.

2. Immunologic Studies

Investigations of humoral or DTH responses to testis autoantigens in T/tw18 mice have not been reported. Thus, there is no direct evidence that the sterility observed in these animals is autoimmune. This is an unfortunate occurrence, since it would be of great interest to ascertain whether the 40% of sterile animals that exhibit orchitis also have autoimmune manifestations and whether the remaining 60% eventually develop a similar condition. To date, there is also no evidence regarding the presence of immune deposits within affected testes, even though this seems an unlikely possibility, since the ultrastructural studies would have revealed electron-opaque deposits. Finally, the phenotype of the lymphocytes present in the inflammatory infiltrates is still undefined.

Indirect evidence of an autoimmune response has been provided by in vitro studies showing that spleen lymphocytes from both fertile (young) and sterile T/tw18 mice are stimulated by germ cells from sterile males, i.e., recognize epitopes on these cells and proliferative vigorously. The same lymphocytes do not respond to germ cells from young fertile males. This evidence has been interpreted as suggesting that germ cells from young animals have the ability to activate suppressor T lymphocytes, but cells from sterile males have lost this ability, a change that correlates with the appearance of orchitis (240). However, one wonders whether this correlation is causal or just coincidental. For example, autoimmune damage to the tubules causes changes in their cell populations, so that Sertoli cells predominate. Thus, preparation of cells from the testes of sterile mice should contain a higher proportion of Sertoli cells than found in similar preparations from fertile animals. In that case, the decrease in suppression could be attributed to the changes in the proportion of germ cells versus Sertoli cells and be considered a consequence, not a cause, of autoimmune disease.

3. Pathogenesis

Obviously, the evidence available does not provide any clues about the mechanisms of testis damage in infertile tailless mice. At this stage, it is premature to consider this condition as autoimmune. However, this natural model is extremely attractive, since it occurs in mice, which are easier and less expensive to maintain than mink, beagles, and monkeys. In addition, markers of lymphocytes and a variety of immunologic procedures have been developed for research in mice that are not available for other species. Therefore, it would be very unfortunate if this natural model were not developed and investigated further.

C. A-Line Beagle Model

The purebred beagle colony at the Argonne National Laboratory has been a closed breeding unit since 1960. The colony population includes two partially inbred lines, one of which, defined as A line, is particularly interesting because of a high incidence of thyroiditis and orchitis (241). The latter condition was discovered because the reproductive performance of A-line beagles is less than that of outbred dogs maintained under identical conditions. The evaluation of semen quality from several A-line males revealed aspermia or greatly reduced numbers of spermatozoa.

The lesions observed in the testes of A-line beagles were lymphocytic infiltration and/or aspermatogenesis. The first was observed in 33% of dogs examined, and 50% had aspermatogenesis. The percentage of dogs with tubular lesions was twice as great in animals with lymphocytic lesions. Lymphocytic infiltration was nodular, diffuse, or in aggregations. Lymphocytes infiltrated the interstitium, surrounded the tubules, and also invaded the tubules and their lumina. In the case of nodular infiltration, sometimes germinal centers were observed in the nodules. Tubular changes included focal degeneration, segmental atrophy, and diffuse atrophy of the seminiferous epithelium. Degenerative changes included aggregation of spermatozoa, cell necrosis, and formation of giant cells. Testes with diffuse tubular atrophy had only Sertoli cells within the tubules.

To date, no immunologic or immunohistopathologic studies of A-line beagle orchitis have been published. Therefore, this model is still at a rather incomplete stage of development, in spite of its obvious interest, because of the association with another autoimmune condition, thyroiditis.

D. Monkey Model

Studies of primates are obviously very important because of the similarities with humans. Unfortunately, little has been done in the area of natural testis autoimmunity in monkeys. Early studies (220) reported the occasional finding of spermatogenic arrest in the testis of rhesus monkeys. Sperm counts revealed decreased numbers of cells, and aspermatogenesis was found in about 50% of seminiferous tubules. More detailed investigations of 13 normal monkeys showed that orchitis, aspermatogenesis, or both were present in 23% of animals (225). Orchitis (defined as mononuclear cell infiltration) was present in 15% and aspermatogenesis in 15%. No epididymal changes were noted. These animals had no detectable circulating antibodies to spermatozoal antigens, but granular deposits of immunoglobulins and C3 were found in 45% of testes, localized at the basement membrane level of the ductuli efferentes and epididymis but never around the seminiferous tubules.

In conclusion, the available evidence regarding "natural" autoimmune responses to spermatozoa and autoimmune orchitis in monkeys is very scarce. It is quite likely that this species can spontaneously develop both autoimmune responses and disease localized to their testes, but we are still at the level of serendipitous findings and no actual model is available.

III. CONCLUSIONS

In 1900, Metalnikoff published his landmark paper, "Studies on spermatoxine," containing a section on autospermatoxine, in which he stated that "when one injects guinea pig spermatozoa subcutaneously or intraperitoneally in another guinea pig, one notices that immediately after the first injection the serum of the inoculated guinea pig becomes weakly toxic, not only to spermatozoa from other guinea pigs, but also to those of the inoculated guinea pig itself. The autotoxicity increases considerably after the second and third injection" (10). After 86 years of research on animal models of testis autoimmunity, the literature on this subject has become overwhelming, often contradictory, and practically impossible to review in its entirety. In our conclusions, therefore, we will try to be selective and highlight those areas that seem more important from the point of view of modern immunology.

First, it is obvious that *antigens and autoantigens of the testis are extremely large in number and very heterogeneous in nature.* They have been detected in spermatozoa, other cells of the seminiferous epithelium, and Sertoli cells, as well as basement membranes. Their characterization is now progressing quite rapidly through the use of monoclonal antibodies, affinity chromatography, SDS-PAGE, and Western blotting. Thus, in a few years we should have a better understanding of the various epitopes involved in testis autoimmunity and infertility.

Second, *autoimmune responses to testis antigens have been demonstrated in a variety of animal species.* Production of autoantibodies as well as delayed-type hypersensitivity reactions occur in animal models of testis autoimmunity, obtained through different methods of induction. More modern methods of detection of these responses have recently been elaborated, but *there is still a need for sensitive, reproducible, and quantitative procedures, especially in the area of cell-mediated immunity.* For example, the quantitation of efferent lymphokine production is still rather rudimentary, an unfortunate circumstance that makes an accurate evaluation of this immune component quite difficult.

Third, *histopathology and immunohistopathology of the reproductive tract in animal models of testis autoimmunity are quite heterogeneous.* This has been noticed since the early studies of Voisin and Freund, and the situation has become more complex over the years. The two major types of testis damage observed in animal models are inflammation and aspermatogenesis. In Waksman's view, the inflammatory process occurs first and is followed by aspermatogenesis. Other investigators have claimed instead that aspermatogenesis occurs first and is followed by inflammation. As suggested by Voisin, both views may be correct; i.e., certain testis antigens may induce aspermatogenesis followed or not by reactive inflammation, and other antigens may cause an inflammatory process that results in aspermatogenesis. The immunohistopathological finding of immune deposits in the testis of certain models and the lack of such deposits in others bring evidence in favor of the heterogeneity of testis autoimmunity. The picture is further complicated by the observation that in some models (e.g., vasectomized rabbits) the deposition of immunoglobulins and complement components does not result in an acute inflammatory process but instead eventuates in the reduplication of basement membranes of seminiferous tubules, similar to what occurs at the level of the renal glomerular basement membranes in membranous glomerulonephritis. The parallel between kidney and testis pathology may be closer than we suspect. It is now well known that immunologically mediated proteinuria occurs not only through complement- and PMN-dependent mechanisms but also independently of the complement-neutrophil system and without glomerular inflammation (242). Perhaps aspermatogenesis may also occur on a similar basis.

Fourth, the debate that has raged over the years regarding the mechanisms of the damage occurring in testis autoimmunity should finally be concluded in a conciliatory way. In part, that debate was an echo of the disputes between "humoral" and "cellular" immunologists (243). Today, immunologists are quite comfortable in recognizing the primary role of cellular elements (T and B lymphocytes and antigen-presenting cells) in the generation of immune and autoimmune responses. However, it is also recognized that *both humoral and cellular mechanisms are involved at the effector level in the production of tissue damage*. The contradictory results of passive transfers of cells and antibodies, often quoted as supporting cell-mediated damage, were most probably caused by differences in the antigens used in the various experiments. As suggested by Voisin, some antigens induce pathogenic antibodies, others induce pathogenic lymphocytes, and others are capable of inducing both pathogenic antibodies and lymphocytes. This is a situation not unlike that occurring in other autoimmune diseases and is schematicaly represented in Fig. 1.. Antibody-dependent cytotoxicity may cause testis damage if antibodies to testis antigens penetrate the reproductive tract through leaky areas of the rete testis, epididymis, and so on, if not the seminiferous tubules themselves. Immune complex-mediated lesions may occur when immune deposits containing antibodies, testis antigens, and

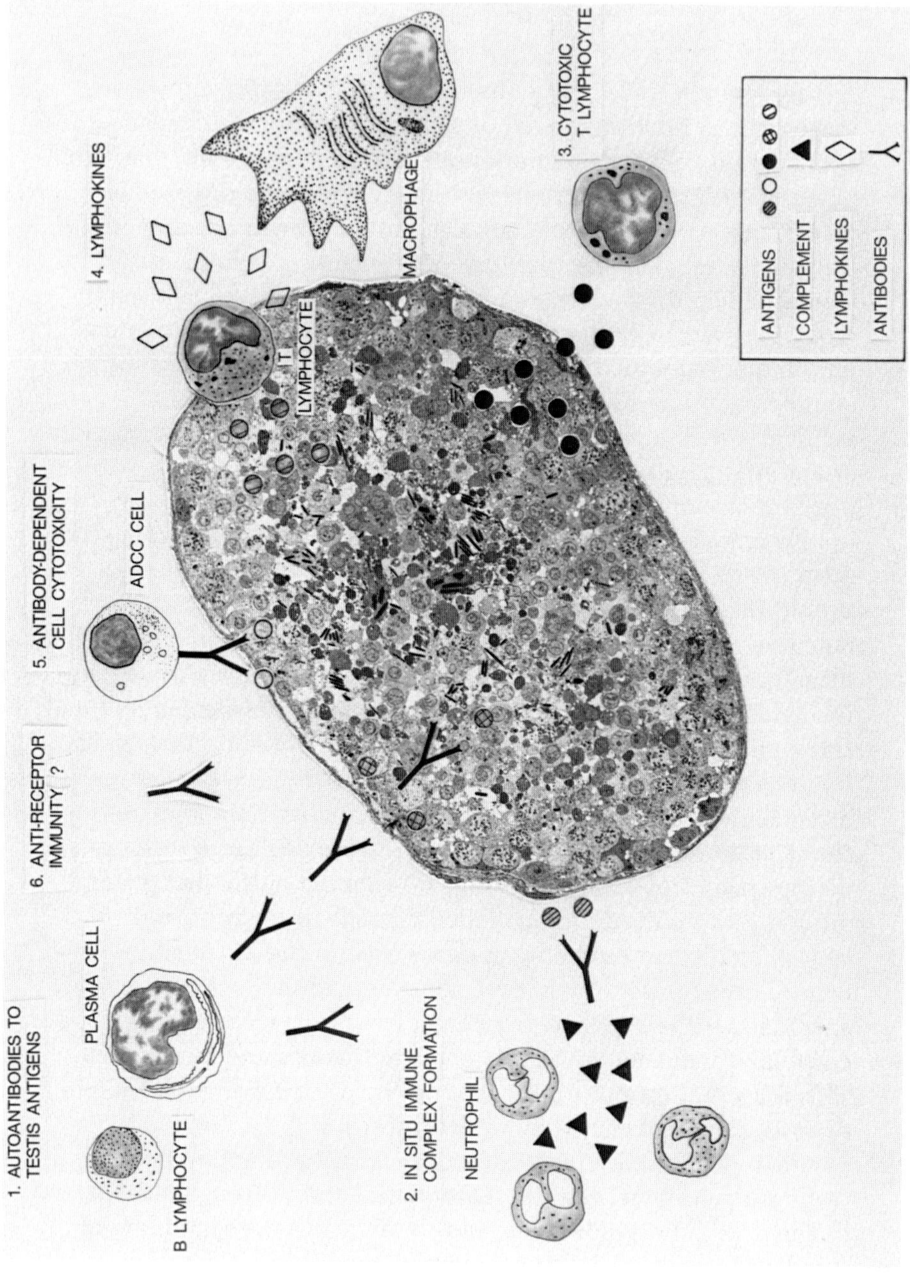

1. AUTOANTIBODIES TO TESTIS ANTIGENS
B LYMPHOCYTE
PLASMA CELL
6. ANTI-RECEPTOR IMMUNITY ?
5. ANTIBODY-DEPENDENT CELL CYTOTOXICITY
ADCC CELL
4. LYMPHOKINES
T LYMPHOCYTE
MACROPHAGE
3. CYTOTOXIC T LYMPHOCYTE
2. IN SITU IMMUNE COMPLEX FORMATION
NEUTROPHIL
ANTIGENS
COMPLEMENT
LYMPHOKINES
ANTIBODIES

complement components are formed at the level of the seminiferous tubules, resulting in a classic inflammatory process or in excessive production of basement membranes. Delayed-type hypersensitivity reactions may produce changes at various levels of the reproductive tract when sensitized lymphocytes react with testis antigens and release lymphokines or act directly as cytotoxic T lymphocytes. An interaction of cells and antibodies may result in antibody-dependent cell-mediated cytotoxicity at the level of the seminiferous tubules or other areas of the excurrent tract. Finally, in this list of pathogenetic mechanisms *one should not forget the possible role of antireceptor immunity*. To our knowledge, there is no published evidence demonstrating autoimmune responses directed against surface receptors of testicular cells (Leydig, Sertoli, and/or germ cells). However, many other organ-specific autoimmune diseases have been recently redefined as the consequence of receptor-specific autoimmune reactions (244), and it would not be surprising if antireceptor immunity were also involved in testis autoimmunity. In conclusion, *damage to the testis may be the result of one or more pathogenetic mechanisms, acting concurrently or in sequence.*

Fifth, *a variety of causes may initiate testis autoimmunity.* The immune system may respond to antigens of bacteria, viruses, and chemicals, cross-reacting with testis antigens. Such a situation might explain the presence of "natural" sperm antibodies in children, in the absence of mature germ cells. It is also possible that the immune system reacts to testis antigens that appear foreign because they have been altered, either naturally or experimentally. Most commonly, since the early days of reproductive immunology it has been assumed that testis autoimmunity results from the release of autoantigens that are normally "sequestered." However, it seems rather naive to imply that most, if not all, testis antigens are isolated from the immune system. Antigens of basement mem-

---

Figure 1 Schematic representation of mechanisms of autoimmune testis damage. Electron microscopy of rabbit testis (original magnification ×1000).

branes or of Sertoli cells are unlikely to be sequestered, but even spermatozoal antigens may come into contact with lymphocytes and macrophages, since it is already known that many areas of the excurrent tract are permeable to a variety of molecules. One should also consider the possibility that *antigens of spermatozoa may actually diffuse from the seminiferous tubules through the Sertoli cell junctions and the seminiferous basement membranes into the interstitial tissue*. Indeed, the concept of the immunologic isolation of spermatozoa (245) should not be interpreted in too rigid a fashion, as did happen in the past, perhaps under the influence of a similarly rigid interpretation of Ehrlich's "horror autotoxicus" paradigm. The blood-testis barrier excludes the passage of certain molecules from the blood into the seminiferous tubules. To our knowledge, it was never demonstrated that testis antigens cannot diffuse in the opposite direction, i.e., from the tubules into the interstitial tissue.

It is possible, therefore, that several testis antigens come into contact with lymphocytes, macrophages, and other antigen-presenting cells at various levels of the reproductive tract. A resident population of intraepithelial lymphocytes has been observed in the terminal portion of the seminiferous tubules near their junctions with the tubuli recti, rete testis, ductuli efferentes, epididymis, and vas deferens of rats and rhesus monkeys (246). In the rat, lymphocytes have been observed in the myoid layer of the limiting membrane of seminiferous tubules (but never within the seminiferous epithelium) (247). The numbers of such lymphocytes increase at the stages of the cycle of seminiferous epithelium when degeneration of cells occurs within the tubules. It has been hypothesized that the breakdown products of the degenerating cells evoke a numerical response of the lymphocytic elements present in the limiting membranes and that the lymphocytes may play a role in segregating sperm antigens from the general circulation (246,247). In terms of modern immunology, it is more likely that spermatozoal antigens react with lymphocytes of the reproductive tract and evoke autoimmune responses, which under normal conditions are immediately down-regulated by suppressive mechanisms. This occurrence would explain the production of so-called natural antisperm antibodies, which since the early periods of reproductive immunology have been observed in most of the animal models summarized in this review as well as in "normal" humans. The low titers of antibodies to spermatozoa often noted when testing control sera could then be explained as resulting from the continuous stimulation of B lymphocytes, which are controlled by T-suppressor cells and/or the idiotype-anti-idiotype network (248). Even the presence of immunoglobulins at various levels of the reproductive tract, which we and others have observed in normal animals, may be explained as the deposition of anti-idiotypic antibodies, not necessarily followed by an inflammatory process. In this view, *autoimmune responses to spermatozoal and other testis antigens may be a normal occurrence* ("physiologic" autoimmunity) (17) *and will cause damage only when they are not kept in check by homeostatic mechanisms* ("pernicious" autoimmunity) (17).

Finally, both natural and experimentally induced animal models indicate that *genetic factors have primary importance in testis autoimmunity*. They may affect the target organ as well as the immune system. For example, leakiness of the blood-testis barrier has been observed in one strain of rats that preferentially exhibit autoimmune responses to spermatozoa (159). Endocrine disturbances on a genetic basis may affect the testis of black mink and cause a secondary autoimmune orchitis (239). Immune responsiveness may also be genetically determined, so that certain strains or individual animals are "good responders" and others are "poor responders" to testis antigens. In addition, *a variety of xenobiotics may be responsible for the induction of autoimmune responses and disease in genetically predisposed individuals*, as demonstrated by recent immunotoxicological investigations (9, 249). These indications are invaluable and should eventually prompt immunogenetic studies of humans, to confirm the data obtained from the models of testis autoimmunity in inbred animals.

In conclusion, after more than 80 years of research on spermatozoal antigens and 35 years of study of experimental autoimmune orchitis, the investigation of animal models of testis autoimmunity has reached a level of maturity and sophistication that is quite exciting. Students of this area have solved many of the questions initially asked in pioneering studies of reproductive immunology and are now poised for modern investigations of basic issues of cellular and molecular immunology.

ACKNOWLEDGMENTS

Our research on animal models of testis autoimmunity was supported by contract NO1-HD-72-2775 and U.S. Public Health Service Grant HD 17546 from the National Institute of Child Health and Human Development of the NIH. We thank Drs. T. Takami and M. Zanetti for their expert collaboration and Ms. Ruth Conrod for excellent secretarial assistance.

REFERENCES

1. R. A. Good, J. Finstad, W. A. Cain, A. Fish, D. Y. Perey, and R. A. Gatti. Models of immunologic diseases and disorders. *Fed. Proc. 28*:191-205 (1969).
2. H. C. Lane, A. S. Fauci. Immunologic abnormalities in the acquired immunodeficiency syndrome. *Annu. Rev. Immunol. 3*:477-500 (1985).
3. P. E. Bigazzi. Immunologic effects of vasectomy in men and experimental animals. *Prog. Clin. Biol. Res. 70*:461-476 (1981).
4. P. E. Bigazzi and N. R. Rose. Spontaneous autoimmune thyroiditis in animals as a model of human disease. *Prog. Allergy 19*:245-274 (1976).
5. W. O. Weigle. Analysis of autoimmunity through experimental models of thyroiditis and allergic encephalomyelitis. *Adv. Immunol. 30*:159-273 (1980).
6. A. N. Theofilopoulos and F. J. Dixon. Murine models of systemic lupus erythematosus. *Adv. Immunol. 37*:269-390 (1985).

7. H. R. Smith and A. D. Steinberg. Autoimmunity—a perspective. *Annu. Rev. Immunol. 1*:175-210 (1983).
8. P. E. Bigazzi. Autoimmune orchitis and thyroiditis. *Methods Enzymol.* in press.
9. P. E. Bigazzi. Mechanisms of chemical-induced autoimmunity. In *Immunotoxicology and Immunopharmacology* (J. Dean et al., ed), Raven Press, New York, 1985, pp. 277-290.
10. S. Metalnikoff. Etudes sur la spermatoxine. *Ann. Inst. Pasteur 14*:577-589 (1900).
11. P. E. Bigazzi and N. R. Rose. Autoimmune thyroid disease. In *The Autoimmune Diseases* (N. R. Rose and I. Mackay, eds.), Academic Press, New York, 1985, pp. 161-199.
12. P. E. Bigazzi Autoimmunity of the adrenals. In *Autoimmunity and Endocrine Disease* (R. Volpe, ed.), Marcel Dekker, New York, 1985, pp. 345-373.
13. B. Noble, J. R. Brentjens, and G. A. Andres. Autoimmune kidney diseases. In *The Autoimmune Diseases* (N. R. Rose and I. R. Mackay, eds.), Academic Press, New York, 1985, pp. 339-370.
14. N. R. Rose, L. D. Bacon, R. S. D. Sundick, Y. M. Kong, P. Esquivel, and P. E. Bigazzi. Genetic regulation in autoimmune thyroiditis. In *Autoimmunity* (N. Talal, ed.), Academic Press, New York, 1977, pp. 63-77.
15. K. W. Beisel and N. R. Rose. Genetics of the autoimmune endocrinopathies: Animal models. In *Autoimmune Endocrine Disease* (T. Davies, ed.), J. Wiley and Sons, New York, 1983, pp. 41-58.
16. C. S. David. H-2 regulation of autoimmune and infectious diseases. In *Immunogenetics: Its Application to Clinical Medicine* (T. Sasazuki and T. Tada, eds.), Academic Press, New York, 1984, pp. 63-74.
17. I. R. Cohen. Autoimmunity: Physiologic and pernicious. *Adv. Intern. Med. 29*:147-165 (1984).
18. F. M. Burnet. *Autoimmunity and Disease*, F. A. Davis Co., Philadelphia, 1972, p. 101.
19. G. A. Voisin, A. Delaunay, and M. Barber. Sur des lesions testiculaires provoquees chez le cobaye par iso- et auto-sensibilisation. *Ann. Inst. Pasteur 81*:48-63 (1951).

20. D. W. Bishop. Aspermatogenesis induced by testicular antigen uncombined with adjuvant. *Proc. Soc. Exp. Biol. Med. 107*: 116-120 (1961).
21. F. T. Rapaport, A. Sampath, K. Kano, R. T. McCluskey, and F. Milgrom. Immunological effects of thermal injury. I. Inhibition of spermatogenesis in guinea pigs. *J. Exp. Med. 130*: 1411-1425 (1969).
22. E. F. Collazo, E. Thierer, and R. E. Mancini. Immunologic and testicular response in guinea pigs after unilateral thermal orchitis. *J. Allergy Clin. Immunol. 49*:167-173 (1972).
23. G. A. Voisin and F. Toullet. Etude sur l'orchite aspermatogenetique autoimmune et les autoantigenes de spermatozoides chez le cobaye. *Ann. Inst. Pasteur 114*:727-755 (1968).
24. S. Shulman. *Tissue Specificity and Autoimmunity*, Springer Verlag, New York, 1974.
25. S. Shulman. *Reproduction and Antibody Response*, CRC Press, Cleveland, Ohio, 1975.
26. A. Hekman and P. H. Rumke. Auto- and iso-immunity against spermatozoa. In *Textbook of Immunopathology* (P. E. Miescher and H. J. Muller-Eberhard, eds.), Second ed., Grune and Stratton, New York, 1976, pp. 947-962.
27. R. E. Mancini and J. A. Andrada. Immunological factors in human male and female infertility. In *Immunological Diseases* (M. Samter, ed.), Third ed., Little, Brown, Boston, 1978, pp. 1308-1329.
28. P. Rumke. Auto- and iso-immune reactions to antigens of the gonads and genital tract. In *Immunology 80. Progress in Immunology IV* (M. Fougereau and J. Dausset, eds.), Academic Press, New York, 1980, pp. 1065-1092.
29. S. K. Tung. Autoimmunity of the testis. In *Immunological Aspects of Infertility and Fertility Regulation* (D. S. Dhindsa and G. F. B. Schumacher, eds.), Elsevier/North Holland, New York, 1980, pp. 33-91.
30. K. S. K. Tung, C. Teuscher, and A. L. Meng. Autoimmunity to spermatozoa and the testis. *Immunol. Rev. 55*:217-255 (1981).
31. K. S. K. Tung and A. C. Menge. Sperm and testicular autoimmunity. In *The Autoimmune Diseases* (N. R. Rose and I. R. Mackay, eds), Academic Press, New York, 1985, pp. 537-590.

32. G. A. Voisin, F. Toullet, and M. D'Almeida. Characterization of spermatozoal auto-, iso- and allo-antigens. *Acta Endocrinol. (Kopern.) 78*(Suppl. 194):173-198 (1975).
33. M. G. O'Rand. Antigens of spermatozoa and their environment. In *Immunological Aspects of Infertility and Fertility Regulation* (D. S. Dhindsa and G. F. B. Schumacher, eds.), Elsevier/North Holland, New York, pp. 151-171.
34. E. Goldberg. Sperm specific antigens and immunological approaches for control of fertility. In *Recent Advances in Reproduction and Regulation of Fertility* (G. P. Talwar, ed.), Elsevier/North Holland, New York, 1979, pp. 281-290.
35. M. Lefroit-Joliy, R. Lebar, and G. A. Voisin. Guinea pig spermatozoal plasma membrane T autoantigen. Attempts at solubilization, purification and characterization. *Mol. Immunol. 16*:327-333 (1979).
36. P. P. Le Bouteiller, F. Toullet, S. Righenzi, and G. A. Voisin. Ultrastructural localization of guinea pig spermatozoal autoantigens on germinal cells by immunoperoxidase techniques. *J. Histochem. Cytochem. 27*:857-866 (1979).
37. P. C. Brown, L. E. Glynn, and E. J. Holborow. The pathogenesis of experimental allergic orchitis in guinea pigs. *J Pathol. Bacteriol. 86*:505-520 (1963).
38. D. W. Bishop and G. L. Carlson. Immunologically induced aspermatogenesis in guinea pigs. *Ann. N.Y. Acad. Sci. 124*: 266 (1965).
39. D. W. Bishop. Sorbitol dehydrogenase: Enzymic antigen and assay for induced aspermatogenesis. In *International Convocation on Immunology, Buffalo, New York, 1968* (N. R. Rose and F. Milgrom, eds.), Karger, Basel, 1969, pp. 334-338.
40. S. Katsh, A. R. Aguirre, F. W. Leaver, and G. F. Katsh. Purification and partial characterization of aspermatogenic antiten. *Fertil. Steril. 23*:644-656 (1972).
41. R. Wellerson, P. Wagstaff, S. Asculai, M. Hudson, and A. B. Kupferberg. Induction of aspermatogenesis in guinea pig through immunization with lactate dehydrogenase-Z isozyme. *Int. J. Fertil. 19*:65-72 (1974).
42. J. J. Jackson, A. Hagopian, D. J. Carlo, G. Limjuco, and E. H. Eylar. Experimental allergic aspermatogenic orchitis. Isolation of a spermatozoal protein (AP1) which induces allergic aspermatogenic orchitis. *J. Biol. Chem. 250*:6141–6150 (1975).

43. A. Hagopian, J. J. Jackson, D. J. Carlo, G. A. Limjuco, and E. H. Eylar. Experimental allergic aspermatogenic orchitis. III. Isolation of spermatozoal glycoproteins and their role in allergic aspermatogenic orchitis. *J. Immunol. 115*:1731-1743 (1975).
44. K. S. K. Tung, L. P. B. Han, and A. P. Evan. Differentiation autoantigen of testicular cells and spermatozoa in the guinea pig. *Dev. Biol. 68*:224-238 (1979).
45. C. Teuscher, G. C. Wild, and K. S. K. Tung. Acrosomal autoantigens of guinea pig sperm. I. The purification of an aspermatogenic protein, AP2. *J. Immunol. 130*:317-322 (1983).
46. C. Teuscher, G. C. Wild, and K. S. K. Tung. Experimental allergic orchitis: The isolation and partial characterization of an aspermatogenic polypeptide (AP3) with an apparent sequential disease-inducing determinant(s). *J. Immunol. 130*: 2683-2688 (1983).
47. C. Teuscher, G. C. Wild, and K. S. K. Tung. Immunochemical analysis of guinea pig sperm autoantigens. *Biol. Reprod. 26*: 218-229 (1982).
48. A. Alonso, J. M. S. De Cerezo, N. Gonzalez, M. P. Bueno, and R. S. Mancini. Immunological responses of guinea pigs sensitized to homologous antigens. *Am. J. Reprod. Immunol. 6*: 14-18 (1984).
49. P. Primakoff and D. G. Myles. A map of the guinea pig sperm surface constructed with monoclonal antibodies. *Dev. Biol. 98*:417-428 (1983).
50. D. G. Myles, P. Primakoff, and D. E. Koppel. A localized surface protein of guinea pig sperm exhibits free diffusion in its domain. *J. Cell Biol. 98*:1905-1909 (1984).
51. D. G. Myles and P. Primakoff. Localized surface antigens of guinea pig sperm migrate to new regions prior to fertilization. *J. Cell Biol. 99*:1634-1641 (1984).
52. P. Primakoff, H. Hyatt, and D. G. Myles. A role for the migrating sperm surface antigen PH-20 in guinea pig sperm binding to the egg zona pellucida. *J. Cell Biol. 101*:2239-2244 (1985).
53. A. E. Cowan, P. Primakoff, and D. G. Myles. Sperm exocytosis increases the amount of PH-20 antigen on the surface of guinea pig sperm. *J. Cell Biol. 103*:1289-1297 (1986).

54. L. S. N. Walsh. Natural auto and homoio spermatoxins in guinea pig serum. *J. Immunol. 10*:803-809 (1925).
55. J. Freund, M. M. Lipton, and G. E. Thompson. Aspermatogenesis in the guinea pig induced by testicular tissue and adjuvants. *J. Exp. Med. 97*:711-726 (1953).
56. S. Katsh and D. W. Bishop. The effects of homologous testicular and brain and heterologous testicular homogenates combined with adjuvant upon the testes of guinea-pigs. *J. Embryol. Exp. Morphol. 6*:94-104 (1958).
57. J. Baum, B. Boughton, J. L. Mongar, and H. O. Schild. Autosensitization by sperm in guinea-pigs. *Immunology 4*:95-110 (1961).
58. P. Le Boutellier, F. Toullet, and G. A. Voisin. Ultrastructural lesions induced in vitro in guinea-pig spermatozoa by a specific autoantibody (anti-T) and complement. *Immunology 28*:983-999 (1975).
59. B. H. Waksman. A histologic study of the auto-allergic testis lesion in the guinea-pig. *J. Exp. Med. 109*:311-324 (1959).
60. P. C. Brown, E. J. Holborow, and L. E. Glynn. The aspermatogenic antigen in experimental allergic orchitis in guinea-pigs. *Immunology 9*:255-260 (1965).
61. K. S. K. Tung and N. J. Alexander. Immunopathologic studies on vasectomized guinea pigs. *Biol. Reprod. 17*:241-254 (1977).
62. T. T. F. Huang, K. S. K. Tung, and R. Yanagimachi. Autoantibodies from vasectomized guinea pigs inhibit fertilization in vitro. *Science 213*:1267-1269 (1981).
63. P. C. Brown, L. E. Glynn, and E. J. Holborow. The dual necessity for delayed hypersensitivity and circulating antibody in the pathogenesis of experimental allergic orchitis in guinea-pigs. *Immunology 13*:307-314 (1967).
64. A. B. Mazzolli. Demonstration in vitro of delayed hypersensitivity in experimental allergic orchitis in guinea-pigs. *J. Reprod. Fertil. 26*:161-166 (1971).
65. Z. H. Marcus, Y. Soffer, A. Ben-David, S. Peleg, and L. Nebel. Studies on sperm antigenicity. I. Delayed hypersensitivity to spermatozoa. *Eur. J. Immunol. 3*:75-78 (1973)
66. V. Toder, Z. H. Marcus, and L. Nebel. Studies on sperm antigenicity. IV. Lymphocyte cytotoxicity in cell-mediated re-

sponse to homologous spermatozoa. *Eur. J. Immunol. 5*:680-683 (1975).
67. Z. Pokorna, J. Pekarek, and J. Svejcar. In vitro production of the factors effective in the transfer of experimental autoimmune aspermatogenesis. *Folia Biol. 21*:139-143 (1975).
68. M. S. Nemirovsky. Effects of antigenic competition between sperm autoantigens and ovalbumin upon humoral and cell-mediated immunity and the development of autoimmune aspermatogenic orchitis (AIAO) in guinea pigs. *Arch. Androl. 3*:43-49 (1979).
69. M. S. Nemirovsky. Role of histoincompatibility on the blastogenic response of lymphocytes from guinea pigs alloimmunized with sperm cells. *Am. J. Reprod. Immunol. 5*:5-8 (1984).
70. V. Y. Muir, J. L. Turk, and H. G. Hanley. Comparison of allergic aspermatogenesis with that induced by vasectomy. I. In vivo studies in the guinea pig. *Clin. Exp. Immunol. 24*:72-80 (1976).
71. V. Y. Muir, J. L. Turk, and H. G. Hanley. Comparison of allergic aspermatogenesis with that induced by vasectomy. II. In vitro studies of cell-mediated immunity to sperm after vasectomy in man and guinea pig. *Clin. Exp. Immunol. 28*:461-466 (1977).
72. V. Y. Muir and J. L. Turk. Immunological unresponsiveness during induction of experimental autoimmune orchitis in guinea-pigs: Studies in vivo and in vitro. *Immunology 36*:95-102 (1969).
73. H. Sanui, S. Yoshida, K. Himeno, and K. Nomoto. Delayed hypersensitivity to syngeneic testicular cells induced by intratesticular bacterial infection in guinea pigs. *Immunolgy 46*: 635-642 (1982).
74. H. Sanui, S. Yoshida, K. Himeno, and K. Nomoto. Experimental allergic orchitis induced by unilateral intratesticular bacterial infection on guinea pigs. *Immunology 49*:45-51 (1982).
75. S. Yoshida, K. Nomoto, K. Himeno, and H. Sanui. Delayed hypersensitivity to syngeneic or xenogeneic testicular cells in guinea-pigs. *Immunology 42*:445-449 (1981).

76. K. A. Laurence, O. Carpuk, A. Lefevre, and D. Mauldin. Allergic aspermatogenesis in the guinea pig. *Int. J. Fertil. 10*: 341-347 (1965).
77. P. C. Brown and L. E. Glynn. The early lesion of experimental allergic orchitis in guinea pigs: An immunological correlation. *J. Pathol. 98*:277-282 (1969).
78. P. C. Brown, J. Dorling, and L. E. Glynn. Ultrastructural changes in experimental allergic orchitis in guinea-pigs. *J. Pathol. 106*:229-233 (1972).
79. K. S. K. Tung, E. R. Unanue, and F. J. Dixon. The immunopathology of experimental allergic orchitis. *Am. J. Pathol. 60*: 313-323 (1970).
80. T. Nagano and K. Okumura. Fine structural changes in allergic aspermatogenesis in the guinea pig. I. The similarity in the initial changes induced by passive transfer of anti-testis serum and by immunization with testicular tissue. *Virchows Arch. Zellpathol. 14*:223-236 (1973).
81. F. Toullet and G. A. Voisin. Induction d'orchi-epididymite aspermatogene auto-immune et de reponses immunes chez des cobayes des lignees consanguines S2 et S13 par immunisation avec des spermatozoides isogeniques et allogeniques et des autoantigenes extraits de spermatozoides homologues. *Ann. Immuno. (Inst. Pasteur) 130C*:373-384 (1979).
82. R.-M. Pelletier, M. S. Nemirovsky, R. Calvert, and J. S. Hugon. Effects of immunization with Freund's complete adjuvant and isologous spermatozoa on the seminiferous epithelium and blood-testis barrier in guinea pigs. *Anat. Rec. 199*:197-211 (1981).
83. W. R. Jones. Immunological aspecst of infertility. In *Immunology of Human Reproduction* (J. S. Scott and W. R. Jones, eds), Academic Press, London, 1976, pp. 375-413.
84. N. J. Alexander. Autoimmune hypospermatogenesis in vasectomized guinea pigs. *Contraception 8*:147-164 (1973).
85. K. S. K. Tung. Pathogenesis of testicular pathology in vasectomized guinea pigs. In *Vasectomy. Immunologic and Pathophysiologic Effects in Animals and Men* (I. H. Lepow and R. Crozier, eds.), Academic Press, New York, 1979.
86. S. H. Stone, E. M. Lerner II, and J. H. Goode, Jr. Adoptive transfer of autoimmune aspermatogenesis in inbred guinea pigs.

In *International Convocation on Immunology, Buffalo, New York, 1968* (N. R. Rose and F. Milgrom, eds.), Karger, Basel, 1969, pp. 339-341.
87. K. S. K. Tung, C. Teuscher, E. H. Goldberg, and G. Wild. Genetic control of antisperm autoantibody response in vasectomized guinea pigs. *J. Immunol. 127*:835-839 (1981).
88. A. L. Meng and K. S. K. Tung. Cell-mediated and humoral immune responses to aspermatogenic antigen in experimental allergic orchitis in the guinea-pig. *J. Reprod. Fertil. 69*:279-288 (1983).
89. D. J. Carlo, A. Hagopian, J. J. Jackson, G. A. Limjuco, and E. H. Eylar. Experimental allergic orchitis and aspermatogenesis. *J. Immunol. 116*:610-622 (1976).
90. F. Toullet and G. A. Voisin. Passive transfer of autoimmune aspermatogenic orchiepididymitis (AIAO) by anti-spermatozoa sera. Influence of the type of autoantigen and the class of antibody. *Clin. Exp. Immunol. 26*:549-562 (1976).
91. F. Toullet, F. Chadenier, J. L. Maillard, and G. A. Voisin. Cellular transfer of autoimmune aspermogenic orchiepididymitis (AIAO) by the i.v. route in the guinea pig. *Clin. Exp. Immunol. 59*:593-603 (1985).
92. G. L. Kantor and F. J. Dixon. Transfer of experimental allergic orchitis with peritoneal exudate cells. *J. Immunol. 108*: 329-338 (1972).
93. K. S. K. Tung. Allergic orchitis lesions are adoptively transferred from vasoligated guinea pigs to syngeneic recipients. *Science 201*:833-835 (1978).
94. C. Hiramine and K. Hojo. Requirement of B lymphocytes in local adoptive transfer of experimental allergic orchitis (EAO) by lymph node cells. *Am. J. Reprod. Immunol. 6*:85-91 (1984).
95. T. S. Kuhn. *The Structure of Scientific Revolutions*, Second ed., University of Chicago Press, Chicago, 1970. p. 17.
96. S. Mudd and E. B. H. Mudd. The specificity of mammalian spermatozoa, with especial reference to electrophoresis as a means of serological differentiation. *J. Immunol. 17*:39–52 (1929).
97. A. J. Weil and A. E. Finkler. Isoantigenicity of rabbit semen. *Proc. Soc. Exp. Biol. Med. 102*:624-626 (1959).

98. K. M. Stevens and C. A. Fost. Sperm and antibody production in rabbits following immunization with sperm and semen. *Proc. Soc. Exp. Biol. Med. 117*:125-127 (1964).
99. L. V. Swanson and H. D. Hafs. Testicular and epididymidal sperm numbers in unilaterally vasoligated rabbits. *Proc. Soc. Exp. Biol. Med. 131*:763-768 (1969).
100. K. Bratanov, V. Dikov, and Y. Popova. On the formation of autospermoantibodies in brood animals. *C.R. Acad. Bulg. Sci. 17*:1117-1119 (1964).
101. K. Bratanov. Reproductive immunology—historical roots, achievements and prospects. In: *Reproductive Immunology 1983* (S. Isojima and W. D. Billington, eds.), Elsevier, New York, 1983.
102. C. Yantorno, M. T. Debanne, and E. Vottero-Cima. Autoimmune orchitis induced by autoimmunization with seminal plasma in the rabbit. *J. Reprod. Fertil. 27*:311-320 (1971).
103. R. J. Ablin and W. A. Soanes. Experimental production of autoimmune aspermatogenic orchitis in the rabbit in consequence of in situ freezing of the testis. *Rur. Surg. Res. 4*: 98-106 (1972).
104. E. Zappi, M. Nemirovsky, and S. Shulman. Cellular and humoral responses of autosensitized rabbits to a testis cryoinjury. *Immunology 26*:477-488 (1974).
105. A. Eyquem and H. Krieg. Experimental autosensitization of the testis. *Ann. N.Y. Acad. Sci. 124*:270-278 (1965).
106. P. E. Bigazzi, L. L. Kosuda, K. C. Hsu, and G. A. Andres. Immune complex orchitis in vasectomized rabbits. *J. Exp. Med. 143*:382-404 (1976).
107. K. S. K. Tung and A. J. Woodroffe. Immunopathology of experimental allergic orchitis in the rabbit. *J. Immunol 120*: 320-328 (1978).
108. M. G. O'Rand and J. P. Porter. Isolation of a sperm membrane sialoglycoprotein autoantigen from rabbit testis. *J. Immunol. 122*:1248-1254 (1979).
109. M. G. O'Rand and J. P. Porter. Purification of rabbit sperm autoantigens by preparative SDS gel electrophoresis: Amino acid and carbohydrate content of RSA-1. *Biol. Reprod. 27*: 713-721 (1982).

110. R. K. Naz, J. M. Saxe, and A. C. Menge. Inhibition of fertility in rabbits by monoclonal antibodies against sperm. *Biol. Reprod. 28*:249-254 (1983).
111. R. K. Naz, B. B. Rosenblum, and A. C. Menge. Characterization of a membrane antigen from rabbit testis and sperm isolated by using monoclonal antibodies and effect of its antiserum on fertility. *Proc. Natl. Acad. Sci. USA 81*:857-861 (1984).
112. P. E. Bigazzi, L. L. Kosuda, L. L. Harnick, R. C. Brown, and N. R. Rose. Antibodies to testicular antigens in vasectomized rabbits. *Clin. Immunol. Immunopathol. 5*:182-194 (1976).
113. N. J. Alexander and K. S. K. Tung. Vasectomy in the rabbit: Immunological and morphological effects. In *Vasectomy. Immunological and Pathophysiologic Effects in Animals and Men* (I. H. Lepow and R. Crozier, eds.), Academic Press, New York, 1979, pp. 355-377.
114. N. J. Alexander and K. S. K. Tung. Immunological and morphological effects of vasectomy in the rabbit. *Anat. Rec. 188*:339-350 (1977).
115. K. S. K. Tung, R. K. Bryson, L.-P. B. Han, and L. C. Walker. Circulating immune complexes in vasectomy. In *Vasectomy. Immunological and Pathophysiologic Effects in Animals and Man* (I. H. Lepow and R. Crozier, eds.), Academic Press, New York, 1979.
116. A. G. Tumboh-Oeri and T. K. Roberts. Immunological and morphological consequences of vasectomy in the rabbit. *Experientia 35*:675-676 (1979).
117. M. G. O'Rand, J. P. Porter, and N. J. Alexander. Isolation of a sperm autoantigen from the kidneys of vasectomized rabbits. *J. Reprod. Immunol. 6*:121-128 (1984).
118. C. J. Flickinger. Fine structure of the rabbit testis after vasectomy. *Biol. Reprod. 13*:61-67 (1975).
119. J. M. Bedford. Adaptations of the male reproductive tract and the fate of spermatozoa following vasectomy in the rabbit, rhesus monkey, hamster and rat. *Biol. Reprod. 14*: 118-142 (1976).
120. R. H. Hooker. Changes in the testes and epididymides of rabbits following long-term vasectomy or vasocystostomy:

Correlation with results of vasovasostomy. *Biol. Reprod. 22*:297-306 (1980).
121. N. K. Lohiya, N. Mathur, S. N. Tiwari, and A. C. Shipstone. Ultrastructural changes in rabbit testis and epididymis following vasectomy: A long-term study. *Acta Eur. Fertil. 14*:141-146 (1983).
122. J. Klein. *Natural History of the Major Histocompatibility Complex*, J. Wiley and Sons, New York, 1986.
123. J. Freund, M. M. Lipton, and G. E. Thompson. Impairment of spermatogenesis in the rat after cutaneous injection of testicular suspension with complete adjuvants. *Proc. Soc. Exp. Biol. Med. 87*:408-411 (1954).
124. K. P. Gunaga, A. R. Sheth, and S. S. Rao. Immunological studies with rat testis: Antigenic characterization. *J. Reprod. Fertil. 23*:263-269 (1970).
125. S. Isojima and T. Shun Li. Stepwise appearance of sperm-specific antigens in rats and their disappearance after fertilization. *Fertil. Steril. 19*:999-1008 (1968).
126. B. Denduchis, L. Lustig, N. N. Gonzalez, and R. P. Puig. Isolation and immunological reactivity of soluble fractions from rat seminiferous tubule basement membrane. *Arch. Androl. 2*:233-240 (1979).
127. B. Denduchis, L. Lustig, N. N. Gonzalez, and R. E. Mancini. Studies on the nature of extracellular components of rat seminiferous tubular wall. I. Isolation and chemical characterization of basement membrane. *Biol. Reprod. 13*:274-281 (1975).
128. L. Lustig, B. Denduchis, and R. E. Mancini. Studies of the nature of extracellular components of rat seminiferous tubular wall. II. Immunological characterization of basement membrane antigen. *Int. J. Fertil. 22*:16-23 (1977).
129. K.-O. Soderstrom, K. Sege, and L. C. Andersson. Expression of histoincompatibility antigens during spermatogenesis in the rat. *J. Immunol. 128*:1671-1675 (1982).
130. J. R. Head and R. E. Billingham. Immune privilege in the testis. II. Evaluation of potential local factors. *Transplantation 40*:269-275 (1985).
131. T. Vanha-Perttula and M. Arya. Lectin staining of rat testis and epididymis after ligation of excurrent ducts at different levels. *Biol. Reprod. 33*:477-485 (1985).

132. P. H. Rumke and M. Titus. Spermagglutinin formation in male rats by subcutaneously injected syngeneic epididymal spermatozoa and by vasoligation or vasectomy. *J. Reprod. Fertil. 21*:69-79 (1970).
133. A. Gupta, R. M. Gupta, I. M. Gupta, and J. P. Thapliyal. Immunologically induced injury in guinea pigs and rats using testis as the target organ. *Indian J. Exp. Biol. 12*:1-4 (1974).
134. G. E. Brannen and D. L. Klein. Immunogenicity of spermatozoa. *Invest. Urol. 12*:193-199 (1974).
135. G. E. Brannen and D. S. Coffey. Immunologic implications of vasectomy. II. Serum-mediated immunity. *Fertil. Steril. 25*:515-520 (1974).
136. G. E. Brannen and D. S. Coffey. Serum-mediated immunoresponses to spermatozoa. *Invest. Urol. 13*:85-89 (1975).
137. P. E. Bigazzi, L. L. Kosuda, and L. L. Harnick. Sperm autoantibodies in vasectomized rats of different inbred strains. *Science 197*:1282-1283 (1977).
138. T. Takami, H. W. Kunz, T. J. Gill III, and P. E. Bigazzi. Genetic control of autoantibody production to spermatozoa in vasectomized rats. *Am. J. Reprod. Immunol. 2*:5-7 (1982).
139. A. Rost, U. Kneppenberg, and U. Fiedler. Nachweis von zirkulierenden Spermatozoen-Antikorpern nach Vasektomie und Epididymektomie mittels der Technik fluoreszierender Antikorper. *Urol. Int. 34*:374-386 (1979).
140. M. H. E. Tonsy, N. R. Rose, M. E. Rehewy, and E. S. E. Hafez. Effect of Freund's complete adjuvant on the immune response of vasectomized rats. *Arch. Androl. 2*:323-329 (1979).
141. M. M. Crissey, M. Srougi, P. E. Bigazzi, J. McDonald, and R. F. Gittes. Correlation of sperm granulomas and sperm autoantibodies in inbred rats. *Fertil. Steril. 33*:328-332 (1980).
142. J. Pedersen, A. Rubenson, and L.-A. Nilsson. Formation of antisperm autoantibodies in rats vasectomized at prefertile age. *Scand. J. Urol. Nephrol. 17*:277-281 (1983).
143. J. Lovett, L. M. Nyberg Jr., S. Brown, and S. Mathur. Suppression of post-vasectomy cytotoxic sperm antibody formation in rats by a short-term pretreatment with cyclosporine. *Am. J. Reprod. Immunol. 11*:65-68 (1986).

144. J. C. Herr, C. J. Flickinger, S. S. Howards, S. Yarboro, D. R. Spell, D. Caloras, and T. N. Gallien. An enzyme-linked immunosorbent assay for measuring antisperm autoantibodies following vasectomy in Lewis rats. *Am. J. Reprod. Immunol. 11*:75-81 (1986).
145. E. Merimsky, R. Orni-Wasserlaug, and I. Yust. Assessment of immunological mechanisms in infertility of the rat after experimental testicular torsion. *Urol. Res. 12*:179-182 (1984).
146. H. L. Lipscomb, P. J. Gardner, and J. G. Sharp. The effect of neonatal thymectomy on the induction of autoimmune orchitis in rats. *J. Reprod. Immunol. 1*:209-217 (1979).
147. L. Lustig, M. L. Satz, M. B. Sztein, and B. Denduchis. Antigens of the basement membranes of the seminiferous tubules induce autoimmunity in Wistar rats. *J. Reprod. Immunol. 4*: 79-90 (1982).
148. G. E. Brannen, A. M. Kwart, and D. S. Coffey. Immunologic implications of vasectomy. I. Cell-mediated immunity. *Fertil. Steril. 25*:508-514 (1974).
149. S. Levine and R. Sowinski. Allergic inflammation, infarction and induced localization in the testis. *Am. J. Pathol. 59*:437-447 (1970).
150. P. J. Gardner and P. D. Shervey. An ultrastructural and histochemical study of autoimmune aspermatogenesis in the rat testis. *Z. Zellforsch. 147*:191-198 (1974).
151. M. Hattori and M. R. Brandon. Infertility in rats induced by neonatal thymectomy. In *Immunological Influence on Human Fertility* (B. Boettcher, ed.), Academic Press, New York, 1977, pp. 311-322.
152. H. Wekerle and M. Begemann. Experimental autoimmune orchitis: In vitro induction of an autoimmune disease. *J. Immunol. 116*:159-161 (1976).
153. L. Lustig, B. Denduchis, N. N. Gonzalez, and R. P. Puig. Experimental orchitis induced in rats by passive transfer of an antiserum to seminiferous tubule basement membrane. *Arch. Androl. 1*:333-343 (1978).
154. B. Denduchis and L. Lustig. Experimental orchitis induced in rats by an antiserum to a noncollagen fraction of seminiferous tubule basement membrane. In *Oligozoospermia:*

Recent Progress and Andrology (G. Frajese, E. S. E. Hafez, C. Conti, and A. Fabbrini, eds.), Raven Press, New York, 1981, pp. 207-218.
155. B. Denduchis, M. L. Satz, M. B. Sztein, R. P. Puig, G. Doncel, and L. Lustig. Multifocal damage of the testis induced in rats by passive transfer of antibodies prepared against non-collagenous fraction of basement membrane. *J. Reprod. Immunol.* *7*:59-75 (1985).
156. R. J. Miller, G. J. Killian, and P. Vasilenko III. Effects of long- and short-term vasectomy on structural and functional parameters of the rat. *J. Androl.* *5*:381-388 (1984).
157. C. J. Flickinger. Ultrastructure of the rat testis after vasectomy. *Anat. Rec.* *174*:477-494 (1972).
158. C. J. Flickinger. Alterations in the fine structure of the rat epididymis after vasectomy. *Anat. Rec.* *173*:277-300 (1972).
159. W. B. Neaves. The effect of vasectomy on the testes of inbred Lewis rats. *J. Reprod. Fertil.* *54*:405-411 (1978).
160. T. L. Lamno-Carvalho, A. L. Favaretto, A. L. Ferreira, and J. Antunes-Rodrigues. Histophysiological study of vasectomized rats. *Braz. J. Med. Biol. Res.* *17*:83-91 (1984).
161. H. M. Torgersen, E. Rovan, M. Steiner, J. Frick, and H. Adam. BCG-induced orchitis: Structural changes during the degeneration of seminiferous tubules of rats and rabbits. *Urol. Res.* *10*:97-104 (1982).
162. J. L. Van Snick and P. L. Masson. Incidence and specificities of IgA and IgM anti-IgG autoantibodies in various mouse strains and colonies. *J. Exp. Med.* *151*:45-55 (1980).
163. C. Teuscher, M. Porter, and K. S. K. Tung. Differential susceptibility to experimental autoimmune orchitis in BALB/c substrains. *Curr. Topics Microbiol. Immunol.* *122*:181-188 (1985).
164. K. A. Laurence, O. Carpuk, and M. Perlbachs. Transfer of testicular lesions by leukocytes from testes-immunized rats. *Int. J. Fertil.* *10*:13-18 (1965).
165. M. B. Sztein, M. L. Satz, and S. A. Serrate. Transfer of cell migration inhibition in vitro with xenogeneic RNA in experimental allergic orchitis. *J. Clin. Lab. Immunol.* *3*:39-43 (1980).

166. J. C. Levaditi, A. Eyquem, and O. Nazimoff. Caracteres non specifiques des lesions histologiques locales observees chez la rat a la suite d'injections intratesticulaires des serum anti-testicule de rat. *C.R.S. Soc. Biol. 160*:1146-1148 (1966).
167. U. Chattopadhyay. Immunological induction of aspermatogenesis. *J. Steroid Biochem. 11*:687-693 (1979).
168. H. Wekerle. In vitro induction of immunological memory against testicular autoantigens. *Nature 267*:357-358 (1977).
169. H. Wekerle and M. Begemann. In vitro induction of experimental autoimmune orchitis. Characterization of a primary T lymphocyte response against testicular self antigens. *Eur. J. Immunol. 8*:294-302 (1978).
170. H. Wekerle. Immunological T-cell memory in the in vitro-induced experimental autoimmune orchitis. *J. Exp. Med. 147*:233-250 (1978).
171. B. Kyewski and H. Wekerle. Increase of T lymphocytes self-reactivity in aging inbred rats: In vitro studies with a model of experimental autoimmune orchitis. *J. Immunol. 129*: 1249-1255 (1978).
172. P. S. Tung and I. B. Fritz. Autoimmune orchitis can be induced by thymic lymphocytes autosensitized against syngeneic Sertoli cells in vitro. *Biol. Reprod. 30*;970-990 (1984).
173. J. R. Head, W. B. Neaves, and R. E. Billingham. Immune privilege in the testis. I. Basic parameters of allograft survival. *Transplantation 36*:423-431 (1983).
174. J. R. Head, W. B. Neaves, and R. E. Billingham. Reconsideration of the lymphatic drainage of the rat testis. *Transplantation 35*:91-95 (1983).
175. G. Gachelin, M. Fellous, J. L. Guenet, and F. Jacob. Developmental expression of an early embryonic antigen common to mouse spermatozoa and cleavage embryos, and to human spermatozoa: Its expression during spermatogenesis. *Dev. Biol. 50*:310-320 (1976).
176. C. F. Millette and A. R. Bellve. Temporal expression of membrane antigens during mouse spermatogenesis. *J. Cell Biol. 74*:86-97 (1977).
177. J. C. Herr and E. M. Eddy. Detection of mouse sperm antigens by a surface labeling and immunoprecipitation approach. *Biol. Reprod. 22*:1263-1274 (1980).

178. F. A. Feuchter, R. B. Vernon, and E. M. Eddy. Analysis of the sperm surface with monoclonal antibodies: Topographically restricted antigens appearing in the epididymus. *Biol. Reprod. 24*:1099-1110 (1981).
179. E. D. Schmell, B. J. Gulyas, L. C. Yuan, and J. T. August. Identification of mammalian sperm surface antigens. II. Characterization of an acrosomal cap protein and a tail protein using monoclonal anti-mouse sperm antibodies. *J. Reprod. Immunol. 4*:91-106 (1982).
180. M. Isahakia and N. J. Alexander. Interspecies cross-reactivity of monoclonal antibodies directed against human sperm antigens. *Biol. Reprod. 30*:1015-1026 (1984).
181. M. Isahakia and N. J. Alexander. Vasectomy-induced autoimmunity: Antisperm and antinucleal autoimmune monoclonal antibodies. *Am. J. Reprod. Immunol. 5*:117-124 (1984).
182. D. N. Crichton and B. B. Cohen. Analysis of the murine sperm surface with monoclonal antibodies. *J. Reprod. Fertil. 68*:497-505 (1983).
183. S. Kohno, E. Ziparo, L. F. Marke, and K. S. K. Tung. Murine Sertoli cells: Major histocompatibility antigens and glycoconjugates. *J. Reprod. Immunol. 5*:339-350 (1983).
184. M. J. Skoskiewicz, R. B. Colvin, E. E. Schneeberger, and P. S. Russell. Widespread and selective induction of major histocompatibility complex-determined antigens in vivo by gamma interferon. *J. Exp. Med. 162*:1645-1664 (1985).
185. Z. Pokorna, M. Vojtiskova, M. Rychlikova, and J. Chutna. An isologous model of experimental autoimmune aspermatogenesis in mice. *Folia Biol. 9*:203-209 (1963).
186. T. H. Tarter and N. J. Alexander. Genetic control of humoral immunity to sperm acrosomal and cell surface antigens. *J. Reprod. Immunol. 6*:213-226 (1984).
187. D. J. Anderson and J. A. Madrigal. Variability in antisperm and antiembryonic humoral immune respones. In *Future Aspects in Contraception. Part 2. Female Contraception* (B. Runnebuam, T. Rabe, and L. Kiesel, eds.), MTP Press Ltd., Boston, 1985, pp. 305-317.
188. K. Ben, N. J. Alexander, and N. Huso. In vitro cell-mediated and complement-mediated cytotoxicity to murine testicular cells. *Am. J. Reprod. Immunol. 12*:33-37 (1986).

189. M. Makooi. Vasectomy and autoimmunity in mice. *Fed. Proc. 33*:289 (1974).
190. T. Samuel, P. R. Crewe, A. H. J. Kolk, P. Rumke, and R. D. Barnes. Cross-reaction of antibodies present in sera of vasectomized mice with human swollen spermheads. *Clin. Exp. Immunol. 25*:80-84 (1976).
191. L. L. Kosuda and P. E. Bigazzi. Autoantibodies to acrosomal antigens of spermatozoa in vasectomized mice. *Invest. Urol. 16*:130-141 (1978).
192. D. J. Anderson and N. J. Alexander. Antisperm antibody titres, immune complex deposition and immunocompetence in long-term vasectomized mice. *Clin. Exp. Immunol. 43*: 99-108 (1981).
193. D. L. Kessler, W. D. Smith, M. S. Hamilton, and R. E. Berger. Infertility in mice after unilateral vasectomy. *Fertil. Steril. 43*:308-312 (1985).
194. G. J. Hoymeyr and A. R. Rabson. Prevention of antisperm autoantibody response in vasectomized Swiss White mice by infusion of heterologous antisperm serum. *Br. J. Urol. 56*: 418-421 (1984).
195. O. Taguchi and Y. Nishizuka. Experimental autoimmune orchitis after neonatal thymectomy in the mouse. *Clin. Exp. Immunol. 46*:425-434 (1981).
196. A. Kojima and C. A. Spencer. Genetic susceptibility to testicular autoimmunity: Comparison between post-thymectomy and post-vasectomy models in mice. *Biol. Reprod. 29*:195-205 (1983).
197. R. D. Allen, K. L. Stevenson, and T. K. Roberts. Analysis of antibodies against mouse spermatozoa using an enzyme linked immunosorbent assay (ELISA). *Am. J. Reprod. Immunol. 10*:26-31 (1986).
198. Z. Pokorna, J. Pekarek, and J. Svejcar. The use of an in vitro test of delayed hypersensitivity for the study of experimental autoimmune aspermatogenesis. *Folia Biol. 19*:1887-1893 (1973).
199. A. G. Tumboh-Oeri and T. K. Roberts. The induction of cell-mediated immunity to spermatozoa following vasectomy in inbred mice. *Int. J. Androl. 1*:81-85 (1981).
200. D. J. Anderson and T. H. Tarter. Immunosuppressive effects

of mouse seminal plasma components in vivo and in vitro. *J. Immunol. 128*:535-539 (1982).

201. S. Kohno, J. A. Munoz, T. M. Williams, C. Teuscher, C. C. A. Bernard, and K. S. K. Tung. Immunopathology of murine experimental allergic orchits. *J. Immunol. 130*:2675-2682 (1983).
202. B. J. Hargis, S. Malkiel, and J. Berkelhammer. Immunologically induced aspermatogenesis in the white mouse. *J. Immunol. 101*:374-375 (1968).
203. K. Sato, K. Hirokawa, and S. Hatakeyama. Experimental allergic orchitis in mice. Histopathological and immunological studies. *Virchows Arch. Pathol. Anat. 392*:147-148 (1981).
204. R. Ichinohasama, K. Hirokawa, and S. Hatakeyama. Spermatogenic disturbance induced in mice by combined local injection of monoclonal antibodies to Sertoli cell and to basal lamina of seminiferous tubule. *Am. J. Reprod. Immunol. Microbiol. 10*:158-165 (1986).
205. D. Boehme. Experimentelle allergische Orchitis und retikuloendotheliales System. I. Funktionelle Veranderungen. *Z. Immunitats-Allergioforsch. 128*:19-30 (1965).
206. D. Boehme. Experimentelle allergische Orchitis und retikuloendotheliales System. II. Histologische Veranderungen. *Z. Immunitats-Allergioforsch. 128*:31-51 (1965).
207. D. Boehme. Response of reticuloendothelial system to experimental allergic orchitis in a genetically susceptible and resistant mouse genotype. *Proc. Soc. Exp. Biol. Med. 118*: 374-376 (1965).
208. J. W. Kille, T. E. Wheat, G. Mitchell, and E. Goldberg. Strain differences in the immune response of mice to homologous sperm-specific lactate dehydrogenase (LDH—C4). *J. Exp. Zool. 204*:259-266 (1978).
209. C. C. A. Bernard, G. F. Mitchell, J. Leydon, and A. Bargerbos. Experimental autoimmune orchitis in T-cell-deficient mice. *Int. Arch. Allergy Appl. Immunol. 56*:256-263 (1978).
210. C. Teuscher, S. M. Smith, E. H. Goldberg, G. M. Shearer, and K. S. K. Tung. Experimental allergic orchitis in mice. I. Genetic control of susceptibility and resistance to induction of autoimmune orchitis. *Immunogenetics 22*:323-333 (1985).

211. C. Teuscher. Experimental allergic orchitis in mice. II. Association of disease susceptibility with the locus controlling *Bordetella pertussis*-induced sensitivity to histamine. *Immunogenetics 22*:417-425 (1985).
212. Z. Pokorna. Induction of autoimmune aspermatogenesis by non-cellular cytophilic material. *Folia Biol. 15*:173-180 (1969).
213. Y. Sakamoto, H. Sanui, S. Yoshida, and K. Nomoto. Local passive transfer of delayed type hypersensitivity to syngeneic testicular cells in mice. *Clin. Exp. Immunol. 56*:353-360 (1984).
214. S. Sakaguchi, K. Fukuma, K. Kuribayashi, and T. Masuda. Organ-specific autoimmune diseases induced in mice by elimination of T cell subset. I. Evidence for the active participation of T cells in natural self-tolerance; deficit of a T cell subset as a possible cause of autoimmune disease. *J. Exp. Med. 161*:72-87 (1985).
215. Y. Sakamoto, K. Himeno, H. Sanui, S. Yoshida, and K. Nomoto. Experimental allergic orchitis in mice. I. A new model induced by immunization without adjuvants. *Clin. Immunol. Immunopathol. 37*:360-368 (1985).
216. B. C. Wentworth and W. J. Mellen. Active immunity induced and spermatogenesis suppressed by testicular antigen in male Japanese quail (*Coturnix coturnix japonica*). *J. Reprod. Fertil. 8*:215-223 (1964).
217. G. J. Losos, A. J. Winter, and K. McEntee. Induction of testicular degeneration in bulls by isoimmunization. *Am. J. Vet. Res. 29*:2295-2306 (1968).
218. L. M. Laird, A. E. Ellis, A. R. Wilson, and F. G. T. Hollday. The development of the gonadal and immune system in the Atlantic salmon (*Salmo salar* L.) and a consideration of the possibility of inducing autoimmune destruction of the testis. *Ann. Biol. Anim. Biochem. Biophys. 18*:1101-1106 (1978).
219. R. E. Mancini, J. A. Andrada, D. Saraceni, A. E. Bachmann, J. C. Lavieri, and M. Nemirovsky. Immunological and testicular response in man sensitized with human testicular homogenate. *J. Clin. Endocrinol. Metab. 25*:859-875 (1965).
220. J. A. Andrada, E. C. Andrada, and E. Witebsky. Experimental autoallergic orchitis in Rhesus monkeys. *Proc. Soc. Exp. Biol. Med. 130*:1106-1113 (1969).

221. N. J. Alexander. Vasectomy: Long-term effects in the Rhesus monkey. *J. Reprod. Fertil. 31*:399-406 (1972).
222. N. J. Alexander. Immunologic and morphologic effects of vasectomy in the Rhesus monkey. *Fed. Proc. 34*:1692-1697 (1975).
223. N. J. Alexander. Vasectomy and vasovasostomy in Rhesus monkeys: The effect of circulating antisperm antibodies on fertility. *Fertil. Steril. 28*:562-569 (1977).
224. N. J. Alexander and K. S. K. Tung. Effects of vasectomy in Rhesus monkeys. In *Vasectomy. Immunologic and Pathophysiologic Effects in Animals and Man* (I. H. Lepow and R. Crozier, eds.), Academic Press, New York, 1979, pp. 423-458.
225. K. S. K. Tung and N. J. Alexander. Monocytic orchitis and aspermatogenesis in normal and vasectomized rhesus macaques (*Macaca mulatta*). *Am. J. Pathol. 101*:17-27 (1980).
226. G. J. Domingue, R. M. Harrison, P. M. Heidger, J. A. Roberts, and J. U. Schlegel. Vasectomy in rhesus monkesy. II. Failure to demonstrate humoral and cellular immune responses specific for sperm. *Urology 9*:645-650 (1977).
227. G. L. Curtis, W. L. Ryan, and S. S. Lacy. Sperm-agglutinating and -immobilizing antibody formation following vasectomy prevented with dexamethasone in cynomolgous monkeys. *Fertil. Steril. 38*:97-99 (1982).
228. B. J. Wilson, N. J. Alexander, G. Porter, and D. L. Fulgham. Cell-mediated immunity in vasectomized rhesus monkeys. *Fertil. Steril. 28*:1349-1355 (1977).
229. N. J. Alexander and T. B. Clarkson. Vasectomy increases the severity of diet-induced atherosclerosis in *Macada fascicularis. Science 201*:538-541 (1978).
230. T. B. Clarkson and N. J. Alexander. Long-term vasectomy. Effects on the occurrence and extent of atherosclerosis in rhesus monkeys. *J. Clin. Invest. 65*:15-25 (1980).
231. N. J. Alexander, T. B. Clarkson, and D. L. Fulgham. Circulating immune complexes in cynomolgous macaques. *Lab. Anim. Sci. 35*:465-468 (1985).
232. T. B. Clarkson, D. M. Lombardi, N. J. Alexander, and J. C. Lewis. Diet and vasectomy: Effects on atherosclerosis in cynomolgous macaques. *Exp. Mol. Pathol. 44*:29-49 (1986).

233. N. H. Lauersen, E. Muchmore, S. Shulman, A. E. Marinescu, Z. R. Graves, Leeds, and S. A. Geller. Vasectomy and atherosclerosis in *Macaca fascicularis*. New findings in a controversial issue. *J. Reprod. Med. 28*:750-758 (1983).
234. J.-C. Monier and M. Lapras. Autoimmunisation et maladies autoimmunes chez les primates. *Sci. Technol. Anim. Lab. 1*: 231-241 (1976).
235. G. Wick, J. Most, K. Schauenstein, G. Kromer, H. Dietrich, A. Ziemiecki, R. Frazier, S. Schwarz, N. Neu, and K. Hala. Spontaneous autoimmune thyroiditis—a bird's eye view. *Immunol. Today 6*:359-364 (1985).
236. W. J. Penhale, A. Farmer, R. P. McKenna, and W. J. Irvine. Spontaneous thyroiditis in thymectomized and irradiated Wistar rats. *Clin. Exp. Immunol. 15*:225–236 (1973).
237. T. Kotani, K. Komuro, T. Yoshiki, T. Itoh, and M. Aizawa. Spontaneous autoimmune thyroiditis in the rat accelerated by thymectomy and low doses of irradiation: Mechanisms implicated in the pathogenesis. *Clin. Exp. Immunol. 45*: 329-337 (1981).
238. K. S. K. Tung, L. Ellis, C. Teuscher, A. Meng, J. C. Blaustein, S. Kohno, and R. Howell. The black mink (*Mustelo vison*). A natural model of immunologic male infertility. *J. Exp. Med. 154*:1016-1032 (1981).
239. K. S. K. Tung, L. E. Ellis, G. V. Childs, and M. Dufau. The dark mink: A model of male infertility. *Endocrinology 11*: 922-929 (1984).
240. G. B. Dooher, K. Artzt, D. Bennett, and U. Hurtenbach. Observations on autoimmune orchitis in sterile mice carrying a recessive lethal mutation at the T/t complex exhibiting spontaneous allergic orchitis. *J. Reprod. Fertil. 62*:505-511 (1981).
241. T. E. Fritz, L. S. Lombard, S. A. Tyler, and W. P. Norris. Pathology and familial incidence of orchitis and its relation to thyroiditis in a closed beagle colony. *Exp. Mol. Pathol. 24*:142-158 (1976).
242. W. G. Couser, D. J. Salant, and M. M. Stilmant. Mechanisms of proteinuria induced by antikidney antibodies in noninflammatory experimental glomerulonephropathy. In *Im-*

mune Mechanisms in Renal Disease (N. B. Cummings, A. F. Michael, and C. B. Wilson, eds.), Plenum Medical Book Company, New York, 1983, pp. 319-335.
243. D. W. Talmage. Beyond cellular immunology. *J. Immunol. 123*:1-5 (1979).
244. L. C. Harrison. Antireceptor antibodies. In *The Autoimmune Diseases* (N. R. Rose and I. R. MacKay, eds.), Academic Press, New York, 1985, pp. 617-668.
245. M. H. Johnson. Physiological mechanisms for the immunological isolation of spermatozoa. *Adv. Reprod. Physiol. 6*: 279-324 (1973).
246. M. Dym and L. J. Romrell. Intraepithelial lymphocytes in the male reproductive tract of rats and rhesus monkeys. *J. Reprod. Fertil. 42*:1-7 (1975).
247. L. Hermo and Y. Clermont. Light cells within the limiting membrane of rat seminiferous tubules. *Am. J. Anat. 145*: 467-484 (1976).
248. P. E. Bigazzi. Anti-idiotypic immunity in autoimmunity. *Ann. N.Y. Acad. Sci. 475*:66-80 (1986).
249. J. H. Michaelson, J. P. McCoy Jr., P. Hirszel, and P. E. Bigazzi. Mercury-induced autoimmune glomerulonephritis in inbred rats. I. Kinetics and species specificity of autoimmune responses. *Surv. Synth. Pathol. Res. 4*:401-411 (1985).

9
Immunology of Testicular Tumors

BIJAY MUKHERJI

University of Connecticut School of Medicine
Farmington, Connecticut

The overwhelming majority of testicular cancers arise from totipotential germ cells. These tumors, therefore, express many characteristics of embryonal cells and tissues. Accordingly, the immunobiology of testicular cancer is of considerable interest. In addition to expressing embryonal characteristics, they may express other transformation-related "neoantigen(s)" that in turn may be immunogenic. Because of their origin, testicular germ cell tumors have been extensively studied from a variety of developmental points of view. The immunology of these interesting tumors has also received a fair amount of scientific attention.

The purpose of this chapter is to review the immunobiology of this tumor as it relates to host-tumor interactions. The review will not be encyclopedic, but all relevant aspects of host-tumor interactions at the immune level will be examined critically to provide state-of-the-art knowledge on the subject. For the purpose of a methodical examination of the topic, and for brevity, the discussion will focus on the following areas:

1. The evidence of host immune response toward testicular cancers, based on studies of histological features at the site of the tumor itself and within the regional lymphoid organs; studies of general evaluation of the immune status of the host as a clinical correlate of immune response against testicular cancers.
2. The cell surgace antigens on testicular cancer cells, unique or otherwise, that bear relevance to immunobiology
3. The available evidence of host immune response, cellular or humoral, against testicular cancers
4. Finally, the mechanisms by which testicular cancer might escape host immune response

I. HISTOLOGICAL FEATURES AND HOST IMMUNE STATUS RELEVANT TO IMMUNOBIOLOGY OF TESTICULAR CANCER

Generally speaking, histological examinations of a given tumor with particular reference to immune response manifested by inflammatory infiltration locally or manifested by perturbations within the draining lymphoid organs have provided useful suggestive clues on the question of the immunogenicity of that tumor in its natural host. Similarly, studies of the general host immune status in correlation with the prognosis, stage of disease, and natural behavior of the tumor have also provided additional suggestive evidence of host immune response. A number of these types of studies on testicular cancer are available to suggest that testicular cancers may also be immunogenic. From a morphological point of view, Dixon first recognized the existence of a characteristic infiltration of lymphocytes within seminomatous tumors and suggested that the good prognosis of seminomatous testicular cancer of germ cell origin may represent a reflection of the inflammatory response (1). In a subsequent study of four different human tumors, including testicular cancer, Marshall and Dayan made similar observations and reported their "prima facie evidence of an immune reaction by the body against the neoplastic cells " (2).

They further suggested that such "evidence . . . lies in the nature of the cellular response in the stroma" (2). The case for the existence of immune response against testis cancer, from morphological studies, could not have been more succinctly put. From an immunobiologic point of view, it is noteworthy that, although the seminomas bearing a good prognosis often exhibit a marked lymphocytic infiltrate within and around the tumor, nonseminomatous germ cell tumors have poor prognosis and usually do not exhibit significant infiltration by mononuclear cells. Understandably, this association between good prognosis and inflammatory infiltration within the tumor mass, as in seminomas, has been assumed to represent a reflection of host immunity.

In some tumor systems, the idea that infiltrating inflammatory cells constitute a reflection of immune response by the host toward the cancer cells has been reinforced by the demonstration that the infiltrating inflammatory cells exhibit appropriate phenotypic and functional characteristics of immune effector cells. In the case of testicular cancers, this author finds no documented evidence that the mononuclear cells infiltrating seminomas or any other testicular cancers are indeed immune effector cells. The inflammatory population infiltrating seminomas, however, has been found by Akaza et al. to be phenotypically a mixutre of both T and B lymphocytes (3). Furthermore, these investigators found that the proportion of T cells and T cells bearing IgG Fc receptors was increased in the tumor tissue in comparison with their relative proportion in the peripheral blood. The investigators suggested that the infiltration of these T cells in the tumor mass might have something to do with the good prognosis of this type of testicular cancer.

Perturbation within the draining lymph nodes, as mentioned earlier, has also been considered to reflect the host immune response to cancer. Jewett et al. (4) have examined draining retroperitoneal lymph node morphology in testicular germ cell tumors and have reported an interesting facet of nonseminomatous testicular cancer from an immunologic viewpoint. These investigators have found no correlation between the prognosis and the cellular morphology of the lymph node. In general, hyperplasia and depletion of cells in lymph nodes are associated with favorable or poor prognosis, respectively. In human teratocarcinoma, no such correlation was found by Jewett et al (4).

Similarly, the state of the immune responsiveness of cancer patients often correlates with prognosis and with the stage of the disease. The generally accepted dogma is that patients showing evidence of immunosuppression or showing inability to respond to a variety of immunologic stimuli do poorly but immunocompetent hosts tend to do well. This association between immune status and prognosis has been construed by many as further evidence of host immune interactions with tumor. In the case of testicular cancers, a number of reports (5–8) dealing with evaluation of the immune status of the host appeared to support the above view. Unfortunately, the number of cases of testicular cancer studied in each of these reports was uncomfortably small. In a larger study of the general assessment of the immune status of patients assayed by dinitrochlorobenzene (DNCB) skin tests and intradermal skin tests to elicit delayed-type hypersensitivity to a variety of common bacterial or fungal antigens, Schellhammer et al. (9), found no major evidence of compromise in the immune status in nearly 50 patients with testicular nonseminomatous germ cell tumors. Any measure of observable depression of immune response was attributed to chemotherapy rather than to stage of disease. Besides evaluations of immunocompetence through skin tests with DNCB or using a panel of microbial antigens, several authors have attempted quantitative as well as qualitative estimations of T cells, activated T cells, or T-cell function measured in lymphocyte proliferation against T-cell mitogens (8–11). These studies, unfortunately, have produced somewhat mixed results, and they do not allow any definitive conclusion or a positive or negative association between the host immune status and stages of testicular cancer or prognosis. Finally, Kakizoe and Ogawas have reported a case of spontaneous disappearance of pulmonary metastasis of testicular cancer (12). Naturally, this observation can be interpreted as yet more evidence of host immune response against this type of tumor.

Although the types of studies mentioned above have provided much useful information, not much more can be said on the subject of immunology of testicular cancers on the basis of these types of data other than that the evidence of host immune response in this type of tumors is, at best, suggestive.

II. ANTIGENS ON TESTICULAR CANCER CELL

Since the issue of immune response toward testicular cancer (or any cancer, for that matter) is contingent on the presence of tumor antigen, it is important that, before proceeding much further, we address the question of whether testicular cancer cells express tumor antigens capable of eliciting immune responses by the host. The author realizes that, for many, the existence of tumor antigens constitutes, essentially, an article of faith. This author also admits that acceptance of the opposite view (i.e., tumor antigen does not exist) leaves no raison d'etre for tumor immunology. An objective inquiry into the question is therefore of special interest, particularly with reference to testicular cancer because of the following two viewpoints.

1. Testicular germ cell tumors, as derivatives of totipotential germ cells, are more than likely to express surface molecules of embryonal character. Not being bonafide members of the repertoire of normal adult cell surface components, these embryonal molecules might thus be viewed by the host as "foreign."
2. Testicular cancer as a progeny of primitive germ cell might possess characteristics of developing embryos. Thus, instead of being a target for rejection they may be immune, like embryos, to host immunity.

In the following sections, the antigens on testicular cancer cells whose presence or absence might have relevance to the immunology of testicular cancer will be reviewed. A number of studies have addressed these issues in human as well as in mouse testicular tumors, and valuable information has been reported. For our purpose, we shall first examine the murine teratocarcinoma system—by far the best studied model.

III. ANTIGENS ASSOCIATED WITH MURINE TERATOCARCINOMA

Teratocarcinomas in mice express a number of embryonal products, such as chorionic gonadotropin, α-fetoprotein, and carcinoembryonic antigen (CEA). Teratocarcinomas are, however, not the only cancers that express these embryonal antigens. In fact, a number of nontesticular tumors also often express these antigens. Although it is not clear whether these embryonic antigens are immunogenetic in their hosts, it is more than likely that they do not present themselves as targets for host immune response.

In addition to CEA, chorionic gonadotropin, or α-fetoprotein, another very interesting embryonal antigen, called F-9, has been identified in murine embryonal cancers (13,14). The F-9 antigen was originally identified on a murine embryonal cell line (14,15). This antigen was found to be capable of inducing a strong immune response in genetically identical strains of mouse. This antigen was subsequently found to be present on all murine embryonal cancer cells and absent on murine cancers of other histological types, as well as the differentiated derivatives of embryonal cancers. Of all cancer cells, only embryonal cancer cells express the F-9 antigen. This antigen, however, is also expressed in significant quantities on embryos at preimplantation stages. Interestingly, the F-9 antigen disappears quickly after implantation and upon further differentiation of the embryo. Finally, the F-9 antigen is expressed by sperm cells of all strains of mouse (13–17). The F-9 protein antigen shows considerable similarity in molecular weight and in subunit structure to the products of the H-2 region of mouse MHC gene (18). The apparent molecular weight of the F-9 protein is approximately 44,000. It has a minor subunit of 12,000 daltons. Although the F-9 protein bears many similarities to the H-2 antigen, the two surface protein antigens seem to map to different regions of chromosome 17. Several investigators have described embryonal antigens, presumably other than F-9 antigen, on teratocarcinoma cell lines (19–21). These investigators have raised antisera using embryonal cancer cell lines other than F-9. Some of these antisera cross-reacted with early postimplantation embryos and, occasionally, with some adult tissue. It is impossible to determine whether these antigens, or groups of antigens, are identical to each other or to the F-9 antigen.

Another type of embryonal antigen expressed by murine embryonal cancer cells, which is somewhat better characterized, is known, as stage-specific embryonic antigens (SSEA). SSEA-1 was initially described as a stage-specific embryonic antigen expressed mostly by embryonal tumor cell lines of mouse and human origin and by early preimplantation stage mouse embryos (22). Subsequently, the distribution of the SSEA-1 was found to be much wider. In addition to embryos and embryonal cancers expressing SSEA-1, this antigen was expressed by other nonembryonal cancers, as well as by many normal cells, such as neutrophils, kidney cell, and epididymis (23–25).

Besides the various embryonal antigens described above, other antigens under the broad category of "onco development" gene products or simply fetal and/or embryonal products have also been referred to in various studies (14,26). Although the distribution of some of these antigens has been fairly well established, none of these antigens has been well characterized.

IV. ANTIGENS ASSOCIATED WITH HUMAN EMBRYONAL CANCER CELLS

A number of human teratocarcinoma cell lines have been established over time, and some of these lines have been studied immunologically. Like murine teratocarcinoma cells, human teratocarcinoma cells are also capable of expressing virtually all the embryonal antigens, including the F-9 antigen and some classes of SSEA, described earlier in referenc to the murine teratocarcinoma cells (27–30). The F-9 antigen on human teratocarcinoma cells is antigenically indistinguishable from that on the murine teratocarcinoma cells. Remarkably, even the distribution of the F-9 antigen in human tissues is identical to that in the mouse (13,28–30). The F-9 antigen is, again, expressed by human embryonal cancer cells and by human sperm cells. The F-9 antigen is, in fact, expressed by sperm cells from a large number of mammalian species (13,14). The F-9 molecule thus appears to represent a fairly well conserved gene product that might serve some yet unidentified but apparently important function(s) in normal embryogenesis. In the strictest sense, F-9 antigen, therefore, is not a true tumor antigen when it reappears in germ cell tumors. As mentioned earlier, SSEA-1 is also expressed by certain human teratocarcinoma cells (22). In humans the SSEA-1 was subsequently, however, found to be expressed by a variety of nonembryonal tumors and normal tissues (31,32). Another SSEA (SSEA-3) has been defined on human teratocarcinoma (but not on murine embryonal cancer) with monoclonal antiserum raised against early embryo (33). SSEA-3 was, again, found on normal human peripheral blood cells. Although neither the SSEA nor the F-9 are true tumor antigens, the question of whether their appearance on germ cell tumors might evoke immune responses will be addressed later. At present, we shall return to the topic of antigens expressed by testicular cancers.

Besides the various embryonal antigens, testicular teratocarcinoma cells have been found to express pregnancy-associated proteins (34,35) that might bear some relevance to immunology, specifically in their potential role in immune escape. Furthermore, using serological techniques, a group of investigators have reported the presence of "common teratoma defined antigen(s)" (36). Other than that this so-called common teratoma defined antigen is present on human and mouse sperm cells and on mouse teratoma cells, the exact nature of this antigen(s) has not been clarified.

Finally, we come to the question of existence of true tumor antigen on testicular cancer. A critical search of the literature by this author did not provide any credible evidence to prove the presence of such antigens on testicular cancers. There are two separate studies, however, that must be mentioned in this connection (37,

38). Orel (37) was able to demonstrate a delayed hypersensitivity reaction in patients with testicular cancer using cell surface proteins extracted from the teratocarcinoma cells. Using a colony inhibition assay, Hellström et al. (38), originally presented evidence of cell-mediated cytotoxicity by lymphocytes from testicular cancer patients that was specifically directed against their autologous testes cancer cells. Based on autologous reactions, both studies thus indirectly suggested the potential existence of some form of tumor antigen on testicular cancers.

Our discussion so far has been occupied with the question of the presence of antigens on testicular cancer cells. An opposing issue, i.e., the absence of certain antigens on testicular cancer cells, from an immunologic viewpoint is of equal interest and equal importance. The antigens referred to are none other than those encoded by the major histocompatibility complex (MHC)—H-2 in mice and histocompatibility leukocyte antigens (HLA) in humans. A substantial body of evidence has been accumulated over the years to suggest that testicular cancer cells express no MHC gene products or express them minimally (39-42). The lack of expression of MHC gene product seems to be a feature shared by both testicular germ cells and sperm cells, considered immunologically highly privileged. In this context, Ostrand-Rosenberg and Cohn (43), have shown that the expression of H-2 antigens on the murine teratocarcinoma cells 402 AX can undergo modulation resulting from an effective host immune response mediated by cells. Through a series of interesting experiments, these investigators have shown that host lymphoid cells regulate H-2 antigen expression by the 402 AX cells passaged in vivo in appropriate susceptible or resistance hosts. Whatever the reason for their lack of expression, the absence of MHC gene product on testicular germ cell tumors may have profound implications with reference to T-cell–mediated immune response. This aspect of the immunology of testis cancer will be examined later.

Finally, this discussion of the antigens on testicular cancer cells, which are of immunologic interest, will be concluded with Table 1, summarizing the current state of our knowledge on the subject.

Table 1 Antigens Expressed by Testicular Germ Cell Tumors[a]

	CEA, CG, α-Fetoprotein	MHC	F-9	SSEA	Pregnancy-associated Ag	Common teratoma Ag	Unique antigen
Mouse	+	–	+	+	+	+	ND
Human	+	–	+	+	+	+	ND

[a]CEA = carcinoembryonic antigen, CG = chorionic gonadotropin.
MHC = major histocompatibility complex, SSEA = stage-specific embryonic antigen.
ND = not yet demonstrated.

V. HOST IMMUNE RESPONSE AGAINST TESTICULAR CANCER

Before we begin our review of the available evidence in favor of host immune response against testicular cancer, it is worth mentioning that host immune response against testicular cancer (like the immune response against any type of cancer) may take several pathways. For example, the host can respond by making antitumor antibody. Alternatively, the host immune response can be mediated through cellular mechanisms. The effector cells involved in cellular immune response include classic T cells, natural killer (NK) cells, activated killer cells, and macrophages. In the following section I shall review the available information on humoral immune response and on the involvement of these effector cells in host immune response against testicular cancer.

A. Humoral Immune Response

The evidence for humoral immune response against testicular cancer is quite limited, whether dealing with this tumor in mouse or in the human. Using a murine teratocarcinoma model (teratocarcinoma 402 AX), Isa and Sanders (44) reported that virtually all 402 AX tumor-bearing mice were capable of producing antibodies against the teratocarcinoma cells. Tumor-bearing mice were found to produce antibodies of all three classes. Interestingly, the sera from these mice bearing 402 AX cells in ascites form contained very little antibody, but the tumor cells in the ascites were found to be coated with antibody. The same tumor cells, when grown in solid form, were not coated with antitumor antibody. Although these studies clearly demonstrated humoral immune response in mice against some tumor cell-associated antigens, the specificities against which the antibodies were directed were not clarified. Using an indirect immunofluorescence technique, Ostrand-Rosenberg et al. (45) detected circulating antibody in the sera from a small percentage of patients with testicular cancer directed against some antigen (5) present on mouse embryonal cancer cells. In another study, Teodorczyk-Injeyen et al. (36), similarly found circulating antibodies in sera from patients with testicular cancer directed against what the authors believed was "teratoma defined antigen." The circulating antibodies, however, shared specificities with murine and human sperm cells. Although the authors used the term "teratoma associated antigen," the study, again, did not clarify the nature of the antigen against which the humoral immune response was directed. It has been previously mentioned that the F-9 antigen is fairly well characterized antigen expressed by testis cancer cells. Although it has been shown that the embryonal antigen F-9 is immunogenic in syngeneic mice, and despite that F-9 antigen is expressed by human germ cell tumors, it is unclear whether patients with germ cell tumors mount a humoral immune response against the F-9 antigen. It is of interest that a serological search for circulating antibody against embryonal antigen(s) in sera from patients with testicular cancer by Artzt et al. (46) has not provided convincing evidence of a humoral immune response toward F-9 or any other well-characterized embryonal antigens. Using both animal and human teratocarcinoma cell lines, Andrews (47) found no definitive evidence for antibodies (in sera from testicular cancer patients) against stage-specific embryonal antigens.

B. Cell-Mediated Immune Response by T Cell

Damjanov and Solter (48) initially observed the phenomenon of marked splenomegaly induced by teratocarcinoma (but not with teratoma) in syngeneic mice. The implication was that the splenomegaly represented a cellular response against the teratocarcinoma cells. Despite that observation, it is still uncertain whether testicular germ cell cancers evoke a classic T-cell–mediated effector response. There is a remarkable consensus that, because testicular germ cell tumors do not express class I MHC-coded antigens, they do not elicit classic T-cell–mediated cytolytic effector function since the expression of cytolytic effector T-cell response follows MHC restriction. Several investigators failed to demonstrate the cytolytic ability of classic T cells against unmodified and chemically or virally modified embryonal cancer cells (49–51), but Wagner et al were able to induce cytotoxic T cells against F-9 cells by immunizing mice with the F-9 cells (52). The cytotoxic T cells thus induced killed a variety of embryonal cell lines and syngeneic spermatogonia. Parietal yolk sac carcinoma or blast cells were not lysed. The authors therefore suggested that the immune cytotoxic T cells specifically killed the F-9 cells. In this regard, it is also worth noting that, in one of the early in vitro studies of cell-mediated cytotoxicity in a variety of autologous and allogeneic human tumor systems, Hellström et al. (38) reported lymphocyte-mediated cytolysis of autologous testicular germ cell tumors. In the light of subsequent methodological development of T-cell isolation, the precise nature of the effector cells used in the early study of Hellström et al. is unclear. We shall soon see that testicular germ cell tumors are sensitive to lysis by NK cells, activated killer cells, and macrophages. Before we leave T-cell-mediated response against testicular cancer, it should be pointed out that Bartlett et al. (53) were able to induce cytostatic (but not cytotoxic) lymphocytes in cocultivation of spleen cells and teratocarcinoma cells in vitro. The cytostatic property was observed across species barriers (53,54).

In a discussion on T-cell-mediated immune response toward testicular cancers, it should be pointed out that, although there are much data in the literature ot support the contention that a T-cell-mediated immune response develops in a wide variety of cancers in mice and humans, classic T-cell-mediated immunity can by no means be definitely implicated in surveillance against cancer. After all, it is now well documented that nude mice, deficient in T-cell-mediated immune apparatus, do not suffer from a higher incidence of spontaneously arising cancers when such mice are kept alive for a long time in a germ-free environment (55). It has been argued by some that nude mice are protected from a higher incidence of cancer by a NK cell-mediated immune response. Indeed, lately the role of NK cells in tumor immunity has received much attention from tumor biologists. Understandably, the topic of NK cell-mediated immune response against testicular cancer was therefore explored by several investigators.

Stern et al. (56) were the first to demonstrate that several murine embryonal cancers were quite efficiently lysed by NK cells. These authors failed to demonstrate any evidence of T-cell–mediated immune response in testicular embryonal cancers. Furthermore, these authors demonstrated that, although primitive embryonal cancer cells were quite sensitive to lysis by murine NK cells, the more differentiated derivative of the same embryonal lines were much less sensitive, or not at all, to lysis by NK cells. More interestingly, Adamson et al. (57) have demonstrated that when the primitive embryonal cancer was subjected to undergo further differentiation under the influence of retinoic acid, the differentiated cells showed a loss of NK sensitivity. Using the murine embryonal cell line F-9, Welsch et al. (58) have subsequently confirmed the susceptibility of murine embryonal cancer to nonclasiic immune effector cells, such as NK cells. Isa and his coinvestigators (44,59) investigated cellular immune response in a murine teratocarcinoma model. They also failed to demonstrate any evidence of T-cell–mediated immunity in lymphoid organs from mice bearing the murine teratocarcinoma cells 402 AX. The murine teratocarcinoma line 402 AX did not express H-2 antigens. Although they failed to demonstrate T-cell–mediated cytotoxicity against the 402 AX target, peritoneal macrophages induced by irradiated 402 AX cells or by thioglycollate were found to be markedly cytotoxic against these murine teratocarcinoma cells.

An interesting exception has been reported by Carroll et al. (60) with reference to the susceptibility of testicular cancer to nonclassic effector cells in a human system. These investigators have failed to demonstrate the NK sensitivity of several human teratocarcinoma cell lines. These human teratocarcinoma cells, however, were found to be quite sensitive to lysis by "killer cells" that were activated in culture in the presence of T-cell mitogen or alloantigen. They also demonstrated that the activated killer cells did not show any MHC-related specificity and speculated that the killing may have been directed against some "unique fetal antigens" that were shared by the human teratocarcinoma cells.

Summarizing the available information on cell-mediated immune response in testicular cancers (Table 2), one appreciates a unique quality in the nature of cellular effector response in testicular cancer. The overwhelming majority of studies suggest a lack of classic T-cell–mediated effector response in this system. On the other hand, experimental evidence for the susceptibility of testicular germ cell cancer to a nonclassic effector mechanism is reasonably good. The biologic significance of such nonclassic immune effector mechanisms against testicular cancer is, however, unclear.

VI. IMMUNE ESCAPE BY TESTICULAR CANCER

A number of mechanisms, such as sneaking through, antigen modulation, receptor blockade, immunoselection, and suppressor cell activity, have customarily been evoked as mechanism by which tumors in general may escape host immunity. Some of these mechanisms may also be involved in the case of testicular cancers. Testicular germ cell cancers, however, appear to be uniquely equipped to escape immune response by an altogether different mechanism. In the following section, I shall briefly mention certain aspects of testicular germ cell tumors that bear particular relevance to this issue. That there might be something unique about embryonal cancer was detected earlier by Arszt and Jacob, who discovered the unusual transplantation behavior of embryonal cancer cells (39). These cancer cells could be transplanted in the mouse across strain barriers. It was therefore believed that the protective immune mechanism against those tumor grafts must have been very inefficient. It was soon discovered that the embryonal cancer cells did not express H-2 antigens, and the interpretation was that the absence of H-2 antigen therefore made it possible to transplant these cells across strain barriers. After the MHC restriction of T-cell effector function was observed by Zinkernagel and Doherty (61), the immunologic implication of the absence of MHC product on testicular germ cell tumor was that the embryonal cancer cell escapes immune destruction because of a lack of T-cell–mediated immunity.

Table 2 Nature of Host Immune Response Against Testicular Germ Cell Tumors[a]

	CTL	NK	Killer cell	Macrophage	Antibody
Mouse	–	+	+	+	+
Human	?	NT	+	?	?

[a]CTL = cytotoxic T lymphocytes, NK = natural killer cell, NT = not tested.

The role of the T cell in immunity against embryonal cancer was examined by Isa (59). This investigator could not demonstrate T-cell–mediated killing of mouse embryonal cancer cells but could, however, induce cytotoxicity in lymphoid organ-derived effector cells depleted of T-cell population. This investigator concluded that the T-cell population had "suppressor activity," as cytotoxic activity in the lymph nodes was observed after the removal of the T cells. Although this study provided an interesting insight into the immunology of testicular cancer, one could argue that the induction of cytotoxicity by a non-T-cell population could have resulted simply from enrichment of non-T-cell population(s), when T cells were removed, rather than from removal of suppressor activity. In addition to the possible existence of suppressor activities in T cells in this murine teratocarcinoma system, the investigator detected a soluable factor in malignant ascites that was lympholytic in the autologous host. This observation was interpreted as a possible mechanism by which the tumor cells may have down-regulated the immune response. In a simlar vein, it should be recalled that circulating factors capable of blocking cytotoxic T-cell responses against testicular cancer have also been demonstrated (62). Despite these reports on suppressor cells or blocking factor, the subject of potential down-regulation of immune response or other mechanisms for immune escape by testicular germ cell tumors unfortunately has not been extensively studied.

It was mentioned earlier that testicular germ cells express a number of embryonal products. In addition, pregnancy-associated proteins have also been detected on these cancer cells. Some of these products may be frankly immunosuppressive. After all, during normal gestation and in early embryongenesis in particular, the embryo readily implants itself in a histoincompatible host and manages to grow. Although this aspect of the immunobiology of testicular germ cell tumors remains unexplored, the possibility that testicular cancers escape immune destruction by masquerading themselves as embryos is intriguing.

VII. SUMMARY

Available data on the immunology of testicular cancer provide suggestive evidence of interactions between the host and the cancer cells at multiple immunologic levels. Clearly, the host immune response is inadequate and its specificities are poorly defined. Much more work is needed to clarify the various issues raised in this review. This author finds intriguing opportunities for further exploration of interactions between host immune apparatus and this tumor whose origin stems from the totipotential germ cells.

REFERENCES

1. F. Dixon, *Cancer 6*:427 (1953).
2. A. H. E. Marshall and A. D. Dayan, *Lancet 2*:1102 (1964).
3. H. Akaza, K. Kobayashi, T. Umeda, and T. Niijima, *J. Urol. 124*:827 (1980).
4. M. A. S. Jewett, S. I. Hadju, R. A. Good, and W. F. Whitmore, Jr., *Br. J. Urol. 49*:335 (1977).
5. W. J. Catalona, P. B. Chretien, and E. E. Trahan, *J. Urol. 111*:229 (1974).
6. W. J. Caralona, J. K. Smolev, and J. I. Harty, *J. Urol. 114*:922 (1975).
7. J. M. Decenzo, R. Allison, and G. W. Leadbetter, *J. Urol. 114*:271 (1975).
8. V. I. Kupin and N. F. Orel, *Vopr. Oncol. 22*:6(1976).

9. P. F. Schellhammer, R. B. Bracken, M. A. Bean, C. M. Pinsky, and W. F. Whitmore, Jr., *Cancer 38*:149 (1976).
10. T. K. Veskova, N. F. Orel, and I. Svezhimina, *Vopr. Onkol. 23*:56 (1977).
11. V. Bek, P. Hausner, J. Kolar, J. Abrahamova, J. Stepan, Z. Hermauska, B. Konopasek, and T. Fucikova, *Neoplasma 28*:223 (1981).
12. T. Kakizoe and A. Ogawas, *Cancer 34*:761 (1974).
13. F. Jacob, *Immunol. Rev. 33*:4 (1977).
14. D. Solter and I. Damjanov, *Methods Cancer Res. 18*:277 (1979).
15. K. Artzt, P. Dubois, D. Bennett, H. Condamine, C. Babinet, and F. Jacob, *Proc. Natl. Acad. Sci. USA 70*:2988 (1973).
16. K. Artzt, D. Bennett, and F. Jacob, *Proc. Natl. Acad. Sci. USA 71*:811 (1974).
17. G. Gachelin, M. Fellous, J. L. Guenet, and F. Jacob, *Dev. Biol. 50*:310 (1976).
18. K. Artzt and D. Bennett, *Nature 256*:545 (1975).
19. P. Stern, G. R. Martin, and M. J. Evans, *Cell 6*:455 (1975).
20. M. J. Dewey, J. D. Gearhart, and B. Mintz, *Dev. Biol. 55*:359 (1977).
21. G. Gachelin, R. Kemler, F. Kelly, and F. Jacob, *Dev. Biol. 57*:199 (1977).
22. D. Solter and B. B. Knowles, *Proc. Natl. Acad. Sci. USA 75*:5565 (1978).
23. D. Solter and B. B. Knowles, *Curr. Top. Dev. Biol. 13*:139 (1979).
24. N. Fox, I. Damjanov, A. Martin-Hernandez, D. Solter, and B. B. Knowles, *Dev. Biol. 83*:391 (1981).
25. I. Damjanov, N. Fox, B. B. Knowles, D. Solter, P. H. Lange, and E. E. Fraley, *Am. J. Pathol. 108*:225 (1982).
26. M. J. Dewey, J. D. Gearhart, and B. Mintz, *Dev. Biol. 55*:359 (1977).
27. B. Hogan, M. Fellows, P. Avnev, and F. Jacob, *Nature 270*:515 (1977).
28. S. Holden, O. Bernard, K. Artzt, W. F. Whitmore, Jr., and D. Bennett, *Nature 270*:518 (1977).
29. P. W. Andrews, P. N. Goodfellow, L. H. Shevinsky, D. L. Bronson, and B. B. Knowles, *Int. J. Cancer 29*:523 (1982).

30. M. H. Buc-Caron, G. Gachelin, M. Hofnung, and F. Jacob, *Proc. Natl. Acad. Sci. USA 71*:1730 (1974).
31. N. Fox, I. Damjanov, B. B. Knowles, and D. Solter, *Cancer Res. 43*:669 (1983).
32. P. Andrews, P. N. Goodfellwo, and I. Damjanov, *Cancer Surveys 2*:41 (1983).
33. L. H. Shevinski, B. B. Knowels, I. Damjanov, and D. Solter, *Cell 30*:697 (1982).
34. S. W. Rosen, N. Javadpour, I. Calvert, and J. Kaminska, *JNCI 62*:1439 (1979).
35. B. E. Rolfe, H. Morton, A. C. Cavanash, and R. A. Gardiner, *Am. J. Reprod. Immunol. 3*:97 (1983).
36. J. Teodorczyk-Injeyan, M. A. Jewett, C. A. Burke, and S. Ostrand-Rosenberg, *Clin. Exp. Immunol. 40*:438 (1980).
37. N. F. Orel, *Vopr. Onkol. 25*:26 (1979).
38. I. Hellström, K. E. Hellström, H. E. Sjorgren, and G. A. Warner, *Int. J. Cancer 7*:1 (1971).
39. K. Artzt and F. Jacob, *Transplantation 17*:632 (1974).
40. W. C. DeWolf, P. H. Lange M. E. Einarson, and E. J. Yums, *Nature 277*:216 (1979).
41. P. W. Andrews, D. L. Bronson, and P. N. Goodfellow, *Tissue Antigens 17*:493 (1981).
42. A. M. Isa, *Transplantation 21*:195 (1976).
43. S. Ostrand-Rosenberg and A. Cohn, *Proc. Natl. Acad. Sci. USA 78*:7106 (1981).
44. A. M. Isa and B. R. Sanders, *Transplantation 20*:296 (1975).
45. S. Ostrand-Rosenberg, M. Eddin, and M. A. S. Jewell, *Dev. Biol. 61*:11 (1977).
46. K. Artzt, personal communication (1986).
47. P. W. Andrews, personal communication (1986).
48. I. Damjanov and D. Solter, *Nature 249*:569 (1974).
49. J. Forman and E. S. Vitetta, *Proc. Natl. Acad. Sci. USA 72*:3661 (1975).
50. R. M. Zinkernagel and M. B. O. Oldstone, *Proc. Natl. Acad. Sci. USA 73*:3666 (1976).
51. P. C. Doherty, D. Solter, and B. B. Knowles, *Nature 266*:361 (1977).

52. H. Wagner, A. Powitz-Starzinski, M. Rollinghoff, P. Golstein, and M. J. Jakob, *J. Exp. Med. 147*:251 (1978).
53. P. F. Bartlett, B. A. Fenderson, and M. Edidin, *J. Immunol. 120*:1211 (1978).
54. K. Sikora, p. Stern, and E. Lenox, *Nature 269*:813 (1977).
55. O. Stuttman, in *The Nude Mouse in Experimental and Clinical Research* (J. Fogh and B. C. Giovanella, eds.), Academic Press, New York, 1978, pp. 411–435.
56. P. Stern, M. Gidlund, A. Örn, and H. Wigzell, *Nature 285*:341 (1980).
57. E. D. Adamson, S. J. Gaunt, and C. F. Graham, *Cell 17*:469 (1979).
58. R. M. Welsh, K. Kane, M. Hansson, A. Kunkel, and R. W. Kiessling, *J. Immunol. 126*:219 (1981).
59. A. M. Isa, in *The Handbook of Cancer Immunology*, Vol. 4 (H. Waters, ed.), Garland, New York, 1978, pp. 297–312.
60. P. G. Carroll and W. C. DeWolf, *J. Immunol. 131*:1007 (1983).
61. R. M. Zinkernagel and P. C. Doherty, *Adv. Immunol. 27*:52 (1977).
62. H. O. Sjorgren, I. Hellström, C. B. Subhas, G. A. Warner, and K. E. Hellström, *Int. J. Cancer 9*:274 (1972).

10
Antigens of the Normal Prostatic Gland

NOEL R. ROSE

The Johns Hopkins University
Baltimore, Maryland

B. K. CHOE*

University of Toronto and Toronto General Hospital
Toronto, Ontario, Canada

**Present affiliation*: The University of Illinois College of Medicine, Chicago, Illinois

Cancer of the prostate and benign prostatic hyperplasia have become increasingly common diseases as the life span of the general population of industrialized countries has been extended during the last few decades. However, the natural history of these two diseases has never been well understood. The last 15 years of intensive research efforts have been directed to the elucidation of basic mechanisms of morphogenesis and distinct functions of prostatic glandular cells in order to develop a logical basis for the diagnosis and treatment of prostatic cancer. Such efforts have resulted in an integrated view of the metabolic, secretory, and proliferative processes and the hormonal interplay of prostatic epithelial cells. Various aspects of prostatic physiology have been reviewed in several monographs (Brandes, 1974a, b; Goland, 1975; Spring-Mills and Hafez, 1980; Murphy et al., 1981).

The morphogenesis, functional activity, and hormonal responsiveness of prostatic glands have been described by earlier investigators, primarily in terms of morphological and biochemical markers. In contrast, the potential of immunologic studies of differentiation antigens in the pathobiologic investigation of the prostate has not been appreciated until recently. Immunologic studies of the prostate propose to characterize the antigenicity of prostate tissue-specific gene products and to describe the temporal relationship of specific gene expression during normal and pathological development by immunochemical and immunohistological methods.

The fibromuscular stroma cells in the prostate not only serve as the sphincteral device but also play complex roles in induction during the differentiation of glandular epithelial cells (Cunha and Lung, 1980). The glandular epithelial cells, as an exocrine gland, contribute several important substances to the ejaculate and also serve as the main site of biosynthesis of dihydrotestosterone in the human (Farnsworth, 1980). Considering the complexities of gene products of differentiated cells in the prostate, immunochemical approaches are expected to improve the resolution obtained from morphological and biochemical markers of prostatic development.

The two soluble prostate-specific antigens known at present are prostatic acid phosphatase and prostate (P) antigen. These prostate-specific proteins are useful markers for morphogenetic and development studies. These marker proteins are often exclusively expressed by malignant cells of prostatic origin. Even though they are not tumor-specific antigens, these prostate-specific antigens may serve as useful markers for the diagnosis of metastatic prostatic cancer. Several surface antigens unique to prostatic glandular epithelial cells have also been described recently.

I. PROSTATIC ACID PHOSPHATASE

A. Biologic and Biochemical Characteristics

Since Gutman's laboratory first reported the elevation of serum acid phosphatase in prostatic cancer patients over 40 years ago, the measurement of serum acid phosphatase levels has been used in the diagnosis of metastic prostatic cancer (Bodansky, 1972; Yam, 1974). During their immunologic studies of male reproductive organs, Shulman and his collaborators (1964) discovered that prostatic acid phosphatase is a tissue-specific antigen and, from an immunologic point of view, it was the first of its kind for the human prostate gland. The antigenic difference between prostatic acid phosphatase (PAPase) and acid phosphatases of other tissue origins has been demonstrated by several investigators, and various forms of immunoassay were introduced thereafter based on this antigenic specificity. Recently, enzymology (Ostrowski, 1980), immunochemistry (Choe and Rose, 1982), and the clinical application of the PAPase immunoassays (Shaw et al., 1982a, b) have been reviewed extensively. Therefore, we will briefly summarize here the application of this enzyme as a marker of prostate cancer.

Human cells are endowed with genetic information for three to five different kinds of acid phosphatases. However, their expression is largely dependent on differentiation of tissue cells. For example, red blood cells synthesize exclusively red cell acid phosphatase, which is a small protein (molecular-weight, 15,000-20,000), coded for by the ACP_2 gene on chromosome 11.

Some differentiated cells in various tissues also synthesize different acid phosphatases as well as lysosomal acid phosphatase. Morphological and functional studies (e.g., reviews by Brandes, 1974a, b; Brandes et al., 1980) have established the presence of two separate forms of acid phosphatase, secretory and lysosomal, in prostatic glandular epithelial cells. The glandular epithelial cells of prostate from fetuses, neonates, or young children do not show secretory activities. Secretory transformation of the epithelium is androgen-dependent. The secretory functions of these epithelial cells develop under the influence of the androgenic surge at puberty. Secretory prostatic acid phosphatase is antigenically and structurally different from lysosomal isozyme. Like other functions in the prostate gland, PAPase synthesis is androgen-dependent; its synthesis is abolished by orchiectomy and hypophysectomy or by antiandrogens. In the adult human prostate gland, basal cells serve as the precursor (stem) cells to the fully differentiated glandular epithelial cell population (Kastendieck and Altenahr, 1979). One of the distinguishing features of basal cells from differentiated glandular cells is the absence of secretory functions, including

PAPase synthesis. The chromosomal location of the PAPase gene and the linkage relationship between the PAPase gene and the lysosomal acid phosphatase gene (ACP2) is not yet established.

Prostatic acid phosphatase is a glycoprotein with a molecular weight of approximately 100,000 with varying amounts of carbohydrate (up to 10%). The variation in carbohydrate content, particularly neuraminic acid residues, gives rise to a few discrete variants that may be distinguished by charge differences in ion-exchange chromatography and electrophoretic analysis. The native enzyme is comprised of two identical subunits with molecular weight of 50,000. Amino acid and carbohydrate compositions are established; however, the amino acid sequence is unknown. Various physicochemical properties of this enzyme have been established by Ostrowski and his collaborators (see review by Ostrowski, 1980).

The antigenic specificity of PAPase resides in the protein portion of the molecular rather than in the neuraminic acid residues. Therefore, electrophoretic or chromatographic variants of PAPase are antigenically identical. To date, anti-PAPase antisera prepared against the enzyme purified from prostate fluid, prostate tissue extracts, or seminal plasma in different laboratories have been indistinguishable (Choe and Rose, 1982). According to our preliminary antigenic mapping study, there are three determinants unique to PAPase and one determinant antigenically cross-reactive with lysosomal acid phosphatase (Lillehoj et al., 1982; Choe et al., 1982).

When malignant glandular epithelial cells arise and proliferate in the prostate, the majority of the cancer cells usually retain their differentiated functions, such as androgen receptor expression and prostatic acid phosphatase synthesis. Although cancer cells synthesize considerably less acid phosphatase than normal or hyperplastic glandular cells, destruction of stromal tissue boundaries by tumor and metastases of tumor causes the appearance of measurable amounts of PAPase in the general circulation in prostatic adenocarcinoma.

Many immunologic assays have been developed and evaluated for their clinical use in the detection of early invasive prostatic carcinoma (see review by Choe and Rose, 1982). Immunochemical assay methods for PAPase are based on either competitive binding or enzymological assays of immune complexes. Radioimmunoassay (RIA) represents a competitive binding assay. Counterimmunoelectrophoresis (CIEP), solid-plane immunoabsorbent assay (SPIA), and immunoenzyme assay (IEA) belong to the latter category. The RIA has been widely applied in clinical investigations. The SPIA and IEA measure the concentration of PAPase by its enzymatic activity after the precipitation of antigen-antibody complexes. Both the competitive binding assay (e.g., RIA) and enzymological immunoassays (e.g., SPIA and RIA) have different advantages and limitations. Both methods seem to have similar specificity (94–100%), and values obtained by both methods correlate well.

B. Clinical Application of PAPase Immunoassays

Accurate staging is the key to the selection of the proper treatment of prostatic carcinoma. The diagnosis of carcinoma of the prostate, suspected by rectal examination or other clinical tests, is established by histopathological examination of the biopsied materials. For the assessment of the extent of disease, pelvic lymphadenectomy, radiological examinations, and radioactive bone scan have been used. The PAPase immunoassays serve as valuable adjuncts to the evaluation of the extent of local disease (stages B_2 and C) or metastases (stage D). The goal of staging is to distinguish "curable" stages (A and B) from "noncurable" stages (C and D) for the choice of therapeutic modalities. The PAPase immunoassays, with their high specificity and sensitivity, may be useful in the detection of early-stage prostatic carcinoma (A and B), but their role in clinical urology has not been clearly defined (e.g., see papers in Shaw et al., 1982a).

The first report of clinical detection of elevated serum acid phosphatase compared with normal levels in patients with localized prostatic carcinoma was made by Foti et al. (1977). The serum level of prostatic acid phosphatase was elevated in 33% of 24 patients with stage A and 79% of 33 patients with stage B prostatic carcinoma. A comparison of the sensitivity of the colorimetric assay in this group showed 12 and 15% in both groups, respectively. Using the radioimmunoassay method 43% of patients from both groups had elevated serum levels of prostatic acid phosphatase.

Studies by other investigators using radioimmunoassay methods are at variance with the studies reported by Foti et al. (1977). Variations also exist within the same groups if the study was done at different institutions. Bruce and his associates (Bruce et al. 1979) reported an elevation of acid phosphatase in 13% of patients with stage A and 26% of patients with stage B prostatic carcinoma. Bruce and Mahan (1982) found that only 8% of 72 patients with stages A and B disease had an elevated enzyme level. A solid-phase fluorescent immunoassay for prostatic acid phosphatase has been developed (Lee et al., 1978), and the initial data in 24 patients showed that 4 of 4 patients with stage A had elevated levels and 2 of 5 patients with stage B had elevated levels. This assay was further modified to a solid-phase immunosorbent assay that uses regular spectrophotometric equipment instead of an expensive spectrophotofluorometer (Lee et al. 1980a). Initial results showed that 19 of 25 patients with localized prostatic carcinoma had elevated serum prostatic acid phosphatase. Lee et al. (1980b), in a series of 33 surgically staged patients with localized prostatic carcinoma (stage A and B), found that 57% had elevated enzyme levels.

Table 1 compares the sensitivities of PAPase immunoassays as reported in the literature for each clinical stage of prostatic carcinoma. All these clinical studies suggest that the appearance of PAPase in sera signifies local invasive cancer or the early lymphatic metastasis of prostatic cancer. The frequency of lymph node metastasis in early prostatic adenocarcinoma is strikingly high and correlates well with the sensitivity of reported PAPase clinical assays (Table 1).

Prostatic acid phosphatase synthesis is under hormonal control and is secreted by differentiated prostatic glandular epithelium. Therefore, poorly differentiated and/or androgen-insensitive

Table 1 Correlation Between Serum PAPase and Metastases

Clinical stage	Frequency of PAPase immunoassay-positive cases (%)[a]	Frequency of lymph node metastases (%)[b]
A_1	–	5
A_2	6–33	25
B_1	12–71	21
B_2	–	35
C	77–83	80
D	86–92	100

[a]Adapted from Foti et al. (1977), Lindholm (1980) Pontes et al. (1981), Bruce and Mahan (1982), Romas et al. (1982) Killiam et al. (1982).
[b]Adapted from Nicholson and Richie (1977), Correa et al. (1981), Kelin (1979).

tumors tend to show decreased PAPase biosynthesis. It is not uncommon to see serum PAPase levels in the advanced metastatic stage of the disease vary from normal to very high concentrations. The reason for this phenomenon is not clear. The underlying mechanisms for the appearance of heterogeneous tumor cell populations may be complex, but PAPase may serve as a useful marker for the androgen sensitivity of these cells.

II. PROSTATE ANTIGEN

A. Characteristics of Prostate Antigen

In 1979, Wang and his collaborators discovered another major secretory protein of the human prostate gland and called it prostate antigen, or P antigen. Its distribution, assay methods, and clinical application have been reviewed by Wang et al. (1982).

The P antigen is a glycoprotein with a molecular weight of 33,000–34,000 as determined by gel filtration on Sephadex-G75 or by sodium dodecyl sulfate-polyacrylamide gel electrophoresis. The isoelectric point of the purified preparation has been found to vary, depending on the extent of glycosylation, from pH 6.8 to pH 7.5. Judging from identical molecular weight estimates obtained under dissociative (sodium dodecyl sulfate-polyacrylamide gel electrophoresis) and nondissociative conditions (gel filtration), the P antigen does not have subunits. Apparently, the P antigen is one of the major secretory proteins of the human prostate gland, although its physiological function is unknown. Papsidero et al. (1981), using immunohistochemical techniques, demonstrated the site of P-antigen synthesis to be the prostatic glandular epithelial cells. The P antigen is strictly localized to the glandular epithelium and has never been observed in the stromal or vascular region of the prostate. Furthermore, the P antigen is not detected in the tissue sections of other organs, including breast, pancreas, colon, stomach, or liver. Nadji et al. (1981) have examined the normal or malignant prostatic tissues, periurethral glands, seminal vesicle, vas deferens, bladder, and various other normal or malignant nonprostatic tissues and did not detect the P antigen in tissues other than normal or malignant prostatic epithelial cells. The P-antigen concentration in seminal plasma is as much as 100 μg/ml.

The P antigen is a highly immunogenic protein in animals, is immunologically distinct from prostatic acid phosphatase, and does not cross-react with proteins in the serum or ejaculate. Thus far, P antigen does not have any known enzyme activity. A purification procedure of P antigen from prostatic tissue or seminal plasma has been described (Wang et al., 1979, 1982).

B. Occurrence of P Antigen in Serum

To assess the possible diagnostic value of P-antigen release in the serum during the early stage of metastatic prostatic cancer, the enzyme-linked immunosorbent assay (ELISA) was developed by Kuriyama et al. (1980). In their model experiment they transplanted two prostatic carcinoma lines, DU145 and LNCaP, into athymic nude mice. In sera of the tumor-bearing mice, the prostate antigen was detected by ELISA and found to have a concentration of 12–22 ng/ml; sera of nude mice carrying various nonprostatic human tumor lines did not show any detectable amount of antigen (Papsidero et al., 1981).

In a series of clinical studies, Kuriyama et al. (1980) have established the normal value of P antigen in sera (0.47 ± 0.66 ng/ml, mean ± SD). The serum P-antigen levels for female, healthy males or patients suffering from nonprostatic disorders were in the range found for normal controls. In most of these subjects the serum P-antigen concentrations were below the detection limits of the ELISA (0.1 ng/ml). Sera from patients with benign prostatic hyperplasia (n = 19) showed a range of P-antigen concentrations from 0.7 to 8.0 ng/ml, with a mean value of 3.4 ng and SD 2.05. The P-antigen concentrations in the sera of prostate cancer patients varied from 0.3 to 270 ng/ml; the mean ± SD for the patient groups were as follows: state A (n = 8), 4.8 ± 4.55; stage B (n = 34), 5.0 ± 4.12; stage C (n = 56), 10.1 ± 15.86; and stage D (n = 344), 24.2 ± 30.62. When the mean ± 2SD of normal value (1.79 ng/ml) was adopted as the upper limit of normal, 68% of BPH, 63% of stage A, 79% of stage B, and over 85% of stages C and D prostate cancer patients showed a significant elevation of the serum P-antigen level. Furthermore, the continuous release of P antigen by growing prostatic cancer cells seems to show a close correlation with the clinical progression of prostatic cancer; therefore the P antigen seems to serve as a useful marker in the diagnosis of prostatic cancer.

III. SURFACE ANTIGEN OF PROSTATIC STROMAL AND EPITHELIAL CELLS

The advent of hybridoma technology opened a new era of immunochemistry for human cell surface proteins, and a large number of surface antigens have been described for lymphocytes and various human tumor cells. The development and characterization of monoclonal antibodies to these cell surface antigens have already been used in biologic and clinical studies as diagnostic and therapeutic tools (e.g., see Kennett et al., 1980). Recently, surface antigens of human prostate stromal and epithelial cells have been investigated by hybridoma methodology in several laboratories, and monoclonal antibodies to a few differentiation antigens have already been reported (Ware et al., 1982; Starling et al., 1984; Frankel et al., 1982). Using a prostatic adenocarcinoma line, PC-3, as the immunogen, Ware et al. (1982) obtained three monoclonal antibodies (Pro-1, 02, and 03) defining prostate-specific differentiation antigen. Wright et al. (1981), also using a prostatic adenocarcinoma line, DU 145, reported one prostate-specific surface antigen. Frankel et al. (1982), using a membrane fraction of tissues of benign prostatic hyperplasia, obtained seven monoclonal antibodies defining prostate-specific and shared differentiation antigens. Of these, two antibodies recognized prostate stromal cell surface proteins as well as proteins of the endothelium of other organs. In the same study, four antibodies recognized three different surface proteins of epithelial cells from many tissues and two antibodies reacted specifically to prostatic epithelial cells. Therefore, some prostatic epithelial cell differentiation antigens seems to be expressed as surface proteins. The general trend in recent years indicates that a large number of surface antigens will continue to be described for normal and malignant human cells. Perhaps more difficult problems remain to establish the structure of these proteins, to interpret the significance of their variations in terms of the pathophysiology of the prostate gland, and to find the application in the diagnosis and treatment of prostatic cancer.

IV. OTHER POTENTIAL MARKERS OF PROSTATE

Hormone receptors are not prostate-specific proteins. However, the growth and development of the prostate gland are regulated by the complex interplay of polypeptide as well as steroid hormones. Therefore, it is worthwhile to point out the potential for immunologic studies of hormone receptor distribution in the stromal and glandular cells of the prostate. The correlations between androgenic and estrogenic stimulation and prostatic cancer has been suggested from experimental carcinogenesis in the rat ventral prostate (Isaacs and Coffey, 1980) and in epidemiologic studies of human prostatic cancer (Rotkin et al., 1980). Increasing evidence associates the inductive (probably hormonal) activities of stromal cells with morphogenetic and functional differentiation of epithelial cells in the prostate gland (Cunha and Lung, 1980). For instance, the induction and perpetuation of abnormal vaginal cytodifferentiation is determined in part by the stromal effects of neonatal exposure to exogenous estrogen (Cunha and Lung, 1980). Such neonatal hormonal conditioning predisposes the vaginal tissues to eventual malignant transformation. Elucidation of the hormonal interactions between stroma and epithelium may provide insight into the development of benign prostatic hyperplasia or prostatic cancer. The current preparative procedures for the analysis of hormone receptor activity or enzymatic activities do not discriminate the localization of such activities among stromal and epithelial cell populations. The task of preparing suitable amounts of purified hormone receptor proteins for the immunochemical studies is formidable. However, the development of immunochemical reagents, such as monoclonal antibodies to hormone receptors, will open new avenues in the physiological studies of male accessory sex glands by immunohistological techniques.

REFERENCES

Bodansky, O. (1972). Acid phosphatase. *Adv. Clin. Chem. 15*: 43–147.

Brandes, D. (ed) (1974a). *Male Accessory Sex Organs: Structure and Function in Mammals*, Academic Press, New York.

Brandes D. (1974b). Hormonal regulation of fine structure. In *Male Accessory Sex Organs: Structure and Function in Mammals.* Brandes, D. (ed.), Academic Press, New York, pp. 184–222.

Brandes, D., Millan, J. C. and Gesell, M. S. (1980). Histochemistry of prostatic carcinoma. In *Prostate Cancer* (R. J. Ablin, ed.), Marcel Dekker, New York, pp. 149–163.

Bruce, A. W., and Mahan, D. E. (1982). The role of prostatic acid phosphatase in the investigation and treatment of adenocarcinoma of the prostate. *Ann. N.Y. Acad. Sci. 390*:110–121.

Bruce, A. W., Mahan, D. E., Morales, A., Clark, A. F., and Belville, W. D. (1979). An objective look at acid phosphatase determinations. Comparison of biochemical and immunological methods. *Br. J. Urol. 51*:213–217.

Choe, B. K., and Rose, N. R. (1982). Prostatic acid phosphatase: A marker for human prostatic adenocarcinoma. *Methods Cancer Res. 19*:199–232.

Choe, B. K., Dong, M. K., Walz, D., Gleason, S., and Rose, N. R. (1982). A single domain of human prostatic acid phosphatase shows antibody-mediated restoration of catalytic activity. *Proc. Natl. Acad. Sci. USA 79*:6052–6055.

Correa, R. J., Jr., Kidd, C. R., Burnett, L., Brannen, G. E., Gibbons, R. P., and Cumming, K. B. (1981). Percutaneous pelvic lymph node aspiration in carcinoma of the prostate. *J. Urol. 126*:190–191.

Cunha, G. R., and Lung, B. (1980). Experimental analysis of male accessory sex gland development. In *Male Accessory Sex Glands* (E. Spring-Mills and E. S. E. Hafez, eds.), Elsevier/North Holland, Amsterdam, pp. 39–59.

Farnsworth, W. E. (1980). Functional biochemistry of the prostate. In *Male Accessory Sex Glands* (E. Spring-Mills and E. S. E. Hafez, eds.), Elsevier/North Holland, Amsterdam, pp. 156–182.

Foti, A. G., Copper, J. F., Herschman, H., and Malvaez, R. (1977). Detection of prostatic cancer by solid-phase radioimmunoassay of serum prostatic acid phosphatase. *N. Engl. J. Med. 297*: 1357–1361.

Frankel, A. E., Rouse, R. V., and Herzenberg, L. A. (1982). Human prostate specific and shared differentiation antigens defined by monoclonal antibodies. *Proc. Natl. Acad. Sci. USA 79*: 903–907.

Goland, M. (ed) (1975). *Normal and Abnormal Growth of the Prostate*, Charles C Thomas, Springfield, Illinois.

Isaacs, J. T., and Coffey, D. S. (1980). Animal models in the study of prostatic cancer. In *Prostate Cancer* (R. J. Ablin, ed.), Marcel Dekker, New York, pp. 61–72.

Kastendieck, H., and Altenahr, E. (1979). Role of basal cells in

non-malignant lesions of the prostate. *Arch. Androl. 2(Suppl. 1)*: 64–70.
Kelin, L. A. (1979). Prostatic carcinoma. *N. Engl. J. Med. 300*: 824–833.
Kennett, R. H., McKearn, T. J., and Bechtol, K. B. (eds.), (1980). *Monoclonal Antibodies*, Plenum Press, New York.
Killiam, C. S., Vargas, F. P., Slack, N. H., Murphy, G. P., and Chu, T. M. (1982). Prostate-specific acid phosphatase versus acid phosphatase in monitoring patients with prostatic cancer. *Ann. N.Y. Acad. Sci. 390*:122–132.
Kuriyama, M., Wang, M. C., Papsidero, L. D., Killan, C. S., Shimano, T., Valenzuela, L. A., Niahiura, T., Murphy, G. P., and Chu, T. M. (1980). Quantitation of prostate-specific antigen in serum by a sensitive enzyme immunoassay. *Cancer Res. 40*: 4658–4662.
Lee, C., Wang, M. C., Murphy, G. P., and Chu, T. M. (1978). Solid phase fluorescent immunoassay for human prostatic acid phosphatase. *Cancer Res. 38*:2871–2878.
Lee, C. L., Killian, C. S., Murphy, G. P., and Chu, R. M. (1980a). A solid-phase immunoabsorbent assay for serum prostatic acid phosphatase. *Clin. Chim. Acta 101*:209–216.
Lee, C. L., Wang, M. C., Killin, C. S., Slack, N. H., Murphy, G. P., and Chu, T. M. (1980b). Solid phase immunogluorescent and immunoabsorbent assays of serum prostatic acid phosphatase. *Prostate 1*:427–439.
Lillehoj, H. S., Choe, B. K., and Rose, N. R. (1982). Monoclonal antibodies to human prostatic acid phosphatase: Probes for antigenic study. *Proc. Natl. Acad. Sci. USA 79*:5061–5065.
Lindholm, G. R., Stirton, M. S., Liedtke, R. J., and Batjer, J. D. (1980). Prostatic acid phosphatase by radioimmunoassay; sensitivity compared with enzymatic assay. *JAMA 244*:2071–2073.
Murphy, G. P., Sandberg, A. A., and Karr, J. P. (eds) (1981). *The Prostatic Cell: Structure and Function*, Parts A and B, Alan R. Liss, New York.
Nadji, M., Tabei, S. Z., Castro, A., Chu, T. M., Murphy, G. P., Wang, M. C., and Morales, A. R. (1981). Prostatic-specific antigen: An immunologic marker for prostatic neoplasms. *Cancer 48*:1229–1232.

Nicholson, T. C., and Richie, J. P. (1977). Pelvic lymphadenectromy for stage B adenocarcinoma of the prostate: Justified or not? *J. Urol. 117*:199-201.

Ostrowski, W. (1980). Human prostatic acid phosphatase: Physiochemical and catalytic properties. In *Male Accessory Sex Glands* (E. Spring-Mills and E. S. E. Hafez, eds.), Elsevier/North Holland, Amsterdam, pp. 197-213.

Papsidero, L. D., Kuriyama, M., Wang, M. C., Horoszewicz, J. S., Leoning, S. S., Valenzuela, L. A., Murphy, G. P., and Chu, T. M. (1981). Prostate antigen: A marker for human prostate epithelial cells. *JNCI 66*:37-41.

Pontes, E. J., Choe, B. K., Rose, N. R., Ercola, C., and Pierce, J. M., Jr. (1981). Clinical evaluation of immunological methods for detection of prostatic acid phosphatase. *J. Urol. 126*:263–265.

Romas, N. A., Shaw, L. M., Hsu, K. C., Ng, P. Y., Pitts, M., Tomashefsky, P., and Tannenbaum, J. (1982). Clinical comparison of immunological assays for determining prostatic acid phosphatase. *Ann. N.Y. Acad. Sci. 390*:104–109.

Rotkin, I. D., Moses, V. K., Kanshal, D., Cooper, J. F., Osborn, W. C., and Benjamin, J. A. (1980). Groups of variables for prevention of prostatic cancer. In *Prostate Cancer* (R. J. Ablin, ed.), Marcel Dekker, New York, pp. 9–25.

Shaw, L. M., Romas, N. A., and Cohen, H. (1982a). Prostatic acid phosphatase measurement: Its role in detection and management of prostatic cancer. *Ann. N.Y. Acad. Sci. 390*:1–45.

Shaw, L. M., Yan, N., Neat, M., and Croop, W. (1982b). Studies of the biochemical and clinical specificity of the immunochemical determination of prostatic acid phosphatase. *Ann. N.Y. Acad. Sci. 390*:73–88.

Shulman, S., Manrod, L., Gonder, M., and Soanes, W. A. (1964). The detection of prostatic acid phosphatase by antibody reactions in gel diffusion. *J. Immunol. 93*:474–480.

Spring-Mills, E., and Hafez, E. S. E. (eds.) (1980). *Male Accessory Sex Glands*, Elsevier/North-Holland, Amsterdam.

Starling, J. J., Beckett, M. L., and Wright, G. L., Jr. (1984). Monoclonal antibodies to prostate adenocarcinoma antigens. In *Monoclonal Antibodies and Cancer* (G. L. Wright, Jr., ed.), Marcel Dekker, New York.

Wang, W. C., Valenzuela, L. A., Murphy, G. P., and Chu, T. M. (1979). Purification of a human prostate specific antigen. *Invest. Urol. 17*:159-163.

Wang, W. C., Kuriyama, M., Papsidero, L. D., Loor, R. M., Valenzeula, L. A., Murphy, G. P., and Chu, T. M. (1982). Prostate antigen of human cancer patients. *Methods Cancer Res. 19*: 179–197.

Ware, J. L., Paulson, D. F., Parks, S. F., and Webb, K. S. (1982). Production of monoclonal antibody. Pro 13 recognizing a human prostatic carcinoma antigen. *Cancer Res. 42*:1215–1222.

Yam, L. T. (1974). Clinical significance of the human acid phosphatase. A review. *Am. J. Med. 56*:604-616.

11
Immunology of Prostatic Tumors

NOEL R. ROSE

The Johns Hopkins University
Baltimore, Maryland,

B. K. CHOE*

University of Toronto and Toronto General Hospital
Toronto, Ontario, Canada

**Present affiliation*: The University of Illinois College of Medicine, Chicago, Illinois

The theory of tumor immunology was first formulated by Ehrlich in 1906. He postulated that immune mechanisms are involved not only with protection against microorganisms but also against aberrant cells arising during cell differentiation within the host. His concept rested on the assumption that cancer cells develop distinctive antigens that are not present on their normal counterparts and that the host immune system can recognize and reject such cancer cells. Early experimental approaches to test this concept utilized tumor transplantation and resulted in the discovery that tumors arising in one animal were rejected when transplanted into another host; however, these early studies were carried out with genetically heterogeneous animals, and it soon became clear that normal tissues were also rejected following such transplantation. This situation led to the eventual development of inbred animals in order to study transplantation genetics. In the 1950s, it became possible to investigate tumors in the syngeneic (genetically identical) animals. Many experimentally induced animal tumors were shown to exhibit determinants (tumor-specific or tumor-associated antigens) that are recognized by the host and led to the immune rejection of the syngeneic tumor (Prehn and Main, 1957; Klein, 1966; Boyse and Old, 1969, Baldwin, 1973; Herberman, 1976). Human studies reached the stage at which in vitro tests for tumor immune reactions (initially developed with well-defined animal systems) were developed for a wide range of human tumor types (Hellstrom and Hellstrom, 1974; Baldwin and Embleton, 1977), although there is considerable controversy as to their function in tumor rejection in vivo (Herberman, 1980). Before considering the special case of immunology of human prostatic cancer, it is necessary to outline the major concepts of tumor immunology.

I. IMMUNE RESPONSES TO TUMOR CELLS

A. Tumor-Specific and Tumor-Associated Antigens

Based on an analysis of experimental tumors in inbred animals, it has been established that tumors induced by chemical carcinogens or oncogenic viruses express novel antigens that differentiate malignant from normal cells. These tumor-specific antigens are often immunogenic so that the existence of such antigens can be demonstrated readily by tumor rejection, by the occurrence of tumor-specific antibodies, or by the in vivo or in vitro generation of tumor-specific, cytotoxic lymphocytes. Other antigens are expressed by tumor cells but only transiently or in small amounts by normal cells. They are usually called tumor-associated antigens (TAA). Many studies concerning biochemical identification of such a tumor-specific or tumor-associated antigen have been published recently; some, but not all, tumor-associated antigens of carcinogen-induced or virally induced tumors are structurally related to glycoproteins of the major histocompatibility complex (MHC) (Law et al., 1980).

Several documented reports of TAA in various human tumors have appeared in the literature (Herberman, 1976). The best-studied human tumor-associated antigens are the carcinoembryonic antigens of gastrointestinal cancers and a α-fetoprotein of primary hepatic cancers. The advent of the Milstein-Kohler hybridoma technique (1975) opened a new era of investigation into TAA of human tumors. A number of antigens characteristic of certain tumors and not detectable on cells in the tissue from which the tumor was initially derived have been identified (Koprowski et al., 1978; Herlyn et al., 1979). However, because of the vast spectrum of clinical changes that accompany tumors, it has been difficult to assess the role of these tumor-associated antigens in neoplastic growth and to identify the crucial alteration(s) leading to malignancy. Moreover, their significance in relation to immune responses of patients to their own tumors are still difficult to demonstrate.

The genetic origins of these TAA is of interest from a theoretical point of view. Recent developments in molecular biology, notably the study of oncogenic viruses and human oncogenes, have provided us with a fundamental theory of oncogenesis (Weinberg, 1982). In spite of the large and heterogeneous spectrum of genes identified to date, all human oncogenes belong to a small number of proto-oncogene families. Apparently, proto-oncogenes are regulating cell-cycle events in normal cells. These cellular proto-oncogene sequences can become activated by one of two routes—by recombination with a retroviral sequence or by nonviral, somatic mutation events. Many of these activated proto-oncogenes code for certain enzymatic functions; it is now known that the *src* gene of retroviruses in murine sarcoma system codes for $p60^{src}$, a tyrosine-specific protein kinase (Collett and Erikson, 1978). Such oncogene-coded enzymes may in turn modify cellular proteins, both structurally and functionally. If this molecular model of oncogenesis holds for all human tumors, TAA should be regarded as highly restricted, modified differentiation antigens. Furthermore, it is now widely accepted that the transition of a normal cell into a neoplastic cell involves a multistep progression (Armitage and Doll, 1954; Barrett and Tso, 1978). The progression from the preneoplastic to the malignant state and clonal expansion of these malignant cells may involve additional functional changes, thereby generating the antigenic diversity of TAA (see review by Ownes et al., 1983).

B. Specific Immune Responses to Tumors

In the tumor-bearing host, tumor-associated antigens can elicit diverse humoral and cellular immune responses. For example, some TAA may elicit the production of specific antibodies. The binding of such antibodies to target cells in the presence of complement may be sufficient to lyse tumor cells. In other tumors, TAA-specific antibodies bind to the target cells, and several types of effector cells, such as K cells or macrophages, which bear Fc receptors, can interact with the tumor cells, eventually producing lysis. This phenomenon, called antibody-dependent cell-mediated cytotoxicity (ADCC), has been studied extensively with experimental murine tumors in vitro, but its in vivo role is uncertain.

As described above, early work in tumor immunology often involved the rejection of transplanted tumors. However, in the mid-1960s the mixed lymphocyte culture (MLC) was introduced as the in vitro analog of the allograft rejection. From numerous experiments involving well-defined virally or chemically induced tumors and animals of highly inbred (syngeneic) strains, the generation of cytotoxic lymphocytes (CTL) was recognized as the cellular basis of tumor rejection. For example, in retrovirus-induced or SV40-induced murine tumor systems, the tumor-specific CTL mediate protective immunity, and the target antigen recognized by such CTL is a tumor-specific transplantation antigen (TSTA). In recent years, a variety of retrovirus-induced or SV40-transformed cell lines has been established from intra-H-2 recombinant mouse strains for the immunogenetic analysis of such TSTA-specific CTL responses (Wagner et al., 1980). The ability of CTL to destroy target tumor cells in cytotoxic reactions appears to require recognition of both TSTA and MHC antigen. Thus, a mouse tumor cell expressing TSTA will be regarded as "foreign" by autologous T cells only if the tumor cell expresses surface H-2 markers identical to those simultaneously expressed by the autologous T cells. This phenomenon, called H-2 or syngeneic restriction, was originally discovered as an important mechanism for the destruction of virally infected cells in the animal (Nabholz and MacDonald, 1983).

Recently, the subpopulation of CTL and their differentiation pathways during the primary and secondary immune responses have been extensively analyzed. The distinction between proliferating T cells and cytotoxic effector T cells have important implications for the elucidation of cellular immune reactions. The major conclusions derived from these studies are that CTL preferentially recognize antigens in the context of gene products of H-2 K, D, or L antigens (Nabholz and MacDonald, 1983), whereas helper T cells (T_H), T cells responsible for delayed-type hypersensitivity reaction (T_{DTH}), and in vitro proliferating T cells in MLC recognize antigens in the context of IA (Moller, 1978). These rules observed in the murine immune system may not be absolute for all species; however, such findings are important in designating and interpreting the experiments of human tumor immunology.

The studies discussed above indicate that highly immunogenic experimental animal tumors elicit strong CTL reactions. It should be recognized that many spontaneous murine tumors are only very weakly immunogenic and that most human tumors belong to this category (Baldwin, 1973). Beginning with the pioneer work of the Hellströms and their collaborators (Hellström and Hellström, 1971), numerous laboratories have undertaken the development of CTL assays for human tumors. Despite initial success, many investigators have recognized technical and theoretical limitations in human CTL assays (Herberman, 1974). Major restrictions include difficulties in obtaining a homogeneous tumor-cell population, the unreliability of tumor cells in the expression of tumor maker antigens in culture, and the low frequencies of tumor-specific CTL precursors in the peripheral blood specimens. In addition, the presence of a subpopulation of lymphoid cells, natural killer (NK) cells, that have ability to lyse a wide variety of tumor targets in the CTL assay became recognized. As will be discussed in the next section, NK cells seem to contribute substantially to protective immunity of the host to its own tumors. The discovery of NK cells poses a challenge to the central dogma of tumor immunology, namely, recognition of tumor-specific antigens by the host immune system.

Measurement of T_H or T_{DTH} cells is far more complicated than the CTL assay; however, the migration of macrophages activated by lymphokines from antigen-stimulated T_{DTH} cells has been used as a measure of cell-mediated immunity to tumors in human tumor immunology (see Thomson, 1982). The specificity of such assays has not been well established; the roles of in vitro proliferating T cells and the D loci (human Ia) particularly need to be clarified. In view of the role of Ia antigens in the autologous mixed lymphocyte reaction (MLR) (Schwartz, 1985), it is desirable to elucidate the contribution of nonspecific factors in this type of assay. Studies of the autologous MLR in humans and animals produced substantial evidence that a subpopulation of T lymphocytes (autoreactive T cells) is stimulated by autologous non-T cells to proliferate, to generate helper and suppressor activity, and, under appropriate conditions, even to develop cytotoxic reactivity. The autologous MLR is thought to be stimulated by the HLA-D loci on autologous non-T stimulator cells. Apparently, immunoregulatory factors are produced during the autologous MLR. Such factors, present the supernatant medium after 48 hr of culture, facilitate the proliferation and differentiation of CTL (Schwartz, 1985).

C. Natural Immunity to Tumors

Cell -mediated cytotoxicity against tumors was first investigated extensively 16 years ago, when the Hellströms introduced the colony inhibition assay. Shortly thereafter, the more convenient ^{51}Cr release assay (Brunner et al., 1968) and microcytotoxicity assay (Takasugi and Klein, 1970) were applied to tumor studies. During this period, the focus was on specific cell-mediated cytotoxicity against tumor-associated antigens; however, it was discovered that nonspecific cytotoxicities against some other tumor targets also occurred by lymphocytes obtained from apparently healthy normal donors. By 1975, the limitations in the search for tumor-specific immunity and the significance of natural effector (NK) lymphocytes were recognized (Herberman, 1980).

Human NK cells are heterogeneous with regard to surface membrane characteristics. NK cells have receptors for a T-cell growth factor and can be propagated in culture in the presence of conditioned medium for phytohemagglutinin-stimulated lymphocytes. Human CTL have high-affinity E receptors for sheep erythrocytes, whereas NK cells have low-affinity E receptors. A major difference between CTL and NK cells is the absence of syngeneic restriction of the NK cells. Furthermore, monoclonal antibodies are able to discriminate between NK and T cells.

NK cells have been found to react with a variety of tumor target cells. In vitro passaged leukemia lines (e.g., K562) are particularly susceptible to lysis, but some carcinoma and sarcoma lines and some in vitro transplanted tumors also lyse rapidly. At least some primary tumor cells are susceptible, and when NK cells are treated with interferon or interferon inducers, their activities are augmented. Most investigators now agree that NK cells specifically recognize their target cells, but the nature of antigens on NK-susceptible target cells is not yet defined. Most evidence available is indirect and circumstantial, but some MHC antigens and certain differentiation antigens are probably the target structures.

The significance of NK cells lies in the fact that they react with many different types of tumors. A wide variety of agents has been shown to increase human and animal NK activity. Since small amounts of homogeneous human leukocyte and fibroblast interferons have been shown to augment NK activity strongly, the effects of most of the other agents are thought to be mediated by interferon induction. Elucidation of the mechanism of NK stimulation will be important for the development of protocols of immunotherapy in the future and warrants further investigation (Herberman et al., 1986).

II. TUMOR-RELATED IMMUNITY IN PROSTATIC CANCER

A. Tumor-Associated Antigens of Prostatic Carcinoma

The occurrence in the sera of prostatic cancer patients of circulating antibodies of varying specificities toward prostatic cancer cells has been demonstrated by Ablin and collaborators (Ablin and Bhatti, 1980). The antibodies were, in general, reactive with the cytoplasmic membrane of secretory epithelial cells of autologous and heterologous prostate tissue (Ablin et al., 1976, 1977). Apparently, some of the antibodies recognized antigenic determinant(s) common to epithelial cells. The prevalence of such antibodies to prostatic epithelial cells was generally low (approximately 10%) among the patients with localized tumors, but the prevalence and the titer of the antibodies were higher among patients with metastatic disease (nearly 92% incidence among stage D patients).

More recently, Webb and her collaborators investigated the antigenic molecules recognized by the circulating antiprostatic epithelial antibodies in the sera of prostatic cancer patients (Webb et al., 1981). They prepared an affinity column by coupling the immunoglobulins of prostatic cancer patients to staphylococcal protein A. Antigens were obtained from autochthonous or allogeneic primary tumor extracts or from a prostatic adenocarcinoma line, PC3, grown in athymic nude mice and radiolabeled. The radioactive antigens recognized by such immunoaffinity columns were analyzed by the SDS-polyacrylamide gel electrophoresis. In a series of control experiments, antibodies reactive to normal human tissues or to tumors of nonprostatic origin were removed by the sequential adsorption of the serum before the preparation of an immunoaffinity column matrix. As one may expect from this type of experiment, the prostatic cancer patients produced antibodies with various specificities, ranging from alloreactive antibodies to histocompatibility antigens to autologous common tissue antigens. However, some patients' sera recognized prostatic tumor-associated antigens of 54 and 48 kD, even after extensive adsorption with normal human tissue extracts. On the basis of such sequential absorption analyses, Webb et al. (1981) have concluded that proteins of 54 and 48 kD are candidates for prostatic cancer-associated antigens.

The same investigators then produced a series of murine monoclonal antibodies specific to human prostatic adenocarcinoma antigens by immunizing mice with an established prostatic carcinoma line, PC3 (Ware et al., 1982), or with a mixture of three cell lines, DU145, PC3, and LNCaP (Webb's group). The monoclonal antibodies, Pro 3 and Pro 5, specifically bound a 54-kD antigen of human prostatic carcinoma tissue. The antigen is expressed as a surface protein on the cancer cell, where it exists as a 175-kD macromolecule. The p54 antigen does not appear to be a tumor-specific antigen; it seems to be a differentiation antigen, the expression of which correlates with malignant transformation of the prostatic epithelial cells (Ware et al., 1982). On the other hand, the monoclonal antibody, Pro 13, showed restricted binding to prostatic carcinoma cells but not to cell lines of bladder, kidney, and pancreatic carcinoma origin or fibroblast cultures. The Pro 13 immunoprecipitates a protein with a molecular weight of approximately 140 kD; under reducing conditions, the protein recognized by Pro 13 dissociates into 30- and 17-kD subunits (Webb's group). The significance of these antigens in malignant transformation of the prostatic epithelial cells and whether the antibodies directed against them have any biologic function in vivo (e.g., cytophilic or cytotoxic) remain to be determined. One of the practical applications of antibodies specific to tumor marker antigens is their use as focusing vehicles for the delivery of cytotoxic agent or for enhancing the imaging of metastatic tumors (Moller, 1982).

Wright and his collaborators (Starling et al., 1984; Campbell et al., 1985) also described a series of murine monoclonal antibodies recognizing surface antigens of prostatic carcinoma cells and bladder cancer cells. Specificity studies indicated that antigens defined by these monoclonal antibodies appear to belong to differentiation antigens of urogenital sinus. Therefore, these immunological markers might become useful for the study of the origins of prostate cancer heterogeneity.

Because of the inability to utilize syngeneic systems, elucidation of the in vivo role of those TAA defined by monoclonal antibodies with the cytotoxic lymphocyte assay has been largely unsuccessful in human tumor immunology. However, indirect evidence suggests the implication of TAA in the sensitization of cytotoxic T lymphocytes. Numerous animal models have shown that the transfer to the tumor-bearing host of relatively large numbers of sensitized lymphoid cells with a high degree of antitumor reactivity can mediate the rejection of established localized and metastatic tumors (Rosenberg and Terry, 1977). Recently, such TAA-sensitized lymphoid cell clones have been successfully amplified in vitro by lymphokins and applied to the treatment of established cancers in humans (Rosenberg and Lotze, 1986). Therefore, it is hoped that these immunological investigations of prostate cancer will find eventually clinical applications in diagnosis and treatment.

REFERENCES

Ablin, R. J., and Bhatti, R. A. (1980). Tumor-associated immunity in prostatic cancer. In *Prostate Cancer* (R. Ablin, ed.), Marcel Dekker, New York, pp. 183–204.

Ablin, R. J., Marrow, C., Guinan, P. D., Bruns, G. R., Sadoughi, N., John, T., and Bush, I. M. (1976). Evaluation of cellular immunologic responsiveness in the clinical management of patients with prostatic cancer. III. Inhibition of leukocyte migration. *Urol. Int. 31*:444–458.

Ablin, R. J., Bhatti, R. A., Bruns, G. R., and Guinan, P. D. (1977). Leukocyte adherence inhibition and immunoreactivity in prostatic cancer. I. Identification of anti-tumor cell mediated immunity and "blocking" factor. *Eur. J. Cancer 13*:699–703.

Armitage, P., and Doll, R. (1954). The age distribution of cancer and multi-stage theory of carcinogenesis. *Br. J. Cancer 8*:1–12.

Baldwin, R. W. (1973). Immunological aspects of chemical carcinogenesis. *Cancer Res. 18*:1–75.

Baldwin, R. W., and Embleton, M. H. (1977). Assessment of cell-mediated immunity to human tumor-associated antigens. *Int. Rev. Exp. Pathol. 17*:49–95.

Barrett, J. C., and Tso, P. O. P. (1978). Evidence for the progressive nature of neoplastic transformation in vitro. *Proc. Natl. Acad. Sci. USA 75*:3761–3765.

Boyse, E. A., and Old, L. J. (1969). Some aspects of normal and abnormal cell-surface genetics. *Ann. Rev. Genet. 3*:269–290.

Brunner, K. T., Mauel, J., and Cerottini, J. C. (1968). Quantitative assay of the lytic action of immune lymphoid cells on ^{51}Cr labeled allogeneic target cells in vitro: Inhibition of isoantibody and by drugs. *Immunology 14*:181–196.

Campbell, A. E., Beckett, M. L., Starling, J. J., Sieg, S. M., and Wright, G. L., Jr. (1985). Antiprostate carcinoma monoclonal antibody (D83.21) crossreacts with a membrane antigen expressed on cytomegalovirus-transformed human fibroblasts. *The Prostate 6*:205–215.

Collett, M. S., and Erikson, R. L. (1978). Protein kinase activity associated with the avian sarcoma virus src gene product. *Proc. Natl. Acad. Sci. USA 75*:2021–2024.

Hellström, K. E., and Hellström I. (1971). Immunologic defenses against cancer. In *Immunobiology* (R. A. Good and D. W. Fisher, eds.), Sinauer Associates, Stamford, Connecticut.

Hellström, K. E., and Hellström, I. (1974). Lymphocyte-mediated cytotoxicity and blocking serum activity to tumor antigens. *Adv. Immunol 18*:209–277.

Herberman, R. B. (1974). Cell-mediated immunity to tumor cells. *Adv. Cancer Res. 19*:207–263.

Herberman, R. B. (1976). In *Mechanisms of Tumor Immunity* (I. Green, S. Cohen, and R. T. McCluskey, eds.), J. Wiley & Sons, New York.

Herberman, R. B. (ed.) (1980). *Natural Cell-Mediated Immunity Against Tumors*, Academic Press, New York.

Herberman, R. B., and Holdne, H. T. (1978). Natural cell-mediated immunity. *Adv. Cancer Res. 27*:305–377.

Herberman, R. B., Reynolds, C. W., and Ortaldo, J. (1986). Mechanism of cytotoxicity by natural killer (NK) cells. *Ann. Rev. Immunol. 4*:651–680.

Herlyn, M., Steplewski, Z., Herlyn, D., and Koprowski, H. (1979). Colorectal carcinoma-specific antigen: Detection by means of monoclonal antibodies. *Proc. Natl. Acad. Sci. USA 76*: 1438–1442.

Klein, G. (1966). Tumor antigens. *Annu. Rev. Microbiol. 20*:223–252.

Kohler, G., and Milstein, C. (1975). Nature: Continuous cultures of fused cells secreting antibody of pre-defined specificity. *Nature 256*:495–497.

Koprowski, H., Steplewski, A., Herlyn, D., and Herly, M. (1978). Study of antibodies against human melanoma produced by somatic cell hybrids. *Proc. Natl. Acad. Sci. USA 75*:3405–3409.

Law, L. W., Roger, M. J., and Appella, E. (1980). Tumor antigens on neoplasms induced by chemical carcinogens and by DNA- and RNA-containing viruses: Properties of the solubilized antigens. *Adv. Cancer Res. 32*:201–235.

Moller, G. (ed.) (1978). Ir genes and T lymphocytes. *Immunol. Rev. 38*:1–280.

Moller, G. (ed.) (1982). Antibody carriers of drugs and toxins in tumor therapy. *Immunol. Rev. 62*:5–216.

Nabholz, M., and MacDonald, H. R. (1983). Cytolytic T lymphocytes. *Ann. Rev. Immunol. 1*:273–306.

Owens, A. H., Jr., Coffey, D. S., and Baylin, S. B. (eds.) (1983). *Tumor Heterogeneity*: Origins and Implications, Academic Press, New York.

Prehn, R. T., and Main, J. M. (1957). Immunity to methylcholanthrene-induced sarcomas. *JNCI 18*:769–778.

Rosenberg, S. A., and Terry, W. D. (1977). Passive immunotherapy of cancer in animals and man. *Adv. Cancer Res. 25*:323–388.

Rosenberg, S. A., and Lotze, M. T. (1986). Cancer immunotherapy using interleukin-2 and interleukin-2-activated lymphocytes. *Ann. Rev. Immunol. 4*:681–709.

Schwartz, R. H. (1985). T lymphocyte recognition of antigen in association with gene products of the major histocompatibility complex. *Ann. Rev. Immunol. 3*:237–261.

Starling, J. J., Beckett, M. L., and Wright, G. L., Jr. (1984). Monoclonal antibodies to prostate adenocarcinoma antigens. In *Monoclonal Antibodies and Cancer* (G. L. Wright, Jr., ed.), Marcel Dekker, New York.

Takasugi, M., and Klein, E. (1970). A microassay for cell-mediated immunity. *Transplantation 9*:219–227.

Thomson, D. M. P. (ed.) (1982). *Assessment of Immune Status by the Leukocyte Adherence Inhibition Test*, Academic Press, New York.

Wagner, H., Pfizenmaler, K., and Rollinghoff, M. (1980). The role of the major histocompatibility gene complex in murine cytoxic T cell responses. *Adv. Cancer Res. 31*:77–124.

Ware, J. L., Paulson, D. F., Parks, S. F., and Webb, K. S. (1982). Production of monoclonal antibody Pro 3 recognizing a human prostatic carcinoma antigen. *Cancer Res. 42*:1215–1222.

Webb, K. S., Ware, J. L., Parks, S. F., and Paulson, D. F. (1981). A serological approach to the definition of human prostatic carcinoma antigens. *The Prostate 2*:369–380.
Weinberg, R. A. (1982). Oncogenes of spontaneous and chemically induced tumors. *Adv. Cancer Res. 36*:149–163.

Index

B

C

G

H

I

T